Pathogenesis of Autoimmune Diseases

Pathogenesis of Autoimmune Diseases

Edited by **Marcy Ward**

hayle
medical

New York

Published by Hayle Medical,
30 West, 37th Street, Suite 612,
New York, NY 10018, USA
www.haylemedical.com

Pathogenesis of Autoimmune Diseases
Edited by Marcy Ward

International Standard Book Number: 978-1-63241-317-8 (Hardback)

Printed in the United States of America.

Contents

Preface   VII

Part 1 Pathogenesis of Systemic Autoimmune Disorders:
        Genetic and Enviromental Contributors   1

Chapter 1 Autoimmune Diseases:
           The Role of Environment and Gene Interactions   3
           Wellington K. Ayensu, Emmanuel O. Keku, Raphael D. Isokpehi,
           Ibrahim O. Farah, Chris A. Arthur and Sophia S. Leggett

Chapter 2 HLA and Citrullinated Peptides in Rheumatoid Arthritis   35
           Iñaki Álvarez

Chapter 3 IRF-5 - A New Link to Autoimmune Diseases   51
           Sujayita Roy and Paula M. Pitha

Chapter 4 Cell Surface Glycans at SLE – Changes During
           Cells Death, Utilization for Disease Detection and
           Molecular Mechanism Underlying Their Modification   69
           Bilyy Rostyslav, Tomin Andriy, Yaroslav Tolstyak, Havrylyuk Anna,
           Chopyak Valentina, Kit Yuriy and Stoika Rostyslav

Chapter 5 Regulatory T Cell Deficiency in Systemic
           Autoimmune Disorders – Causal Relationship
           and Underlying Immunological Mechanisms   91
           Fang-Ping Huang and Susanne Sattler

Chapter 6 Postinfectious Autoimmune Syndrome as a
           Key Factor in Chronization of the Infectious Disease   107
           Natalia Cherepahina, Murat Agirov, Jamilyia Tabaksoeva,
           Kusum Ahmedilova and Sergey Suchkov

Chapter 7 Contribution of Peroxynitrite, a Reactive Nitrogen
           Species, in the Pathogenesis of Autoimmunity   121
           Rizwan Ahmad and Haseeb Ahsan

Chapter 8   Gut Microbiota - "Lost in Immune Tolerance"   137
            Serena Schippa and Valerio Iebba

Chapter 9   Immunological Effects of Silica and
            Related Dysregulation of Autoimmunity   153
            Naoko Kumagai, Hiroaki Hayashi, Megumi Maeda,
            Yoshie Miura, Hidenori Matsuzaki, Suni Lee,
            Yasumitsu Nishimura, Wataru Fujimoto and Takemi Otsuki

Part 2   Pathogenetic Aspects
            of Organ Specific Autoimmune Diseases   171

Chapter 10 Immunogenetics of Type 1 Diabetes   173
            Rajni Rani

Chapter 11 Tolerance and Autoimmunity in Type 1 Diabetes   197
            Valentina Di Caro, Nick Giannoukakis and Massimo Trucco

Chapter 12 Autoimmunity in Vitiligo   225
            E. Helen Kemp, Sherif Emhemad,
            David J. Gawkrodger and Anthony P. Weetman

Chapter 13 Graves' Disease
            - The Interaction of Lymphocytes and Thyroid Cells   249
            Ben-Skowronek Iwona

Chapter 14 Hashimoto's Thyroiditis – Interactions of
            Lymphocytes, Thyroid Cells and Fibroblasts   261
            Ben-Skowronek Iwona

            Permissions

            List of Contributors

Preface

This book was inspired by the evolution of our times; to answer the curiosity of inquisitive minds. Many developments have occurred across the globe in the recent past which has transformed the progress in the field.

Autoimmune Disorders refers to a heterogeneous and multifaceted group of diseases which can affect virtually any organ system of the human body. This book intends to present currently accessible manifestations by providing an etiopathogenetic overview of both systemic and organ detailed autoimmune diseases, comorbidities of autoimmune disorders, growth as well as new findings in the thrilling fields of osteoimmunology and immunology of pregnancy.

This book was developed from a mere concept to drafts to chapters and finally compiled together as a complete text to benefit the readers across all nations. To ensure the quality of the content we instilled two significant steps in our procedure. The first was to appoint an editorial team that would verify the data and statistics provided in the book and also select the most appropriate and valuable contributions from the plentiful contributions we received from authors worldwide. The next step was to appoint an expert of the topic as the Editor-in-Chief, who would head the project and finally make the necessary amendments and modifications to make the text reader-friendly. I was then commissioned to examine all the material to present the topics in the most comprehensible and productive format.

I would like to take this opportunity to thank all the contributing authors who were supportive enough to contribute their time and knowledge to this project. I also wish to convey my regards to my family who have been extremely supportive during the entire project.

Editor

Part 1

Pathogenesis of Systemic Autoimmune Disorders: Genetic and Enviromental Contributors

1

Autoimmune Diseases: The Role of Environment and Gene Interactions

Wellington K. Ayensu[1,3], Emmanuel O. Keku[2], Raphael D. Isokpehi[1,3], Ibrahim O. Farah[1], Chris A. Arthur[4] and Sophia S. Leggett[4]
[1]College of Science, Engineering & Technology, Jackson State University, Jackson,
[2]Department of Public Health and Preventive Medicine, School of Medicine,
St. George's University, St. George, Grenada,
[3]Bioinformatics Section; Jackson State University, Jackson,
[4]School of Health Sciences, College of Public Service, Jackson State University, Jackson,
[1,3,4]USA
[2]West Indies

1. Introduction

Data from epidemiological studies indicate global increase in the incidence and prevalence of numerous autoimmune diseases (AD) as seen in the United States (Jacobson et al.1997). According to estimate from the US National Institute of Health (NIH) the prevalence of AD is in the range of 23.5 billion. From 1996 to date at least 237,203 cases per year of AD are diagnosed in the US; and of this, 42,137 are new cases of primary glomerulonephritis, multiple sclerosis, polymyositis/dermatomyositis and systemic lupus erythematosus (SLE). Early in 1996 alone 6,722,573 women and 1,789,273 men suffered from varieties of diseases that had components of autoimmunity. Currently up to 150 autoimmune based diseases have been identified and approximately 40 more are awaiting confirmation. Similarly the incidence of several autoallergic diseases, type 1 insulin dependent diabetes mellitus (IDDM), rheumatoid arthritis, and Graves' disease, hyperthyroidism included are on the increase. Of the 1.2 million new cases of AD diagnosed every 5 years, at least one or more cases will include these autoimmune disease components. (Jacobson et al.1997)

The global incidence and prevalence for each AD is currently lacking and that calls for improvement on data collection and reporting. Nearly 10% of developed world's population suffer from AD and contribute significantly to chronic diseases and mortality. Women are three times more likely to be at risk than men in acquiring these diseases with non-Caucasians at higher risk. We are also seeing global prevalence of allergic respiratory diseases on the increase for the past 20-30 years. Over 15 million people in US suffer from asthma alone; approximately 50 million are diagnosed with some form of allergic diseases (Smith et al, 1997). Presently the direct annual health care cost for AD in US is in excess of $100 billion US dollars as compared to $57 billion for cancer. Hospitalization alone takes over half the cost of the direct expenditures. Almost 20% of the population classified as 'high-cost patients' consume more than 80% of the resources. Consequently the cost to public health from clinical management of these conditions is on the increase. All indications point to future better management of asthmatics through research and interventional efforts directed at communities, hospitalizations and high-cost patients in order to decrease health care resource use and provide cost savings. This calls for rigorous investigations into the role of environmental xenobiotics/substances and/or pollutants that are risk factors in the development of autoimmune diseases. In this chapter we intend to survey the public health concerns imposed by pollutants of the air, water and the food chain with concentration on typical examples of the effects of mercury on health to demonstrate the likelihood of dangers imposed through environmental and genetic disturbances in health.

2. Environmental chemicals and autoimmune diseases

Many scientists concur that several species within mammals to amphibians, birds, reptiles, and fish so far under monitoring systems are close to total extinction; well over 30,000 plant and animal species are estimated to be lost each year, a morbidity rate generally agreed to be much faster than at any time. Loss of species seems to be explained in most cases through the global weather changes as well as pollutional activities of man. But industrial activities seem to play major role in this problem; the latest data emanating from the industrial front estimate that at least 85,000 possible pollutants are currently being released into the environment through industrial activities alone http://www.epa.gov/glnpo/lmmb/substs.html (FDA/EPA).

2.1 Chemicals and substances of public health concern
These pollutants cover the heavy metals like thallium, aluminium, cadmium, lead, gold and mercury as well as pesticides, herbicides, preservatives, dyes, plastics, bisphenol A and rubber products. The Environmental Working Group indicated from studies in 2005 that a cocktail of 287 pollutants are measured in new born US fetal cord blood (http://www.ewg.org/reports/bodyburden2/execsumm.php). Perfluorooctanoic acid (*PFOA or* C8), and perfluorooctanoate, a synthetic but stable perfluorinated carboxylic acid and fluorosurfactant PFOA's were included in the findings as well as pesticides, dioxins, flame retardants. Recently another concern has been brought to the limelight by the internal Florida Department of Environmental Protection (DEP) Workgroup. It is stated that the current update of the American Chemical Society's Abstract Service reveals that as of August 2007 over 98% of the commercially available compounds are not under regulatory practices as they should be. This amounts to about 15 million out of over 32 million substances commonly referred to as Emerging Substances of Concern, or ESOC that have been registered for regulation (Chemical Abstract Service [CAS] website): http://www.cas.org/cgi-bin/cas/regreport.pl.
Much uncertainty surrounds the outcome from releases of these substances into the environment. No information about the pharmacokinetics or pharmacodynamics interactions among life forms on these substances are available. No available information on transport and toxicological effects are on record. Within two years between 2005 and 2007 over 5 million new chemicals have been reported to be registered and 5 million more chemicals became commercially available. Currently CAS informs that within each week more than 50 new substances or additions to existing substances to the database is the norm; http://www.cas.org/index.html. Apparently the ratio of unregulated to regulated chemicals keeps growing exponentially. The ESOC chemicals fall under various categories of organic groups encompassing from flame retardants (PBDEs), pharmaceuticals to endocrine-modulating chemicals (EMCs), nanoparticles to biological metabolites as well as newly discovered Industrial chemicals and toxins. They are constantly being discharged into

the environment where they find their way into our water bodies posing an unknown level of risk to life forms including humans, animals, and plants.

Regulatory Agencies are therefore challenged to find answers to solve what may be an unknown outcome of these ESOC substances being continually released into the biosphere. In the absence of detail knowledge on the environmental outcome and without effective regulation no useful assessment can be made on the environmental risk posed. Thus vast majority of ESOC substances have to be non-traditionally managed by other means such as prevention and effects-based environmental assessment methods. That effort is even more tasking and presents difficulties in monitoring the trends of the etiology of diseases now becoming prevalent in the environment under such practices. ESOC substances are now recognized to be of global concern; among these are included polybromina -teddiphenyl ethers (PBDEs), perfluorooctanoic acid (PFOA), siloxanes, perfluorooctanesulfonate (PFOS) and hexa- bromocyclododecanes (HBCDs). PBDEs and HBCDs come under flame-retardant chemicals that are moderately long-lived and volatile; readily released to the atmosphere because they do not strongly bind to substrates. Once in the atmosphere they are globally transported and readily bioaccumulate in biological tissues.

2.1.1 Nanoparticles

Human activities now have added sources of environmental contaminants. Human-originated nanomaterials are naturally man-made structures that differ in size range from 1 to 100 nanometers (nm). They are commonly used in drug delivery nanotherapeutic pharmaceuticals, cosmetics, personal care products, energy storage products, fabrics, lubricants and equipments like golf balls. The use of nanomaterials has been on the increase and now it is ubiquitous. Their minuscule sizes allow traversing not only biological membranes but also the blood/brain barrier (BBB) and display physical and chemical properties different from parental compounds. Examples are gold or silver metals known to be inducers of autoimmunity but also possess magnetic properties.

The intrinsic stereospecificity of these substances allow these molecules to play significant toxicological role in the environment (Donaldson et al 2004) and are therefore of public health concern. Carbon black displays enhanced severe effect than titanium dioxide (Renwick et al 2004), while the nanoparticle sizes of both chemicals are inducers of increased lung inflammation and destruction of the epithelial linings than their larger size. Adsorptions onto the surface of nanoparticles may play synergistic role in the reactivity; in vitro studies with fractions of diesel exhaust particles showed effects on cells (Xia et al 2004). Atmospheric nanoparticles may be complex enough to form interactions with organics and metals capable of higher levels of toxicity; metallic iron potentiates the effect of carbon black nanoparticles resulting in enhanced reactivity displayed as oxidative stress (Wilson et al 2002). Conversely other combinations with pullulan (polysaccharide polymer of maltotriose units, also known as α-1,4- ;α-1,6-glucan) and dextran tend to reduce toxicity of the respective nanoparticles (Gupta and Gupta 2005, Berry et al 2003).

Some nanoscale materials may be catalytic or behave as semiconductors, properties that can only increase the likelihood that nanomaterial could produce unanticipated toxicological effects. Nonbiodegradable ceramics, metals and metal oxides within nanomaterials are quite environmentally stable and persistent (EPA, 2007) and therefore undergo bioaccumulation in the food chain (Biswas and Wu, 2005). They are currently implicated in the induction of acute and chronic biological toxicity (Oberdörster, 2004a and 2004b; Lovern and Klaper, 2005; Lam et al., 2004; Shvedovaet al., 2005; Fortner et al., 2005) of unknown physiological mechanisms and hence consequences.

2.1.2 Particulate matter
Nanoparticles compare with particle pollution or particulate matter (PM), a group of complex mixture of extremely small air-borne particles and liquid droplets in air suspensions. There are a number of components covering acids (nitrates and sulfates, organic chemicals, metals, soil or dust and sulfates, organic chemicals, metals, soil or dust or mold spores). Particles less than 10 micrometers in diameter (PM_{10}) pose an even worse health concern because of their inhalation properties that allow for accumulation in the respiratory system; they are found in all types of combustion (motor vehicles, power plants, wood burning, etc.) and some industrial processes. Severe health risks are posed among fine particles less than 2.5 micrometers in diameter ($PM_{2.5}$). Fine particles easily lodge and penetrate deeply into the bronchial tree and into the deepest alveolar areas of the lung upon inhalation. Coarse particles measuring between 2.5 and 10 micrometers are derived from crushing or grinding operations, and dust from paved or unpaved roads.
Properties of PM link them to a variety of significant health problems starting from offensive asthma to early mortality of exposed patients who suffer from cardiac and bronchial diseases. Exposures to PM result in high rate of respiratory symptoms involving irritation of the airways, coughing, or difficulty breathing, decline in lung functions, aggravated asthma, and development of chronic bronchitis, irregular heartbeat and nonfatal heart attacks. Individuals with a variety of health issues particularly those with prior heart or lung diseases tend to suffer premature deaths on exposure to PM. Children and older adults are the most likely to be affected by particle pollution exposure but healthy individuals are found to experience temporary symptoms from exposure to elevated levels www.epa.gov/asthma; and plays esthetic role by significantly effecting visibility impairment in the nation's cities and national parks. To protect public health and welfare, EPA has continually issued National Ambient Air Quality Standards (NAAQS) since 1971 for six criteria pollutants among which are particulate matter and Sulfur Dioxide (SO_2), Ozone (O_3), Nitrogen Dioxide (NO_2), Lead (Pb), and Carbon Monoxide (CO). The NAAQS from EPA has undergone revisions in 1987 and 1997 and again in September 2006 and it is helpful to familiarize oneself; there is an urgent need for studies to unravel the pharmacokinetics and pharmacodynamics of these particles to help disclose the role played in disease pathogenesis especially concerning the autoimmune state- asthma being one of the priorities.

3. Autoimmune diseases: etiologies and mechanisms

All indications show that tissue burdens of PBDE in life forms including humans are doubling in every two to five years. Human breast milk has been found to contain as much as 419 ng/g lipid weight of PBDE (Schecter et al., 2003). The question then arises whether these molecules contribute to what we measure in the increases in the incidence of ADs. These substances are known to interfere with the reproductive and developmental stages of mammals as well as in birds and invertebrates (McKernan *et al.*, 2006, Wollenberger 2005); they are carcinogenic, endocrine-modulating, and have neurotoxicological effects (Birnbaum, 2005). Autoimmune diseases present a major affront to the health of Americans as well as of global concern. Vast arrays of diseases come under auto-allergic/–immunity; these cover maladies that may present as localized to be organ specific or systemically distributed to the extremities to involve all organ systems typically noted in systemic lupus erythematosus (SLE). In health the Immune System guards us against invasion of foreign substances including harmful bacteria, viruses, and parasites quite well without any perturbation. At times, however this machinery loses control and begins to attack even the self itself. Hypersensitivity responses resulting from direct attack of body components by antibodies or immune cells instead of attacking foreign substances alone generally come under autoimmunity or autoallergic responses. Autoimmune state becomes apparent with rise of demonstrable presence of autoantibodies or complexes of these with body substances or the presence of cells, T lymphocytes that attack self-constituents. Minor and harmless autoimmune states exist in normal persons in general; it is part component of the defense system as envisaged by Jerne's hypothesis (<http://www.enotes.com/microbiology encyclopedia/). In the disease state, however, autoimmunity becomes defined when the benign state results rather in pathology; it sets in motion homeostatic deterioration. The process is dependent on both genetic influences and environmental triggers.

For the past decades it has been conclusively demonstrated that alleles of the major histocompatibility complex (MHC) contribute to the susceptibility to autoimmunity but relatively recently there is an unparalleled discovery of novel genes in molecular pathways implicated in autoimmunity. Some of the variants identified clearly participate in the modulation of T-lymphocyte (T-cell) activation and do contribute to many different forms of human autoimmunity. Other genes tend to have restricted roles, with susceptibility apparently confined to one autoimmune condition or to a specific ethnic group. To gain insight into the initiation mechanisms of autoimmune diseases requires identification of the genetic determinants underlying disease pathogenesis and this implicates new biochemical pathways. The Autoimmune state may be either the direct originator of disease itself or arise as a secondary disease from perturbations from other chronic diseases. Direct autoimmune states are phenotypically demonstrated in patients that have antibodies in the active disease phase: examples are represented by idiopathic thrombocytopenia (ITP), Grave's disease and myasthenia gravis, pemphigus vulgaris and bullous pemphigoid, diseases that can be transferred among species through antibody transfers.

Disease transfer through T lymphocytes exchanges have not conclusively been demonstrated to lead to pathology but with the aid of cytokines may rather alleviate or exacerbate disease state. Indirect cause of autoimmunity has been defined by Rose and Bona, 1993 as when disease can be induced in an animal model. SLE is well represented by several genetically determined mouse models which, while not exactly clinical replica of the human disease do very closely replicate pathological and serological characteristics clinically seen to occur. Hashimoto's thyroiditis and multiple sclerosis can be reproduced by immunizing animals with an antigen analogous to the putative autoantigen of the human disease. Absence of direct and indirect evidence with markers describing the state of autoimmunity become circumstantial: positive family histories for disease, presence of certain MHC class II alleles are examples.

Currently it takes a great effort to assess accurately the initiation levels of these diseases in humans; the very initiating factors are difficult to focus on and in which stage/s or area of the metabolic processes gets initially disturbed becomes challenging to screen and allow for therapeutic management. Majority of ADs such as multiple sclerosis (MS), insulin-dependent diabetes mellitus (IDDM), rheumatoid arthritis (RA), systemic lupus erythematosus (SLE), and thyroiditis one finds representative spectrum of autoimmune diseases that appear to have etiological background in dysregulated immune system. Enough supporting evidence exist to confirm the autoimmune nature of many of these disorders but still it is gravely challenging to decipher their precise etiology and/or the initiating factors. Of late a small fraction of the T cells, the regulatory T cells are among the focal area of studies and have become recognized as particularly crucial for control of autoreactive immune responses. Normally the processing of a self antigen by the antigen presenting cells (APC) allow binding of processed antigenic fragments to the MHC molecules within the APC followed by display of these MHC-peptide complexes on APC's membrane surface for presentation to the appropriate T cells; this eventually terminates in activation of antigen-specific T cells. These T cells are then capable of attacking the self tissues expressing that particular self antigen. The process is believed to be the critical steps in the initiation of anti-self T cell responses.

Genome wide studies indicate that costimulatory signals examplified by CTLA4 or PD1 and the modulators of T-cell receptor signaling (LYP, encoded by *PTPN22*), somehow must be confirmatory key checkpoint for human autoimmunity as happens in the T-cell during the period of T-cell receptor training to eliminate self-antigen carrying T cells in the thymus. This notion of the crypticity of self antigenic determinants (Sercarz et al., 1993; Moudgil and Sercarz, 2005) takes strength from the premise that rely on potentially immunogenic regions (determinants/epitopes) within a self antigen that are processed and presented by the MHC molecule to T cells at different levels of immunogenecity. This means that certain 'dominant self' epitopes are well processed and presented, whereas others, the (cryptic or recessive self) (Sercarz et al., 1993) ones are poorly or never processed and presented. Thus this type of staging of determinants (dominance/crypticity) in turn plays a critical role in thymus gradation of the T cell repertoire: the T cells specific for dominant self epitopes are tolerized with ease while those purportly aimed at cryptic self epitopes evade tolerance induction and become part of the mature T cell repertoire (Gammon and Sercarz, 1989; Cibotti et al., 1992; Sinha et al., 2004).

T cells that evade tolerance induction are capable of being activated in the periphery under certain stressful inflammatory circumstances such as occur during infection; this has the consequence of enhanced processing and presentation of once latent (cryptic) determinants (Lehmann et al., 1992; Lanzavecchia, 1995). These activated T cells at times are capable of escaping appropriate constraint from regulatory T cells and permitted to execute their effector function of initiating autoimmune damage. The unveiling of previously cryptic determinants leading to activation of self-reactive T cells that escaped tolerance induction during thymic selection, owing to the crypticity of self determinants is considered a primary cornerstone of a theory of autoimmunity (Moudgil and Sercarz, 2005). The idea of determinant hierarchy provides a vital link between the thymic selection of potentially autoreactive T cells and the subsequent activation of these T cells in the periphery under conditions that facilitate the revelation of previously cryptic determinants. Peripheral ongoing immune tolerance of the mature immune system also attracts attention as another source of autoimmune initiation. This idea is supported by variations seen in the expressions of "self-antigen" in the thymus (e.g., insulin in T1D); in this instance T-cells are selected for survival according to the affinity of their cell surface receptors for self-antigen. This may represent a major key step in the genesis of autoimmune disease.

Other means of autoimmune genesis stem from APCs. These cells play crucial role in antigen processing and presentation to the T-helper (Th) cells. Dendritic cells for example are key cells in the initiation and perpetuation of immune responses. Highly polymorphic genes within the *MHC*, with links to autoimmune inductions, encode proteins to which antigens bind and presented directly to T-cells by APCs. Another source of autoimmune initiation focus on the cell surface marker CD4-positive Th cells; they are the conductors of the adaptive immune response and many genes with an established role in autoimmune disease have their expression in this cell type.

Autoimmune diseases present specific issues that need attention. Drugs used to manage known chronic and acute diseases are implicated in triggering and are therefore thought to be indirect causes of various autoimmune diseases following administration. Many of the prescription drugs commonly used for highly prevalent diseases come under this category: these inexhaustively include drugs like Alferon N, Allopurinol, Atenolol, Atorvastatin, captopril, Penicillin, Carbamazepine, chlorpromazine, Chlorthalidone, cimetidine, Ethosuximide, gold salts, griseofulvin, Hydralazine, Interleukins, Infergen, Interferons, Interferon Alfa, Hydrochlorothiazide, Intron A, Isoniazid, Levodopa, Lithium, Lovastatin, Mesantoin, Methimazole, Methyldopa, Methylsergide, Metoprolol, Minocycline, Minoxidil, Ophthalmic timolol, Nitrofurantoin, Oral contraceptives, Quinidine, Phenytoin, PegIntron, P-aminobenzoic, Penicillamine, Perphenazine, Trimethadione, Pravostatin, Phenylbutazone, Procainamide, Valproic acid, Propylthiouracil, Simvastatin, sulfasalazine, sulfonamides, streptomycin, Sulfonamide antimicrobials, Tetracyclines, Tiotropium Bromide inhaler and Tumor Necrosis factor.

The concern here can well be summarized with the incidence and/or prevalence of asthma, one of the most common chronic diseases of childhood estimated to affect 6 million children. More than 22 million Americans are diagnosed with asthma, and approximately 50 million of individuals are diagnosed with some form of allergic diseases. Presently in US the annual direct health care cost for AD in general is in excess of $100 billion US dollars as compared to $57 billion for cancer. Hospitalization alone takes over half the cost of the direct expenditures. "High- cost patients" that form about 20% of the population spend more than 80% of the resources. As a result, the cost to public health from clinical management of these conditions is on the increase.

4. Global problems associated with asthma and COPD

Epidemiological data following the natural history of asthma reveal that in 1999 mortality rates from the disease declined in comparison to previous years. This was followed by a surge in recent decades in asthma prevalence also in the United States and other Western countries; data suggest this trend may also be reaching a plateau. The general trend of global asthma incidence is rising worldwide but looking at US data we see increased morbidity and mortality from asthma from 1980s -1990s with plateau in the 1990s. This finding is the reverse of what was seen in the 1978-1980 where an increase in mortality due to asthma was measured: from 1990-1999 mortality declined. Commencing from 1995 the rate of outpatient visits for asthma increased; whereas the rates of hospital admissions declined *from 19.5 per 10,000* of the population in 1995 to *15.7 in 1998* attributed to enhanced rates of dispensed steroid prescriptions for inhaled medications. This finding has been interpreted as due to the improved treatment of asthma responsible for these favorable developments.

The implication, if it holds supports explanations of certain changes in environmental chemicals releases. Recent increases in asthmatic conditions in the population may be linked to many causes the cardinal one being the amount and types of substances that are being released increasingly into the biosphere. Releases of substances most of which have an unknown effect and still others closely linked to inductions of asthmatic features in the ever increasing population with genetic predispositions present ominous threat to the very survival of several species including man himself.

Exposures to environmental factors early on in childhood play significant role in the risk in developing asthma. Clinicians have known for quite a while that asthma is not a single disease. Risk to asthma stems from early environmental factors as well as the presence of susceptibility genes; subsequent disease induction and progression from inflammation as well as response to therapeutic agents plays big roles in disease etiology. It is a typical consequence of environmentally induced autoallergic disease known to be heterogeneous (Asosingh et al 2007, Dompeling et al, 2000, Dweik et al, 2001, Kharitonov and Barnes, 2001, Weiss, 2002, Pascual and Peters 2005, Salvato, 2001, Wu et al, 2000) existing in many forms. The immunologic profile of the asthmatic airways presents as proliferation and activation of helper T lymphocytes (CD4+) of the subtype T_H2 responsible for the allergic inflammation in atopic asthmatics. Upon stimulation these cells release a number of cytokines covering IL-4, agent for IgE synthesis, IL-5, essential for eosinophils' maturation, and IL-3 and granulocyte-macrophage colony-stimulating factor, GMCSF (Bolland and Ravetch 2000, Candore et al, 2002, Lang et al, 2010, Pollard et al 1997).

In allergic as well as nonallergic individuals we observe populations of eosinophils in the airways with increased levels in asthmatics with allergies http://www. clevelandclinicmeded .com/ medical pubs/disease management/allergy/ bronchial-asthma/that have higher rates of asthmatic attacks. These cells serve as the source of mediators that exert damaging effects on the airways. Ultimately, mediators lead to degranulation of effector/proinflammatory cells in the airways that release other mediators and oxidants, a common final pathway that culminates in chronic injury and inflammation commonly seen in asthma. Chronicity of the asthmatic condition has been confirmed by several parameters. Low pH and high output of reactive oxygen and nitrogen species (ROS) during asthmatic exacerbations are specific biomarkers in expired air reflecting altered airway redox problems (Clynes et al, 1988, Comhair et al, 2000, De Raeve et al, 1997, Dweik et al 2001). Superoxide, hydrogen peroxide, and hydroxyl radicals are among ROS agents that are responsible for the inflammatory changes in the asthmatic airway (Candore et al 2002, Bolland and Ravetch 2000, Pollard et al, 1997). These ROS originate from the lungs of asthmatic patients induced by activated inflammatory cells (ie, eosinophils, alveolar macrophages, and neutrophils) (Holgate et al, 2000).

Pathogenicity in asthma in particular is portrayed by overall interactions between neural mechanisms, inflammatory cell mediators such as leukotrienes and prostaglandins, and intrinsic abnormalities of the arachidonic acid pathway and smooth muscle; all these cells play significant roles in the initial as well as disease progression. Inflammation is the most likely etiological basis of airway hyperreactivity and variable airflow obstruction.

Asthma usually persists into later childhood and adulthood from early childhood in the presence of the appropriate genetic background. Tolerance to allergens is a normal security that prevents such responses, but the specific immunological events that mediate tolerance in this setting are still under scrutiny. Despite the explosion of information about asthma, the nature of the basic pathogenesis has not been established. However, asthma clearly does not result from a single genetic abnormality, but is rather a complex multigenic disease with a strong environmental contribution. For example, asthmatic children and adults sensitive to inhalant allergens such as dust mites, mold spores, cat dander, etc portray such reactions right from childhood compared with adult-onset asthmatics. Local epithelial environment within the connective tissue is believed to be actively involved in regulation of events and the relation between the airway epithelium and the subepithelial mesenchyme is proposed to be a key determinant in the concept of *airway remodeling* (Davies et al, 2003; Weiss, 2002; Li and Wilson 1997, Pascual and Peters, 2005, Salvato 2001). Difficulties and/or problems underlying diagnosis and classification of these diseases are simply due to the fact that most of the ADs become apparent only at variable phases of several chronic stages of organic ailments. Some ADs present as auto allergies covering several fields of diseases: the incidence of several of these diseases is also on the increase and covers type 1 insulin dependent diabetes mellitus (IDDM), rheumatoid arthritis, and Graves' disease, hyperthyroidism included. There is scarcity of information on the global incidence and prevalence for each AD. Some autoimmune/allergic diseases (AD) can be seen in cases of chronic obstructive pulmonary diseases (COPD). As such the incidence of these disorders has not been well defined. However, sharp global increases in the prevalence have been observed in the United States.

Etiological initiators of and pathogenesis of most ADs are obscure; they are presumed to be numerous with cigarette smoking a typical COPD-associated. Cigarette smoking is clearly the major risk factor for COPD but exposures to other noxious substances including dusts and chemicals found under occupational settings are known to contribute to the development of the disease (Pauwels et al, 2001).The attributable fraction contributing to COPD cases caused by occupational exposures is estimated to be in the range of less than 15% to as high as 31% among those who never smoked (Hnizdo et al, 2004). We find that minority groups have been historically overexposed to hazardous industrial substances and are candidates with increased risk for work-related airflow obstruction putting them highly in the AD group as well; making it necessary to improve on data collection and reporting. Estimation shows, however that nearly 10% of developed world's population suffer from AD and contribute significantly to chronic diseases and mortality. Women are three times more likely at risk than men in acquiring these diseases with non-Caucasians in the higher risk groups. The global prevalence of allergic respiratory diseases including COPD has been also on the increase for the past 20-30 years.

5. Mercury as environmental inducer of autoimmunity

Psychoneuroimmunological studies demonstrate in various ways that homeostatic regulation of the internal milieu links the soma with the neural pathways; stressors effects relate the two in bidirectional pathways. Current Naturopathic Medical view of diseases also links the involvement of the genes to autoimmune proneness. In this wise the authors concentrate on the metal mercury as a representative highly reactive toxic agent within the body as a means of gaining an insight into the problem of etiologies of autoimmune diseases. Mercury has a high affinity binding to *sulfhydryl* as well as to *hydroxyl, carboxyl,* and *phosphoryl* functional groups very commonly displayed on macromolecules, proteins and the genetic materials. It is widely distributed as an environmental and industrial pollutant. No known beneficial metabolomic effect is assigned to mercury in the physiology of humans, yet a 70 kg man is loaded with an equivalent of 13mg mercury (Pier, 1975) distributed in the skin, nails, hair, and kidneys. The net outcome of exposure to mercury is dose-dependent and at low concentrations mercury is the agent for the induction of several diseases that affect most systems of the body.

The central nervous system (CNS), the brain and the kidneys suffer most where Mercury Induced Autoimmunity (MeIA) can be particularly threatening in onset and severe among especially non-Caucasians that manifest *defined* major histocompatibility complex (MHC) haplotypes. Several data confirm that mercury is also associated with polyclonal cell stimulation. Mercury Induced Autoimmunity (MeIA) engages helper T lymphocytes in the induction of disease process in responder animals (Jiang YG, Möller G 1995, Horwitz and Stohl, 1993; Puck JM, Sneller MC. 1997) and in humans (Liossis et al 1996). It is suggested there is a genetic basis for airway hyperresponsiveness with linkage to chromosomes 5q, 11q (Li and

Wilson1997) and 12q24 in Hispanic subgroups (Salvato 2001). While MeIA is well characterized into different arrays of disease susceptibility in animal studies (De Raeve et al 1997) and in humans (Holgate et al, 2000, Li and Wilson 1997,) the role of mercury in the pathogenesis of autoallergic/immune syndromes like asthma and SLE is not well characterized.

Our Microarray data resulting from low doses (1-3 µg/mL) exposures of human cell lines to mercury indicate differential expressions of several genes located on many human chromosomes. Most genes affected were expressed more than twice the control level; several genes were also down-regulated with mercury treatment. We found close to a total of two hundred highly up-regulated genes with greater than a two-fold change difference (p ≤ 0.002) in the lowest mercury concentration (1µg/mL); 12 genes were moderately over-expressed with an increase of more than one fold (p ≤ 0.005); and a total of more than two thousand genes were down-regulated albeit most repressions were not statistically significant (p>0.05) according to the Wilcoxon's Signed Rank test. Only forty of these genes were down regulated to statistically significant levels at p≤0.05 according to the Welch's ANOVA/- Welch's test. Clear distinctions were seen in the gene expression profiles of the experimental versus controls. Affected genes distributed among almost all of human chromosomes with higher than normal effects on genes associated with chromosomes 1-10, 12, 14-18, 20 (sex-determining region Y), 21 (splicing factor and ATP-binding), X (including BCL-co-repressor). Genes affected include potassium voltage-gated channel–subfamily H member 2 (KCNH2), stress responses, G-protein signal transduction, putative MAPK activating protein (PM20, PM21), *ras* homolog gene family, cytokine receptor activity and polymerase (DNA directed), regulatory subunit (50kDa), leptin receptor involved in hematopoietin/interferon-class (D200-domain), and thymidine kinase 2, mitochondrial TK2 (HGNC) and related genes. Closely associated genes on a chromosome tend to be influenced for expression perhaps due to the availability of close and adjacent *phosphorylation* receptors found by bioinformatics tools.

Identified genes of interest that were over- or under-expressed operate in several pathways including principally the immune and cell cycle (cyclin-dependent kinases) pathways, apoptosis, and cytokine expressions (Figs 1-3) as well as the TGF-beta and the GABA, NMDA receptor subtypes. We have since confirmed that mercury has significant effect on GABA receptors in microarray experimentations in murine cell lines (unpublished data). Our lab results reinforce the capability of mercury exerting significant influence in most metabolic processes probably generating ROS (Kavuru et al 1998; Lang 2000, 2006, Montuschi and Barnes 2002, Wu et al 2000) that participate in the degree of disease outcome of the autoallergic/asthmatic syndromes. The auto allergic phase is the body's adverse response to the onslaught resulting in signs and symptoms invariably difficult to definitively differentially diagnose early on in disease. Estimates from the National Institute of Health (NIH) data indicate that in US alone the prevalence of AD to be about 23.5 billion (Jacobson et al, 1997); in 1996 approximately 1 in 31(3.13%) or 8.5 million people were afflicted with one form or other of AD. Since then at least 237,203 cases of AD are diagnosed annually; of this 42,137 are new cases of primary glomerulonephritis, multiple sclerosis, polymyositis/ dermatomyositis and systemic lupus erythematosus (SLE). Of the total 6,722,573 are women and 1,789,273 men suffering from varieties of diseases that had autoimmune components (Jacobson et al, 1997, Smith et al, 1997). Currently almost 100 types of AD have been identified and approximately 40 more autoimmune-based diseases are awaiting clarification and confirmation.

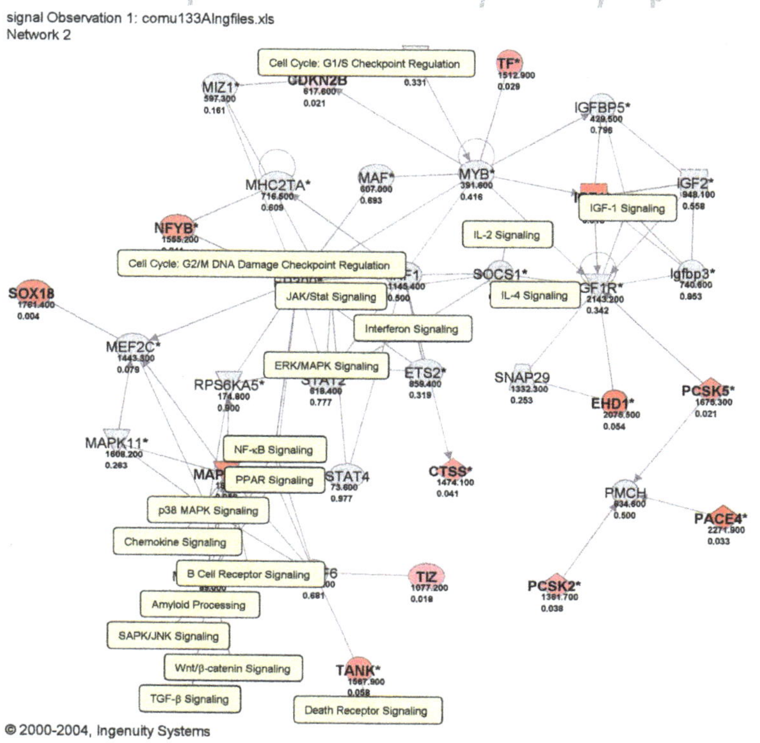

Fig. 1. Results: HepG2 Genes affected by Mercury exposure

5.1 Mercury toxicity: evidence for autoimmunity and neural problems

Mercury (Hg) has long been recognized as a neurotoxicant; however, many experiments with murine models have conclusively implicated this heavy metal as inducer of autoallergies as well as immunotoxicant. In particular Hg has consistently been shown to induce autoimmune disease in susceptible animals with phenotypic consequence of autoantibodies overproduction and pathophysiological signs of lupus-like diseases. This finding has been endorsed by epidemiological studies demonstrating links between occupational Hg exposure and lupus. Mercury rather may interact with triggering events, such as genetic predisposition, exposure to antigens, or infection, to exacerbate disease. Non mercury-susceptible mice that are exposed to mercury do succumb to mercury-induced autoimmune disease (MeIA) with very low doses and short term exposures of inorganic Hg (20-200 µg/kg) exacerbates disease and accelerates mortality in the graft versus host disease model of chronic lupus in C57Bl/6 x DBA/2 mice.

Furthermore, low dose Hg exposure increases the severity and prevalence of experimental autoimmune myocarditis (induced by immunization with cardiac myosin peptide in adjuvant) in A/J mice. Immunosuppression as well as immuno-stimulatory signals results from exposure to the metal in many species humans and rodents included (Pollard et al., 1999). MeIA is prominent among some genetically predisposed individuals that carry syntenic genes as haplotypes in linkage disequilibrium. Some of these individuals are

signal Observation 1: comu133AIngfiles.xls
Network 1

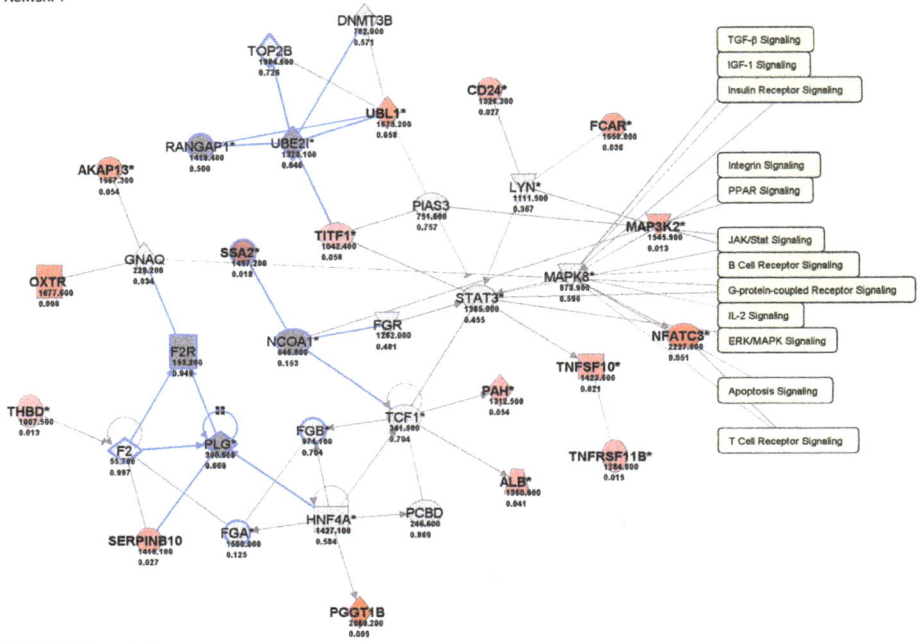

© 2000-2004, Ingenuity Systems

Fig. 2. Results: HepG2 Genes affected by Mercury exposure

genetically prone to develop spontaneous autoimmune diseases. The etiology and pathogenicity of these, mostly systenic, autoimmune states have been difficult to trace. Immunological findings support the notion that the origins of majority of these idiopathic autoimmune diseases can be traced to environmental contaminants of the biosphere with xenobiotic compounds like silver, gold and mercury strongly implicated. *Exposure to* low levels of mercury (<40μg/kg body weight) in susceptible persons may be unsafe; predisposed individuals develop all types of AD typically systemic lupus erythematosus (SLE). Evidence is derived not only from experiments of nature as happened in Miamata in Japan but also from many strains of inbred mice described below. These strains of animals do develop lupus-like disease that imitate closely a simplified version of human systemic lupus erythematous (SLE), with the production of autoantibodies and the subsequent development of immune-complex mediated glomerulonephritis (Theofilopoulos et al., 1985).

The general consensus is that the dose of mercury, duration of exposure as well as the genetic background of the exposed animal (Hanley et al., 2002; Hultman et al., 1992, 1993; Jiang and Möller, 1995; Kono et al., 1998; Pollard et al., 2002) contributes to disease outcome. The H-2 haplotype plays important role in the specificity of resulting autoantibody as well as susceptibility to immune complex generation; but there is a role for involvement of non-MHC genes in MeIA susceptibility also. Acute renal tubular lesions and immunosuppression follow exposure to large doses, whereas chronic administration of smaller doses of mercury leads to the development of SLE (Bariety et al., 1971; Kasturi et al., 1995; Roman-Franco et al., 1978). Mercury-induced autoimmunity shares the same pathogenicity and clinical

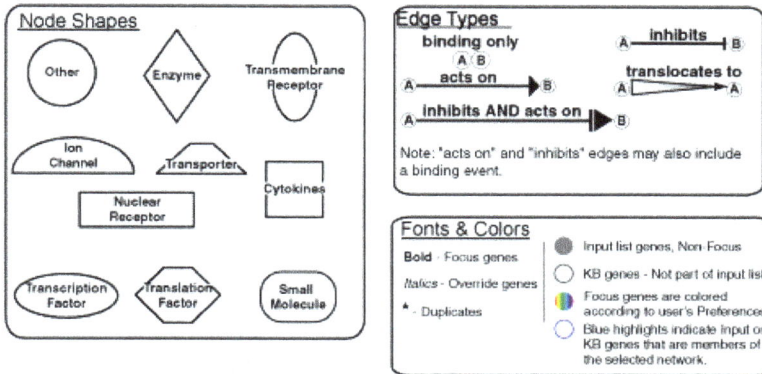

Fig. 3. Key for Both Figs 1 and 2

manifestations seen in patients suffering from clinically diagnosed systemic lupus erythematosus (SLE) (Dubey et al., 1991; Hirsch et al., 1982; Mathieson et al., 1992); the symptomatology is also the same (Biancone et al., 1996; Jiang and Möller, 1995; Kono et al., 1998) with very minor differences.

In humans most of the genes participating in immunity are located on the major histocompatibility complex (MHC) on chromosome 6 with its equivalent on the H-2 region on chromosome 17 in mice. The complexity of the interactions leading to disease state are reflected in the arrays of disease manifestations. Various susceptibility modes are demonstrated by different combinations of gene haplotypes in different strains of animals. BALB/c mice of H-2^d haplotype are highly susceptible to MeIA phenotypically demonstrated as lymphoproliferation without accompanying immune-complex glomerulonephritis (ICGN) (Jiang and Möller, 1995). Mice with $B10.D2$ haplotype specificity are capable of lymphoproliferation but with less severe ICGN than BALB/c mice on exposure to mercury. The H-2^d haplotype $DBA/2$ strain of mice is however, resistant to both lymphoproliferation and ICGN (Hultman et al., 1992; Jiang and Möller, 1995; Kono et al., 1998; Takeuchi et al., 1995). RT-1^n rats are susceptible, whereas RT-1^1 haplotypes are resistant (Eneström and Hultman, 1995; Sapin et al., 1984). An H-2^s haplotype carrying A.SW mice and others show high susceptibility to Hg-induced autoantibodies, whereas $C57BL/6$ strains (H-2^b) are less susceptible. DBA/2 mice strains bearing H-2^d haplotypes are not responsive while H-2^k–bearing mice show intermediate susceptibility (Dubey et al., 1991; Hultman et al., 1993; Jiang and Möller, 1995; Kono et al., 1998).

Most SLE susceptibility loci have been mapped in New Zealand hybrid models; at least 12 of them are located outside the H-1, the murine major histocompatibility complex, H-2. Three regions commonly noted by linkage studies in New Zealand models are found on murine chromosomes 1, 4, and 7 (Drake 1995, Kono et al., 1994, Morel et al., 1994); these have equivalent syntenies in human loci (Duits et al., 1995; Moser et al., 1998; Salmon et al., 1996) that seem to be *ethnically* distinct (Duits et al., 1995: Salmon et al., 1996). Another region along both *H-2 class II* and *TNF-_* gene polymorphisms have been described to act as H-2-linked predisposing genetic elements for the development of SLE; a very strong evidence suggests the contribution of *TNF-* polymorphism that may be the modulator of the initial steps of disease development (The *Wbw2* locus (telomeric to H-2)) which was not linked with autoantibody production might play a role in determining lupus susceptibility; this reaffirms the clustering of functionally related H-2 and non-H-2 genes in the H-2 region on chromosome 17 to be active players in the induction of SLE, a typical example of AD usually quoted. Genetic variants do exist in autoimmune susceptibility that may be a basis for health disparity among races and forewarns that in dealing with xenobiotics like mercury, susceptibility among different racial groups may exhibit differences enough to be taken into account in therapeutic managements.

It has been determined that mercury is immunologically processed uniquely in disease pathogenesis. The process involves the antinuclear autoantibody, (AnoA Abs) response directed against fibrillarin. The AnoA Abs response directed against fibrillarin is one of the most representative manifestations of MeIA that is linked to H-2^s (Hanley et al., 2002; Hultman et al., 1992; Hultman et al., 1993; Pollard et al., 2002) and, more specifically, to the class II I-A^s molecule, by analysis of H-2 congenic mice (Pollard et al., 2002) and is described below. The discovery of potential SLE inducibility on mercury exposure in humans offers the opportunity for comparison with data from murine models of SLE. This means that identification of potential SLE susceptibility loci in humans offers the chance to compare data from murine models of SLE induced by xenobiotics such as mercury.

Mercury-induced cell death (MeICD) is processed through proteolytic breakdown of fibrillarin, a 34kDa MWt macrophage degradable protein component of small nucleolarribonucleoprotein particles (snRNPs); the generation of a unique (19kDa) proteolytic fragment required no pre-interaction between mercury and fibrillarin (Pollard et al, 1997, 2002).

MeICD was associated with a novel protease transiently synthesized and that stimulate *self-reactivity* quite differently from that elicited by full-length protein. Above all *xenobiotic-induced autoimmunity characterized by autoantibody responses against native self-Ag did not require pre-interaction between xenobiotic and Ag*. The genetically restricted anti-fibrillarin autoantibody response of MeIA was not found directed against a fibrillarin-Hg complex as expected of MHC-dependent antigen processing although a metal-protein interaction occurred (Pollard et al., 1997, 2002). This finding endorses a longstanding belief that SLE-prone patients could generate self-autoantibodies spontaneously even without any physical presence of observable inducers of auto-antigens. Cell demise through MeICD was found to be mediated through both nonapoptotic and apoptotic protease activities but the processing pathway of fibrillarin was different enough to suggest the action of different *proteases* (Casiano et al., 1996; Pollard et al., 1997, 2002). It was surmised that the cleavage patterns for a number of auto-antigens must differ between non-apoptosis ($HgCl_2$, heat, ethanol) and apoptosis (anti-Fas) induced cell death (Casiola-Rosen et al., 1995; Pollard et al., 1997). Apparently an MHC-restricted autoantibody response and interaction with $HgCl_2$ are characteristics that differentiate fibrillarin as an autoantigen in $HgCl_2$-induced autoimmunity. The observation that specific cleavage fragments of fibrillarin result from $HgCl_2$ induced death and not other forms of cell death means that *novel* cleavage fragments probably act as *autoimmunogens*. Besides other effects of mercury on the immune system including specific cytokine requirements (Gillespie et al., 1995; Ochel et al., 1991; Van Vliet et al., 1993), inhibition of Fas-mediated cell death are possible means of terminating self-tolerance leading to the equivalent of the SLE state (Whitekus et al., 1999).

As detected in Asthmatic states MeIA is one of the autoimmune models in which T_H1/T_H2 imbalance play critical roles (Biancone et al., 1996; Dubey et al., 1991; Hirsch et al., 1982; Jiang and Möller, 1995; Mirtcheva et al., 1989; Sapin et al., 1984). Although the mechanism by which mercury modifies the immune system is obscure, cationic mercury has a high affinity for *sulfhydryl* groups as the principal site for binding and also has a substantial affinity for *amines, phosphoryl, carboxyl, and hydroxyl groups* (ATSDR, 1999). Mercury is capable of linking with macromolecules including the genetic materials and proteins to form complexes that can activate the immune system. Some of the modified proteins may have epitopes closely resembling self-immunogens (*cryptic antigens*) easily leading to autoimmune disorders in predisposed individuals (Pollard et al., 1997, 2002; Takeuchi et al., 1995). The activation of CD4+ and CD8+ T cells requires a prior induction of antigen presenting cells (APC) (Jiang and Möller, 1995). Mercury binds to molecules on accessory APC cells and transforms molecules on these cells to superantigens capable of activating T cells with a particular set of Vβ Ag-binding receptors (Jiang and Möller, 1995). The mechanism of MeIA can therefore be differentiated from mechanisms induced by polyclonal cell-activators (PCA) such as pokeweed mitogen, PWM. These PCA do not require helper T cells assistance in antibody/cellular inductions.

The presence or absence of IFN-γ on the responder or the non-responder T_H1/T_H2 cell types respectively is thought to be prerequisite in the response to or failure of response respectively (Kono et al., 1998). The balance between the T_H1/T_H2-type responses does not contribute directly to autoimmune susceptibility. Rather IFN-γ has been found to be necessary for the activation of the immune system to respond to poor epitopes, including both self and non-self Ags leading to humoral and cellular auto responses. Dose differentials of IFN-γ appear to directly contribute to disease proneness. High dose immunization with Ag and a strong adjuvant tend to override the IFN-γ requirement (Ferber et al., 1996; Jones et al., 1997). Similarly, a strong genetic predisposition may decrease the threshold for susceptibility enough to overcome the IFN-γ requirement (Abbas et al., 1996). Susceptibility to autoimmune diseases therefore is generally considered a multi-process with many stages or focal barriers evidenced by clinical observations in SLE patients (Andre et al., 1996; Hultgren et al., 1996; Manoury-Schwartz et al., 1997; Vermeire et al., 1997). Lupus is therefore not inherited as a simple Mendelian trait but inherited as a multifactorial and complex trait.

Latest information confirms that the steps to disease state are characterized by unknown, but a large number of susceptibility alleles that give rise to quantitative phenotypic effects. Dose effect allows each of the susceptibility alleles to have partial contribution to probability of increased disease severity. Still nongenetic factors do contribute to disease susceptibility. Recent linkage analyses have revealed over 100 large genomic regions, each represented as a quantitative trait locus (QTL)http://www.discoverymedicine.com/tag/quantitative-trait-locus/ that are associated with increased susceptibility to lupus in mice (Kono et al., 2006) and at least 8 validated QTLs in families of lupus patients (Tsao, 2003) that partially overlap with the mouse QTLs. Some of the genes contribute to the murine lupus QTLs and participate in human SLE. Analysis of these genes is providing insight into pathogenesis of human SLE. Use has been made of linkage analyses on some model murine species that spontaneously get the lupus; these have involved analyses using 129, MRL-*Fas^{lpr}*, BXSB.*Yaa*, and the F_1 hybrid between NZB and NZW (BWF1) and their recombinant inbred derivatives, NZM2410 and NZM2328.

Statistically significant associations between over 100 genomic regions and a lupus-related phenotype covering most commonly lupus nephritis or anti-nuclear autoantibody (ANA) synthesis have been analyzed. Through substitution techniques whereby for example a QTL located in a lupus susceptible strain was replaced with the corresponding genomic interval from a resistant strain only 35 of the 100 genomic regions have been so far confirmed (Morel, 2010). Substitution of the *Adnz1* region (in NZM.C57Lc4 congenic strain) in lupus-prone NZM2328 mice with the appropriate genomic interval from a non-autoimmune genome led to the predicted and expected milder form of glomerulonephritis (Waters et al., 2004). Conversely when the susceptible QTL was bred into a non-autoimmune genome such as B6.NZM2410.*Sle1* mice, which carry the NZM2410-derived*Sle1* QTL that showed the strongest association with lupus nephritis, produced the expected high levels of ANA (Mohan et al., 1998). The implication was that none of the susceptibility loci was sufficient for the induction of full-blown lupus pathology; each of these loci directed the expression of typical phenotypes such as ANA or increased lymphocyte activation (Morel et al., 1997). Therefore each of these component phenotypes itself has an independent genetic basis, at least in the mouse.

In human SLE, risk haplotypes of some of the susceptibility genes such as *STAT4* (Sigurdsson et al., 2008) or *IRF7/PHRF1* (Salloum et al., 2010) correspond to production of specific autoantibody profiles, suggesting that, as in mice, component phenotypes have unique genetic basis also. Confounders make the human analyses harder and difficult to explore due to the unavoidable co-expressivity of all other susceptibility alleles. Intersections of gene-function properties have been identified among the 35 validated murine susceptibility loci. High overlaps have been detected on chromosomes 1, 4, 7, and 13; longer areas are seen on chromosome 1; where 16 independent loci have been identified in 6 strains. The overlap is very conspicuous in the telomeric portion of chromosome 1 with its equivalent region localized in the human *1q23-42* site, a region identified to have many known linkages to human SLE (Tsao, 2003). These results tend to imply that at least some lupus-prone genes are shared among lupus-prone mouse strains and humans as well in that region.

Characterization of the original QTLs lupus congenic strains corresponded to a cluster of susceptibility loci best demonstrated for *Sle1*: this corresponds to at least 7 independent loci. Phenotypic expressions of *Sle1*, ANA synthesis have been linked with 3 independent sub-loci, *Sle1a*, *Sle1b*, and *Sle1c* (Morel et al., 2001). Further studies demonstrated that ANA production was feasible by the way of various distinct paths in each of these 3 sub loci. *Sle1a* regulates inducement of activated, nucleosome-reactive CD4$^+$ T cells and inhibits the number of CD4$^+$ Foxp3$^+$ http://www.discoverymedicine.com/tag/foxp3/regulatory T cells (Chen et al., 2005a; Cuda et al., 2007) with contribution from two independent sub-loci within *Sle1a*, *Sle1a1* and *Sle1a2* (Cuda et al., 2010). Findings indicate *Sle1b* function to regulate tolerance in immature B cells (Kumar et al., 2006; Wandstrat et al., 2004). *Sle1c*, with its two subloci, *Sle1c1* affects germinal center B-cell responses, and *Sle1c2*, that induces appearance of autoreactive CD4$^+$ T cells respectively (Boackle et al., 2001; Chen et al., 2005b). *Sle1d*, sandwiched between*Sle1b* and *Sle1c2*, enhances the severity of glomerulonephritis when mice carrying this allele are crossed with NZW mice (Morel et al., 2001). Also interlocked between *Sle1a* and *Sle1b* is the *Fcgr2b* the presence of which reduces expression on germinal-center B cells and plasma cells (Rahman et al., 2007): a phenotype known to have links with lupus patients (Mackay et al., 2006). The obvious deduction is that other lupus-prone strains may express identical state of genetic complexity in that region and at other loci and therefore is an avenue of either common or strain-specific genes, possible determinant of individual gene level and hence probable disparity among races.

Synergistic interactions between specific loci were also found to be linked with co-expressivity found in *Sle1* and *Yaa* on a B6 background that led to severe lupus nephritis (Croker et al., 2003); the co-expression of either *Sle2* or *Sle3* with *Yaa* achieved only the phenotypes of either parent strains. In humans genetic interactions have been harder to identify for SLE (Harley et al., 2009) partly due to the extreme genetic diversity co-segregating with any gene or locus of interest. Additive effects have, however, been identified between risk variants of*STAT4* and *IRF5* (Abelson et al., 2009; Sigurdsson et al., 2008), suggestive of specific genetic interactions in human SLE. The co-expression of *Sle1*, *Sle2*, and *Sle3* on a B6 background has been seen to give rise to fully penetrant lupus nephritis (Morel et al., 2000).

A clear demonstration of mercury's possible influence on several metabolic pathways is seen in the number of possible pathways affected Figures 1-3: red coloration indicates upregulated genes and blue coloration indicates inhibition of gene expression on exposure to mercury. Mercury exposure leads to effects on several of biochemical pathways involving products of genes in cell cycle signaling: G2/M checkpoint regulation, TGF-β, IGF-1, insulin receptor activity, chemokine, Wint/ β-catenin, integrin, PPAR, SAPK/JNK, JAK/Stat, B and T cell receptor, G-protein-coupled receptor, IL-2, ERK/MAPK, death receptor signaling such as apoptosis, NF-κB, cell cycle and above all immune responses regulated by most of these genes. Pathways indicated are examples of mercury's potential to affect susceptible individuals that carry MHC haplotype combinations and who are prone to develop not only autoimmune and/or cancerous diseases but risk factors for obesity and other chronic associated diseases yet to be evaluated through mercury toxicity.

Our studies confirm that several genes in haplotype combinations are subjected to pronounced changes on exposure to environmental mercury. Among these genes we mention the transforming factor beta (TGF-β) superfamily of cytokines. This group of family genes is associated with regulating the cell cycle essentially for maintenance of normal immunological homeostasis and lymphocyte proliferation. Proteins synthesized from these genes play important roles in regulating essential cellular functions such as differentiation and apoptosis. TGF-β superfamily of cytokines is over expressed on mercury exposure. Some cells, lymphocytes among them are known to respond to TGF-β by undergoing apoptosis. Apoptosis may lead up to accumulation of self-antigens within a localized part of the body and break the body's immunological tolerance to give rise to the autoimmune state. The mechanisms regulating this process are yet to be clarified. Over expression of TGF-β cytokines induced by mercury may lead to transcription of Smad6 and Smad7; these molecules act as inhibitors of TG apoptosis is necessary for maintenance of tolerance. Failure to eliminate immature B cells has the consequence of autoimmune diseases and cancer development. Several aberrant functions associated with many pathways involving the cell cycle and the immune responses are therefore possible through intoxication with mercury. Such wide effects of mercury translate to risk associations when disease susceptibility is our prime concern. This means that it is only at the right genetic combinations and the appropriate line-up of associated genes that disease susceptibility ensues. That goes to argue for severity of disease as well. Mercury-exposed individuals carrying the appropriate allelic-combinations located on specific haplotypes are prone to develop autoimmune diseases.

Not only do some metals induce autoimmunity but can also affect the nervous system when present during fetal development. Mercury readily crosses the human placenta and accumulates in fetal tissue during gestation (David et al., 1972). Mercury can concentrate in umbilical cord blood significantly more than in the maternal blood (Sakamoto et al., 2004). This could affect various developmental processes (Clarkson, 1997; Hassett-Sipple et al., 1997; Pendergrass et al., 1997) leading to behavioral dysfunctions associated with autism (Bernard et al., 2001) and others. Arrhythmias and cardiomyopathies have also been associated with mercury toxicity. Mercury intoxication can result in mental retardation, cerebral palsy, seizures and ultimately death (WHO, 1990). For the early protection of children, it becomes necessary to come up with reliable and relevant tools that identify chemicals with developmental neurotoxicity potential. Once identified, these neurotoxicants need to come under regulatory practices in order to restrict their use and to control exposure as, for example in the case of lead (Silbergeld, 1997).

5.2 Spontaneous lupus: who are at risk

To date genetic mappings endorse genetic susceptibility to autoimmunity and confirms it to be highly associated with individuals with certain combinations of genes in MHC-haplotype linkages: *Fasl* (CD95/L), *Sap* (serum amyloid P-component), *Fcγr2b* (FcγRIIB), *Cr2* (CD21/CD35) and *Ptprc* (CD45) amongst them. Deficiency in individuals of Fcer1g (FcRγ-chain) results in resistance to autoimmunity. These genes are not by any means exhaustive. As mentioned above gene type and dosage seem to determine severity of autoimmune diseases. This indicates that susceptibility and/or initiation factors operate via multiple pathways subjected to regulatory or focal checkpoints that finally give rise to the pathological state. The situation is exemplified by SLE, type 1 diabetes, IDDM and RA patients. In genetically predisposed patients the synthesis of autoantibodies and/or the generation of cellular attack of self-antigens may follow different pathways. Such mechanisms are known to be influenced by gene dosage and contributions from *ethnic* and environmental background. Clinical management or treatment schedules need to vary accordingly.

Thus lupus susceptibility genes are now of deep interest to immunologists/allergists and are being identified in the mouse and their contribution to the disease state is being actively sought through analysis of rare or common variants. Discoveries of the roles of the susceptible lupus genes mainly in the mouse have given insights and critical lead to links with human SLE disease patterns. However the molecular mechanisms by which they contribute to autoimmune pathogenesis are yet to be clearly defined. The multifactorial complex nature of lupus disease susceptibility is currently thought to operate via a combination of common genetic variants that result in small phenotypic effects; rare variants end in large phenotypic effects (Cirulli et al., 2010). So far identified common variants in lupus susceptibility genes include the PTPN22 or *IRF5* among others. Genome wide Association studies (GWAS) and analysis also reveals scarce variants such as C4 and TREX (Graham et al., 2009). Rare *SIAE* variants responsible for the loss-of-function have been linked with autoreactive B cells (Surolia et al., 2010); the *lpr* and *gld* in humans represented in lupus-prone murine strains lead to a functional decline in CD95 or C95L, respectively (Cohen et al., 1992); the *Yaa* mutation, an equivalent of a *Tlr7* gene duplication (Pisitkun et al., 2006), and a mutation in the Coronin A1 gene in the B6.Fas[lpr]/Scr strain that regulates CD4[+] T cell activation (Haraldsson et al., 2008) have all been located.

The murine equivalent of humans common variant genes have now been identified for SLE. NZB and NZW allele of *Fcgr2b* encode a negative regulator of B-cell signaling and predicates an autoimmune phenotype (Rahman et al., 2007; Xiu et al., 2002). Studies currently endorse links between *FCGR2B* variants and human SLE (Lee et al., 2009). *Cr2* polymorphism that function to encode the complement receptor type 2, a B-cell co-receptor known to contribute to the *Sle1c1* phenotypes (Boackle et al., 2001; Chen et al., 2005b). SLE patients do carry a common *CR2* haplotype more frequently than in healthy controls; and follicular dendritic cells (FDC) express a novel CR2 splice variants of SLE patients (Douglas et al., 2009; Wu et al., 2007). *Sle1b* corresponds to polymorphisms in four signaling lymphocytic activation molecule (SLAM) family member genes (Wandstrat et al., 2004), including *Ly108* directly implicated in the regulation of B-cell tolerance (Kumar et al., 2006). Variants of *SLAMF3* (*LY9*) and *SLAMF4* (*CD244*) have also been linked with human SLE (Graham et al., 2008; Suzuki et al., 2008). For the *Sle1* sub-loci, *Sle1a.1* corresponds to the expression of a novel splice isoform of the *Pbx1* gene that is associated with increased CD4[+] T cell activation in both mice and humans (Cuda et al.,2007, 2010). Searches are still going on to reveal the mechanisms linking *Pbx1* expression and T cell phenotypes. Complex phenotypic expressions are associated with *Sle3* locus that includes myeloid cell-induced CD4+ T-cell activation (Zhu et al., 2005) and mild glomerulonephritis (Mohan et al., 1999). Kallikrein (*Klk*) polymorphic genes, serine esterases that regulate a wide spectrum of biological functions in the kidney including inflammation, apoptosis, redox balance, fibrosis, and local blood pressure located in the *Sle3* interval have been linked with increased susceptibility to nephritis in SLE mice and SLE patients (Liu et al., 2009).

To date close to 22 identified and validated loci with confirmed associations with SLE susceptibility (Graham et al., 2009) have been mentioned in the literature. These loci are placed in one of four groups on the basis of mouse characteristics (Morel, 2010). Group one genes are thought to be directly implicated in lupus pathogenesis through their capacity to either induce or modulate disease in the mouse. A representative one is *STAT4*, a transcription factor linked with signal transduction of the IL-12 and IL-23 receptors that has a critical role in regulating the effector functions of helper T cells (Korman et al., 2008). In addition, *Stat4* deficiency modifies disease severity in the NZM lupus models (Jacob et al., 2003; Xu et al., 2006). The *IRF5* whose risk alleles are associated with an increased production of interferon alpha (IFNα) in SLE patients (Niewold et al., 2008) is a puzzling piece. In two different murine models (Richez et al., 2010; Savitsky et al., 2010) *IRF5* however, failed to establish a link between IRF5 and IFNα, pointing instead to a transcriptional control of the IgG2a locus. It is still not clarified if these discrepancies reflect species-specific functions of IRF5 or whether the association between *IRF5* polymorphisms and IFNα production does not involve a direct mechanistic link between the two genes. The second group covers GWAS-identified SLE susceptibility genes with known functions in the murine immune system but without current established link with lupus pathogenesis in man. For example, tumor necrosis factor alpha-induced protein 3 (TNFAIP3) and its binding partner TNFAIP3-interacting protein 1 (TNIP1) are negative regulators of nuclear factor κB signaling and tumor necrosis factor (TNF)-mediated apoptosis (Vereecke et al., 2009).

These findings imply that overexpression of TNFAIP3 would inhibit pathogenesis in lupus-prone mice; its deficiency would exacerbate disease. Newly discovered genes without a known function are placed in the third category of genes associated with SLE in GWAS. The *JAZF1* in this group has now been associated with multiple human phenotypes (Gateva et al., 2009) still awaiting detailed basic functions workout. *FCGR2A* belongs to the fourth group of genes and is associated with SLE risk in GWAS but has no equivalent ancestral gene in the mouse, and therefore cannot yield information for human SLE analysis.

6. Conclusions

The Biosphere is gradually being overwhelmed with several substances from industrial and other activities that has direct role in changes in the incidence and prevalent measures in various diseases. Among these diseases the autoimmune state seems to be a major avenue that impacts and disrupts the homeostatic mechanisms. Autoimmune diseases like asthma are excellent representation of environmental problems acting as indicators of atmospheric as well as the air, the soil and water bodies that are affected by pollutional activities. Thus rises in the incidence and the prevalence of AD within the communities count as direct role of the environmental pollution affecting the gene pool and becomes public health concern. It is important to follow the effects of these substances and the pathways of disease pathogenesis. Currently GWAS is becoming a powerful tool or vehicle that is helping in the understanding the functional roles of the polymorphic alleles particularly those alleles prevailing across ethnic groups. Analyses of population differences in autoimmune state is a first and important step *in* unraveling the complexity of these genes affected by environmental pollutants represented by mercury. It is common knowledge now that environmental contaminants through the food chains occur; pesticides are found in fruits, vegetables and cereals of European origin estimated to contain about 300 biocides in food products (Commission of the European Communities, 2007, Suñol, 2009), also seen in the urine in majority of US population (Mage *et al.*, 2004); and human adipose tissue, serum, and placenta in agricultural areas (López-Espinosa *et al.*, 2007).

Studies in the laboratory reveal increasing concern as to whether pesticides currently used can cause neurodevelopmental toxicity (Bjorling-Poulsen *et al.*, 2008). Similar concerns go for several substances released into the environment. Regulatory checks help to determine the role they play in diseases seen in the population. We are at a time that full-genome association analyses can produce equivocal array of data, some of which are likely to provide vital new biological insights into autoimmunity that may hold the key to novel therapies. The state of the matter is that susceptibility alleles of autoimmune diseases are now believed to fall into two general groups: (1) those genes that confer susceptibility to multiple autoimmune phenotypes (*CTLA4, TPN22, PDCD1, FCRL3*); and (2) those that confer tissue specificity to autoimmunity (*INS* in T1D, *PADI4* in RA). Of note also is that allelic diversity within the *MHC* is also a major determinant of tissue specificity. Having a clear understanding of the genetic basis of autoimmunity and the application of this knowledge to appropriate clinical therapies may provide clinical social medicine benefits in several ways. It may be possible to have early diagnostic tools to detect high risk individuals at the highest genetic risk in prospective longitudinal studies aimed at defining the role of manageable/preventable environmental influences on disease. Also the identification of genetically susceptible individuals will enable targeting of preventive therapy once it becomes available at or evasion of detrimental environmental influences. It may also be helpful to align genetic profiles with prognosis as seen in degrees of disease severity in SLE, RA, IDDM etc or response to specific therapies so that more appropriate or aggressive treatments can be selectively targeted. This will particularly be of unimaginable use in health disparity studies.

7. Acknowledgments

This work was supported in part by the Mississippi IDeA Network for Biomedical Excellence, (NIH-NCRR-P20RR0 16476); Arkansas IDeA Network for Biomedical Excellence (NIH-NCRR-P20RR016460); Research Centers in Minority Institutions (RCMI) — Center for Environmental Health at Jackson State University (NIH-NCRR G12RR013459); Pittsburgh Supercomputing Centre's National Resource for Biomedical Supercomputing (T36GM095335); and National Center for Integrative Biomedical Informatics, University of Michigan (NIH-U54DA021519).

Disclaimer: The views and conclusions contained in this document are those of the authors and should not be interpreted as necessarily representing the official policies, either expressed or implied, of the funding agencies.

8. References

Abbas, A.; Murphy, K, & Sher, A. (1996). Functional diversity of helper T lymphocytes. *Nature* 383:787-796.

Abelson, A.; Gado-Vega, A, Kozyrev, S, Sanchez, E, Velazquez-Cruz, R, Eriksson, N, Wojcik, J, Reddy, L, Lima, G, D'Alfonso, S, Migliaresi, S, Baca, V, Orozco, L, Witte, T, Ortego-Centeno, N, Abderrahim, H, Pons-Estel, B, Gutierrez, C, Suarez, A, Gonzalez-Escribano, M, & et al (2009). STAT4 associates with systemic lupus erythematosus through two independent effects that correlate with gene expression and act additively withIRF5 to increase risk. *Ann Rheum Dis* 68:1746-53.

Andre, I.; Gonzalez, A, Wang B, Katz, J, Benoist, C, & Mathis D. (1996). Checkpoints in the progression of autoimmune disease: lessons from diabetes models. *Proc Natl Acad Sci USA* 93:2260- 2274.

Asosingh, K.; Swaidani, S, Aronica, M , & Erzurum, S, (2007)Th1- and Th2-dependent endothelial progenitor cell recruitment and angiogenic switch in asthma. *J Immunol*, 178: 6482-6494.

ATSDR, (1999). Toxicological Profile for Mercury: TP-93/10. Agency for Toxic Substances and Disease Registry. Centers for Disease Control, Atlanta, Georgia.

Bariety, J.; Druet, P, Laliberte, F, & Sapin, C. (1971) Glomerulonephritis with γ and β1C globulin deposits induced in the rat with mercuric chloride. *Am. J. Pathol.* 65, 293.

Bernard, S.; Enayati A, Redwood, L, Roger, H, & Binstock T, (2001) Autism: A novel form of mercury poisoning. *Med.Hypotheses* 56: 462-471.

Berry, C.; Adam, S, & Curtis, (2003) Functionalisation of magnetic nanoparticles for applications in biomedicine, *J. Phys. D: Appl. Phys* 36 R198 doi: 10.1088/0022-3727/36/13/203 Journal of Physics D: Applied Physics

Biancone L.; Andres, G, Ahn, H, Lim, A, Dai, C, Noelle, R, Yagita, H, De Martino C, & Stamenkovic, I, (1996) Distinct regulatory roles of lymphocyte costimulatory pathways on T helper type-2 mediated autoimmune disease *J. Exp Med* 183 (4), 1473-1481

Birnbaum, L. (2005). PBDEs: Toxicology update. In: *Proceedings of the 2005 National Forum on Contaminants in Fish, Section III: Presentations*, September 18–21, Baltimore, Maryland: *U.S. Environmental Protection Agency*. EPA-823-R-05-006. Available: http://epa.gov/waterscience/fish/forum/2005/proceedings2005.pdf)

Biswas, P, & Wu, C,(2005)Nanoparticles and the Environment – A Critical Review Paper, *J. Air Waste Ma.*, 55, 708-746.

Bjorling-Poulsen, M.; Andersen, H, & Grandjean P. (2008),Potential developmental neurotoxicity of pesticides used in Europe. *Environ. Health*, 7:50-72.

Boackle, S.; Holers, V, Chen X, Szakonyi, G, Karp, D, Wakeland, E, & Morel, L, (2001) Cr2, a candidate gene in the murine Sle1c lupus susceptibility locus, encodes a dysfunctional protein. *Immunity* 15: 775-85.

Bolland, S & Ravetch, J. (2000). Spontaneous autoimmune disease in Fc(γ)RIIB-deficient mice results strain-specific epistasis. *Immunity* 13:277-289.

Candore G.; Lio, D, Colonna-Romano, G, &Caruso, C. (2002) Pathogenesis of autoimmune diseases associated with 8.1 ancestral haplotype: effect of multiple gene interactions. *Autoimmun Rev*, 1, 313-317.

Casiano, C.; Martin, S, Green, & Tan, E. (1996). Selective cleavage of nuclear autoantigens during CD95 (Fas/Apo-1)- mediated T cell apoptosis. Journal of Experimental Medicine 184, 765-770.

Casciola-Rosen, L, Anhalt, G, & Rosen, A. (1995). DNA-dependent protein kinase is one of a subset of autoantigens specifically cleaved early during apoptosis. *J Exp Med* 182, 1625-1634.

Chen, Y.; Cuda, C, & Morel L. (2005a), Genetic determination of T cell help in loss of tolerance to nuclear antigens. *J Immunol* 174:7692-702.

Chen,Y.; Perry, D, Boackle, S, Sobel E, Molina, H, Croker, B, & Morel L. (2005b) Several genes contribute to the production of autoreactive B and T cells in the murine lupus susceptibility locus Sle1c. *J Immunol*175:1080-9.

Cibotti, R.; Kanellopoulos, J, Cabaniols, J, Halle-Panenko, O, Kosmatopoulos, K, Sercarz, E, &Kourilsky, P. Tolerance to a self-protein involves its immunodominant but does not involve its subdominant determinants. *Proceedings of the National Academy of Sciences USA* 89(1):416-420, 1992.

Clarkson, T (1997). The toxicology of mercury. Crit Rev Clin Lab Sci 34:369-403 Clynes, R.; Dumitru, C, & Ravetch, J. (1988). Uncoupling of immune complex formation and kidney damage in autoimmune glomerulonephritis. *Science* 279:1052-1063.deficiency of Fcer1g (FcRγ-chain) ends up in resistance to autoimmunity.

Comhair, S, Bhathena, P, Dweik, R, Kayuru, M, & Erzurum, S. (2000) Rapid loss of superoxide dismutase activity during antigen-induced asthmatic response. *Lancet* 355-624

Commission of the European Communities. (2007). Commission Staff Working Document: Monitoring of Pesticide Residues in Products of Plant Origin in the European Union, Norway, Iceland and Liechtenstein. 2005. SEC 1411.

Croker, B.; Gilkeson, G, & Morel, L (2003). Genetic interactions between susceptibility loci reveal epistatic pathogenic networks in murine lupus. *Genes Immun* 4:575-85.

Cuda C.; Wan, S, Sobel, E, Croker, B, & Morel L. (2007). Murine lupus susceptibility locus Sle1a controlsregulatory T cell number and function through multiple mechanisms. *J Immunol* 179:7439-47.

Cuda, C.; Zeumer, L, Sobel, E, Croker, B, Morel, L. (2010) Murine lupus susceptibility locus Sle1a requires the expression of two subloci to induce inflammatory T cells. *Genes Immun*, epub, May 6.

David, O.; Clark, J, & Voeller, K. (1972) *Lead* and hyperactivity. *Lancet.* 2:900-903. MedlineWeb of Science

De Raeve.; Thunnissen, F, Guo, F, Lewis, M, Kavuru, M, Secic, M, Thamassen, M, & Erzurum, S (1997). Decreased superoxide dismutase activity in asthmatic airway epithelium: correction by inhaled corticosteroid in vivo. *Am J Physiol.* 272: L148-L154.

Dompeling E.; Jobsis, R , & van Schayck, O. (2000) Siblings, day-care attendance, and the risk of asthma and wheezing.*N Engl J Med.* 343:(26) 1967-1968.

Donaldson, K.; Stone, V, Tran, C, Kreyling, W, & Borm, P, (2004). Nanotoxicology. *Occup Environ Med* 61:727-728

Douglas, K.; Windels, D, Zhao, J, Gadeliya, A, Wu, H, Kaufman, K, Harley, J, Merrill, J, Kimberly, R,Alarcon, G, Brown, E, Edberg, J, Ramsey-Goldman, R, Petri, M, Reveille, J, Vila, L, Gaffney P,James, J, Moser K, Alarcon-Riquelme, M, & et al.

(2009). Complement receptor 2 polymorphisms associated with systemic lupus erythematosus modulate alternative splicing. *Genes Immun* 10:457-69.

Drake, C..; Rozzo, S, Hischfeld, H, Smarnworawong, N, Palmer, E, & Kotzin, B (1995). Analysis of the New Zealand Black contribution to lupus-like renal disease: multiple genes that operate in a threshold manner. *J. Immunol.* 154, 2441-7.

Dubey, C.; Bellon, B, Hirsch, F, Kuhn, J, Vial M, Goldman M, & Druet, P. (1991), Increased expression of class II major histocompatibility complex molecules on B cells in rats susceptible or resistant to HgCl2-induced autoimmunity. Clin Exp Immunol. Oct;86 (1):118-23.PMID:1914225 PMCID: PMC1554158

Duits, A.; Bootsma, H, Derksen, R, Spronk, P, Kater, L, Kallenberg, C, Capel P, Westerdaal, N, Spierenburg, G, & Gmelig-Meyling, F. (1995). Skewed distribution of IgG Fc receptor IIa (CD32) polymorphism is associated with renal disease in systemic lupus erythematosus patients. Arthritis Rheum.Dec; 38(12):1832-6.

Dweik, R.; Comhair, S, Gaston, B, Thunnissen, F, Farver, C, Thomassen, M, Kavuru, M, Hammel, J, Abu-Soud, H, & Erzurum, S. (2001). Nitric oxide chemical events in the human airway during the immediate and late antigen induced asthmatic response. *Proc Natl Acad Sci USA.* 2001;98:2622- 2627.

Economic Costs of Asthma (1997) *Am. J. Respir. Crit. Care Med.*, 156(3), 787-793.

Eneström S, & Hultman P (1995) Does amalgam affect the immune system? A controversial issue. *Int Arch Allergy Immunol.* Mar, 106(3):180-203.

EPA's (2007) Report on the Environment: Science Report (SAB Review Draft) *The EPA's* 2007 Report on the Environment:

Fortner, J.; Lyon D, Sayes, C, Boyd, A, Falkner, J, Hotze, E, Alemany, L, Tao, Y, Guo, W, Gateva K, Sandling, V, Hom, J, Taylor G, Chung, S, Sun, X, Ortmann, W, Kosoy, R, Ferreira, R, Nordmark, G, Gunnarsson, I, Svenungsson, E, Padyukov, L, Sturfelt, G, Jonsen, A, Bengtsson, A, Rantapaa-Dahlqvist S, Baechler, E,

Brown, E, Alarcon, G, & et al.(2009) A large-scale replication study identifies TNIP1, PRDM1, JAZF1, UHRF1BP1 and IL10 as risk loci for systemic lupus erythematosus.*Nat Genet* 41:1228-33.

Fortner, J.; Lyon, D, Sayes, C, Boyd, A, Falkner, J, Hotze, E, Alemany, L, Tao, Y, Guo, W, Ausman, K, Colven, V, & Hughes J. (2005). C60 in Water: Nanocrystal Formation and Microbial Response *Environ. Sci. Technol.*, 39 (11), pp 4307–4316

Gammon, G.; & Sercarz, E (1989). How some T cells escape tolerance induction. *Nature* 342(6246):183-185.

Gateva ,V.; Sandling, J, Hom, G, Taylor, K, Chung, S, Sun, X, Ortmann, W, Kosoy, R, Ferreira, R, Nordmark G, Gun- narsson I, Svenungsson E, Padyukov L, Sturfelt G, Jonsen A, Bengtsson AA, Ranta- paa-Dahlqvist S, Baechler EC, Brown EE, Alarcon GS, et al (2009). A large-scale replication study identifies TNIP1, PRDM1, JAZF1, UHRF1BP1 and IL10 as risk loci for systemic lupus erythematosus. *Nat Genet* 41:1228-33.

Gillespie, K.; Qasim, F, Tibbatts, L, Thiru, S, Oliveira, D, & Mathieson, P. (1995) Interleukin-4 gene expression in mercury-induced autoimmunity. Scand J Immunol. Mar; 41(3):268-72. PMID:7871386

Graham, D.; Vyse, T, Fortin, P, Montpetit, A, Cai, Y, Lim, S, McKenzie, T, Farwell, L, Rhodes, B, Chad, L, Hudson, T, Sharpe, A, Terhorst, C, Greenwood, C, Wither, J, & Rioux, J. (2008) CNIOSGES Investig- ators. Association of LY9 in UK and Canadian SLE families. *Genes Immun* 9:93-102.

Graham, R.; Hom, G, Ortmann, W, & Behrens, T. (2009) Review of recent genome-wide association scans in lupus. *J Intern Med* 265:680-8, 2009.

Gupta, A; and Gupta, M. (2005) Review: Synthesis and surface engineering of iron oxide nanoparticles for biomedical applications, BiomaterialsVolume 26, Issue 18, Pages 3995-4021.

Hanley, A.; Karter, A, Festa, A, D'Agostino, R, Wagenknecht, L, Savage, P, Tracy, R, Saad, M, & Haffner, S. (2002) Factor analysis of metabolic syndrome using directly measured insulin sensitivity: The Insulin Resistance Atherosclero- sis Study.Diabetes.Aug;51(8):2642-7.PMID:12145182

Haraldsson, M, Louis-Dit-Sully, C, Lawson, B, Sternik, G, Santiago-Raber, M, Gascoigne, N, Theofilopoulos, A, & Kono, D (2008) The lupus-related Lmb3 locus contains a disease-suppressing Coronin-1A gene mutation. *Immunity* 28:40-51.

Harley, I, Kaufman, K, Langefeld, C, Harley, J, Kelly, J. (2009). Genetic susceptibility to SLE: new insights from fine mapping and genome-wide association studies. *Nat Rev Genet* 10:285-90.

Hassett-Sipple, B.; Swartout, J, Schoeny, R, Mahaffey, K, & Rice, G. (1997) Mercury Study Report to Congress Volume V: health Effects of Mercury and Mercury Compounds. United States Environmental Protection Agency. EPA-452/R-97-007

Hirsch, F.; Couderc, J, Sapin, C, Fournie, G & Druet, P (1982). Polyclonal effects of HgCl2 in the rat: its possible role in an experimental and immune disease. *Eur. J. Immunol.* 12, 620.

Hirsch, F.; Kuhn, J, Ventura, M, Vial, M-C, Fournie, G, & Druet, P. (1986). Autoimmunity induced by HgCl₂ in Brown Norway rats I. Production of monoclonal antibodies. *J. Immunol.* 36, 3272-3276.

Hnizdo, E, Sullivan, P, Bang, K, & et al, (2004). Airflow obstruction attributable to work in industry and occupation among US race/ethnic groups: a study of NHANES III data. *Am J Ind Med* 46:126–35

Holgate, S.; Davies, D, Lackie, P, Wilson S. & et al (2000). Epithelial-mesenchymal interactions in the pathogenesis of asthma. J Allergy Clin Immunol. 2000; 105: 193-204.

Horwitz, D. & Stohl W. (1993). Abnormalities in T lymphocytes. In Dubois Lupus Erythematosus. Wallace DJ and Hahn BH, eds. Lea & Febiger, Philad4elphia. 83-86.

http://www.cas.org/cgi-bin/cas/regreport.pl.

http://www.cas.org/index.html.

http://www. clevelandclinicmeded.com/

http://www.discoverymedicine.com/tag/foxp3/

http://www.discoverymedicine.com/tag/quantitative-trait-locus/

http://www.enotes.com/microbiology -encyclopedia/

www.epa.gov/asthma

(http://www.ewg.org/reports/bodyburden2/execsumm.php).

http://www.epa.gov/glnpo/lmmb/substs.html(FDA/EPA)
http://www.discoverymedicine.com/tag/major-histocompatibility-complex/
http://www.discoverymedicine.com/category/medical-specialties/immunology/
    autoimmunity-immunology-medical-specialties/
http://www.discoverymedicine.com/tag/autoimmunity/
http://www.discoverymedicine.com/category/medical-specialties/neurology/multiple-
    sclerosis/
http://www.discoverymedicine.com/category/medical-specialties/endocrinology/
    diabetes/
http://www.discoverymedicine.com/tag/iddm/
http://www.discoverymedicine.com/category/medical-specialties/rheumatology/
    rheumatoid-arthritis/
http://www.discoverymedicine.com/category/medical-specialties/rheumatology/
    systemic-lupus-erythematosus/
http://www.discoverymedicine.com/category/species-and-cell-types/human/immune-
    system/lymphocyte/tcell/

Hultgren, S,Jones, C, & Normark, S. (1996). Bacterial adhesins and their assembly. In Neidhardt,F.C. (ed.), *Escherichia coli and Salmonella; Cellular and Molecular Biology.* ASM Press, Washington, DC, pp. 2730–2756.

Hultman, P.; Bell, L, Enestrom, S, & Pollard, K. (1992). Murine susceptibility to mercury. I. Autoantibody profiles and systemic immune deposits in inbred, congenic and intra-H-2 recombinant strains. *Clin Immunol Immuno-Pathol* 65:98-108.

Hultman, P.; Bell, L, Enestrom, S, & Pollard, K. (1993). Murine susceptibility to mercury. II. Autoantibody profiles and renal immune deposits in hybrid, backcross, and H-2d congenic mice. Clin Immunol Immunopathol 68:9-20.

Jacob, C.; Zang, S, Li, L, Ciobanu, V, Quismorio, F, Mizutani, A, Satoh, M, & Koss, M. (2003) Pivotal role of Stat4 and Stat6 in the pathogenesis of the lupus-like disease in the New Zealand mixed 2328 mice. *J Immunol* 171:1564-71, 2003.

Jacobson, D.; Gange, S, Rose, N, & Graham, N. (1997) Epidemiology and estimated population burden of selected autoimmune diseases in the United States. *Clin Immunol Immunopath* , 84, 223- 243.

Jiang, Y. & Möller, G. (1995) In vitro effects of HgCl$_2$ on murine lymphocytes. I. Preferable activation of CD4$^+$ T cells in a responder strain. *J Immunol* 154: 3138-3146.

Jones, P.;Osborn, T, & Briffa, K. (1997). Estimating sampling errors in large-scale temperature averages. *Journal of Climate* 10:2548-2568.

Kasturi,L.; Eshleman, J, Wunner, W, & Shakin-Eshleman, S. (1995) The hydroxy amino acid in an Asn-X-Ser/Thr seq-uon can influence N-linked core glycosylation efficiency and the level of expression of a cell surface glycoprotein. *J. Biol. Chem.*, 270, 14756–14761

Kavuru, M.; Dweik, R & Thomassen, M. (1999) Role of bronchoscopy in asthma research. Clin Chest Med. 1999; 20:(1) 153-189.

Kavuru, M.; Lang, D, & Erzurum, S (2005) Asthma The Cleveland Clinic Disease Management Project, Allergy & Immunology.

Kharitonov, S, & Barnes, P (2001) Exhaled markers of pulmonary disease. *Am J Respir Crit Care Med.* 1693-1722. Kono, Y., Yoshinaga, M., Oku, S., Nomura, Y., Nakamura, M. and Aihoshi, S. (1994) Effect of obesity on echocardio-graphic parameters in children. *International Journal of Cardiology 446*, 7-13.

Kono, D.; Balomenos, D, Pearson, D, Park, M, Gildebrandt, B, Hultman, P, Pollard, K. (1998).The prototypic TH2 auto immunity induced by mercury is dependent on IFN- γ and not T_H1/T_H2 imbalance. *J Immunol. 161*:234-240.

Kono, D. & Theofilopoulos, A. (2006). Genetics of SLE in mice. *Springer Semin Immunopathol* 28:83-96.

Korman, B.; Kastner, D, Gregersen, P, & Remmers E. (2008). STAT4: genetics, mechanisms, and implications for auto-immunity. Curr Allergy Asthma Rep. Sep;8(5):398-403.PMID:18682104[PubMed indexed for MEDLINE] PMCID: PMC2562257

Kumar, K.; Li, L, Yan, M, Bhaskarabhatla, M, Mobley, A, Nguyen, C, Mooney, J, Schatzle, J, Wakeland,E, & Mohan, C. (2006). Regulation of B cell tolerance by the lupus susceptibility gene Ly108.*Science* 312:1665-9.

Lam, C.; James J, McCluskey, R & Hunter R (2004). Pulmonary toxicity of single-walled carbon nanotubes in mice 7 and 90 days after intratracheal instillation. *Toxicol. Sci.* 77:126-134.

Lang, D. (2000). Anti-leukotriene agents and aspirin-sensitive asthma – Are we removing the second bassoonist or skating to where the puck is gonna be?. *Ann Allergy Asthma Immunol,* 85: 5-8.

Lang, D. (2006). The long acting beta agonist controversy: A critical examination of the evidence. Cleve *Clin J Med*; 73 973-992.

Lang, S.; Butterfield, D, Schulted, M, Kelley, D, & Lilley, M, (2010). Elevated concentrations of formate, acetate and dissolved organic carbon found at the Lost City hydrothermal field Geochimica et Cosmochimica Acta 74, 941–952

Lanzavecchia, A(1995). How can cryptic epitopes trigger autoimmunity? *Journal of Experimental Medicine* 181(6): 1945 -1948.

Lehmann PV, Forsthuber T, Miller A, Sercarz EE. Spreading of T-cell autoimmunity to cryptic determinants of an autoantigen. *Nature* 358(6382):155-, 1992.

Lee, Y.; Ji, J, & Song, G, (2009) Fcγ receptor IIB and IIIB polymorphisms and susceptibility to systemic lupus erythe-matosus and lupus nephritis: a meta-analysis. Lupus 18:727-34.

Li, X.; & Wilson, J. (1997). Increased vascularity of the bronchial mucosa in mild asthma. Am J Respir Crit Care Med. 156: 229-233.

Liossis S-NC.; Kovacs, B, Dennis, G, Kammer, G. & Tsokos G. (1996). B cells from patients with systemic lupus eryth-ematosus display abnormal antigen receptor-mediated signal transduction events. J Clin Invest 98:2549-2557.

Liu, K.; Li, Q, gado-Vega, A, Abelson, A, Sanchez, E, Kelly, A, Li, L, Liu, Y, Zhou, J, Yan, M, Ye, Q, Liu, S, Xie, C, Zhou, X, Chung, S, Pons-Estel, B, Witte, T, de Ramon, E, Bae, S, Barizzone, N, & et al.(2009) Kallikrein genes are associated with lupus and glomerular basement membrane-specific antibody-induced nephritis in mice and humans. *J Clin Invest* 119:911-23.

Lopez-Espinosa, M.; Granada, A, Carreno, J, Salvatierra, M, Olea-Serrano, F, & Olea, N. (2007). Organochlorine pesticides in placentas from Southern Spain and some related factors. *Placenta.* Jul;28(7):631-8. Epub 2006 Nov 15. PMID:17109956 [PubMed - indexed for MEDLINE]

Lovern, S.; & Klaper R. (2005). Impact of titanium dioxide and carbon nanoparticles on Daphnia magna. Society of Environmental Toxicology and Chemistry, Midwest Regional Chapter Annual Meeting. Abstract.

Mackay, M.; Stanevsky, A, Wang, T, Aranow, C, Li, M, Koenig, S, & Ravetch, J, (2006) Diamond B. Selective dysregulation of the FcγIIB receptor on memory B cells in SLE. *J Exp Med* 203:2157-64.

Mage, D.; Allen, R, Gondy, G, Smith, W, Barr, D & Needham, L.(2004). Estimating pesticide dose from urinary pesticide concentration data by creatinine correction in Third National Health and Nutrition Examination Survey (NHANES- III). *J Expo Anal Environ Epidemiol.* Nov;14(6):457-65.

Manoury-Schwartz, B.; Chiocchia, G, Bessis, N, Abehsira-Amar, O, Batteux, F, Muller, S, Huang, S, Boissier, M, & Fournier C. (1997). High susceptibility to collagen-induced arthritis in mice lacking IFN-γ receptors. *J Immunol* 158:5501- 5506.

Mathieson, P.; Thiru, & D, Oliveira, D. (1992). Mercuric chloride-treated Brown Norway rats develop widespread tissue injury including necrotizing vasculitis. *Lab Invest* 67:121-132.

McKernan, M.; Rattner, B, Ackerson, B, Barton, M, Schoen, K, Hale R. & Ottinger, M. (2006). Comparative toxicity of polybrominated flame retardants in avian embryos. Poster at (2006) Society of Environmental Toxicology and Chemistry Meeting.

Mirtcheva, J.; Pfeiffer, C, De Bruijn, J, Jacquesmart, F, & Gleichmann, E. (1989).Immunological alterations inducible by mercury compounds. III. H-2A acts as an immune response and H-2^e as an immune "suppression" locus for HgCl$_2$-induced antinuclear autoantibodies. *Eur J Immunol* 19:2257- 2268.

Mohan, C.; Alas, E, Morel, L, Yang, P, Wakeland, E, (1998). Genetic dissection of SLE pathogenesis - Sle1 on murine chromosome 1 leads to a selective loss of tolerance to H2A/H2B/DNA subnucleosomes. *J Clin Invest* 10 11362-72.

Mohan, C.; Yu, Y, Morel, L, Yang, P & Wakeland, E. (1999). Genetic dissection of Sle pathogenesis: Sle3 on murine chromosome 7 impacts T cell activation, differentiation, and cell death. *J Immunol* 162:6492-502.

Monroe, R. & Halvorsen S. (2006). Mercury abolishes neurotrophic factor–stimulated Jak-STAT signaling in nerve cells by oxidativestress. Toxicological Sciences 94, 129-138.

Montuschi, P. & Barnes, P. (2002). Exhaled leukotrienes and prostaglandins. *J Allergy Clin Immunol.* 109: 615-620.

Morel, L.; Rudofsky, U, Longmate, U, Schiffenbauer, J, & Wakeland, E. (1994). Polygenic control of susceptibility to murine systemic lupus erythematosus. *Immunity* 1:219.

Morel, L.; Mohan, C, Yu, Y, Croker, B, Tian, N, Deng, A, & Wakeland, E (1997). Functional dissection of systemic lupus erythematosus using congenic mouse strains. *J Immunol* 158:6019-28.

Morel, L.; Croker, B, Blenman, K, Mohan, C, Huang G, Gilkeson, G, & Wakeland, E. (2000) Genetic reconstitution of systemic lupus erythematosus immunopathology with polycongenic murine strains. *Proc Natl Acad Sci USA* 97:6670-5.

Moser, K.; Neas, B, Salmon, J, Yu, H, Gray-McGuire, C, Asundi, N, Bruner, G, Fox, J, Kelly, J, Henshall, S, Basino, D, Dietz, M, Hogue, R, Koelsch, G, Nightingale, L, Shaver, T, Abdou, N, Albert, D, Carson, C, Petri, M, Tread- well, E, James, J, & Harley, J. (1998). Genome scan of human systemic lupus erythematosus: evidence for linkage on chromosome 1q in African-American pedigrees. *Proc Natl Acad Sci USA* 95(25):14869-14874.

Morel, L.; Blenman, K, Croker, B, & Wakeland, E. (2001). The major murine systemic lupus erythematosus susceptibi-lity locus, Sle1, is a cluster of functionally related genes. *Proc Natl Acad Sci U S A* 98:1787-92.

Morel, L. (2010) Genetics of SLE: Evidence from mouse models. *Nat Rev Rheumatol* 6:348-57.

Moudgil, K.; & Sercarz, E. (2005). Understanding crypticity is the key to revealing the pathogenesis of autoimmunity. *Trends in Immunology* 26(7):355-359, 2005.

Niewold, T.; Kelly, J, Flesch, M, Espinoza, L, Harley, J, & Crow, M. (2008). Association of the IRF5 risk haplotype with high serum interferon-alpha activity in systemic lupus erythematosus patients. *Arthritis Rheum* 58:2481-7.

Oberdörster. E. (2004). Manufactured Nanomaterials (Fullerenes, C_{60}) Induce Oxidative Stress in the Brain of Juvenile Largemouth Bass. *Environ Health Perspect* 112:1058-1062.

Oberdörster, G.; Sharp, Z, Atudorei, V, Elder, A, Gelein, R, & et al. (2004). Translocation of inhaled ultrafine particles to the brain. *Inhal Toxicol* 46:437–445.

Oberdorster, E. (2004b). Toxicity of nC60 fullerenes to tow aquatic species: Daphnia and largemouth bass. American Chemical Society, Anaheim, California. March 27–April 2004. Abstract IEC21.

Ochel, M.; Vohr, H, Pfeiffer, C, & Gleichman, E (1991). IL-4 is required for the IgE and IgG1 increase and IgG1 auto-antibody formation in mice treated with mercuric chloride. J Immunol. May 1;146(9):3006-11.

Pascual, R. & Peters, S. (2005) airway remodeling contributes to the progressive loss of lung function in asthma: an overview. *J Allergy Clin Immunol.* 116: 477-486.

Patrick, L. (2002). Mercury toxicity and antioxidants: Part 1: Role of glutathione and alpha-lipoic acid in the treatment of mercury toxicity. *Altern. Med. Rev.* 7, 456–471.

Pauwels, R.; Buist, A, Calverley, P, & et al. (2001). Global strategy for the diagnosis, management, and prevention of chronic obstructive pulmonary disease. NHLBI/WHO Global Initiative for Chronic Obstructive Lung Disease (GOLD) Workshop summary. *Am J Respir Crit Care Med* 163: 1256–76

Pendergrass, J.; Haley, B, Vimy, M, Winfield, S, Lorscheider, F, (1997) Mercury vapor inhalation inhibits binding of GTP to tubulin in rat brain: similarity to a molecular lesion in Alzheimer diseased brain. *Neurotoxicology* 18:315-324.

Pier, S. M. (1975). The role of heavy metals in human health. *Texas Rep Biol Med. 33*(1), 85-106.

Pisitkun, P.; Deane, J, Difilippantonio, M, Tarasenko, T, Satterthwaite, A, & Bolland, S. (2006) Autoreactive B cell responses to RNA-related antigens due to TLR7 gene duplication. *Science* 312:1669-72.

Pollard, K, Lee, D, Casiano, C, Blüthner, M, Johnson, M, & Tan EM. (1997). The autoimmunity-inducing xenobiotic mercury interacts with the autoantigen fibrillarin and modifies its molecular and antigenic properties. *J Immunol* 158:3521-3528.

Pollard, K.; Pearson, D, Hultman, P, Hildebrandt, B, & Kono, D. (1999). Lupus-prone mice as models to study xenobiotic-induced acceleration of systemic autoimmunity. *Environ Health Perspect* 107(5):729-735.

Pollard, K, Pearson, L, Blüthner, M, Tan, E. (2002). Proteolytic cleavage of a self-antigen following xenobiotic-induced cell death produces a fragment with novel immunogenic properties. *J Immunol* 165(4):2263-2270.

Puck, J. & Sneller, M. (1997). ALPS: an autoimmune human lymphoproliferative syndrome associated with abnormal lymphocyte apoptosis. *Semin Immunol* 9:77-81.

Rahman, Z.; Niu, H, Perry, D, Wakeland, E, Manser, T, & Morel, L (2007). Expression of the autoimmune Fcgr2b NZW allele fails to be upregulated in germinal center B cells and is associated with increased IgG production *Genes Immun* 8:604-12.

Renwick, L.; Brown, D, Clouter, A, & Donaldson, K. (2004). Increased inflammation and altered macrophage chemo-tactic responses caused by two ultrafine particle types. *Occup Environ Med* 61:442 447 doi:10. 1136/ oem. 2003 .00 8227

Richez, C.; Yasuda, K, Bonegio, R, Watkins, A, Aprahamian, T, Busto, P, Richards, R, Liu, C, Cheung, R, Utz, P, Marshak-Rothstein, A, & Rifkin, I, (2010). IFN regulatory factor 5 is required for disease development in the FcγRIIB-/-Yaa and FcγRIIB-/- mouse models of systemic lupus erythematosus. *J Immunol*184:796-806.

Roman-Franco, A.; Turiello, M, Albini, B, Ossi, E, Milgrom, F, & Andres, G. (1978). Anti-basement membrane anti-bodies and antigen-antibody complexes in rabbits injected with mercuric chloride. *Clin Immunol Immun- opathol* 9:464-472.

Rose, N. & Bona, C. (1993). Defining criteria for autoimmune disease (Witebsky's postulate revisited). Immunol Today, 14(9), 426-430.

Sakamoto, M.; Kubota, M, Liu, X, Murata, K, Nakai, K, & Satoh, H, (2004) Maternal and fetal mercury and n-3Poly-unsaturated fatty acids as a risk and benefit of fish consumption to fetus. *Environ. Sci.Technol.* 38: 3860-63

Salloum, R.; Franek, B, Kariuki, S, Rhee, L, Mikolaitis, R, Jolly, M, Utset, T, Niewold, T (2010). Genetic variation at the IRF7/PHRF1 locus is associated with autoantibody profile and serum interferon-alpha activity in lupus patients. *Arthritis Rheum* 62:553-61.

Salmon J.; Millard S, Schachter L, Arnett F, Ginzler E, Gourley M, Ramsey-Goldman R, Peterson M & Kimberly R. (1996). FcγRIIA alleles are heritable risk factors for lupus nephritis in African –Americans. *J Clin Invest* 97: 1348-1354.

Sapin, C.; Hirsch, F, Delaporte, J, Bazin, H, & Druet, P. (1984). Polyclonal IgE increase after HgCl$_2$ injections in BN and LEW rats: a genetic analysis. Immunogenetics 20;227-234.

Salvato, G. (2001) Quantitative and morphological analysis of the vascular bed in bronchial biopsy specimens from asthmatic and non-asthmatic subjects. *Thorax*. 56: 902-906.

Savitsky, D, Yanai, H, Tamura, T, Taniguchi, T, & Honda, K. (2010). Contribution of IRF5 in B cells to the develop -ment of murine SLE-like disease through its transcriptional control of the IgG2a locus *PNAS* 107:10154-9.

Schecter, A.; Pavuk, M, Päpke, O, Ryan, J, Birnbaum, L, & Rosen, R. (2003) Polybrominated Diphenyl Ethers (PBDEs) in U.S. Mothers' Milk Polybrominated Diphenyl Ethers (PBDEs) in U.S. Mothers' Milk *Env Health Perspec- tive* 111(14) Nov.

Sercarz, E.; Lehmann, P, Ametani, A, Benichou, G, Miller, A, Moudgil, K.(1993) Dominance and crypticity of T cell antigenic determinants. *Annual Review of Immunology*11:729-766, 1993.

Shvedova, A.; Kisin, E, Mercer, R, Murray, A, Johnson, V, Potapovich, A, Yulia, Y, Gorelik. T, Arepalli, S, Schwegler -Berry, D, Hubbs, AF, Antonini, J., Evans D.E, Ku, B-Ki, Ramsey,D Maynard, A., Kagan V E., Castranova J,& Baron, P. (2005); Unusual inflammatory and fibrogenic pulmonary responses to single-walled carbon nanotubes in mice. *Am Cellular and Molecular Physiology.Lung Cell Mol. Physiol.* 289:L698-L708

Sigurdsson, S.; Nordmark, G, Garnier, S, Grundberg, E, Kwan, T, Nilsson, O, Eloranta, M, Gunnarsson, I, Svenungsson, E, Sturfelt, G, Bengtsson, A, Jonsen, A, Truedsson, L, Rantapaa-Dahlqvist, S, Eriksson, C, Alm, G, Goring, H, Pastinen, T, Syvanen, A &, et al. (2008) A risk haplotype of STAT4 for systemic lupus erythemaatosus is over-expressed, correlates with anti-dsDNA and shows additive effects with two risk alleles of IRF5. *Hum Mol Genet* 17:2868-76.

Silbergeld, E. (1997) Preventing lead poisoning in children 1997 *Annu. Rev. Public Health* 1997; 18:187-210.

Sinha P, Chi HH, Kim HR, Clausen BE, Pederson B, Sercarz EE, Forster I, Moudgil KD. Mouse lysozyme-M knockout mice reveal how the self-determinant hierarchy shapes the T cell repertoire against this circulating self antigen in wild-type mice. *Journal of Immunology* 173(3):1763-1771, 2004.

Smith, H.; Malone, C, Lawson, A, Okamoto, J, Battista, C, Saunders, B. A national estimate of the economic costs of asthma, (1997). *Am J. Respir Crit Care Med* (156): 787-793.

Smith, J.; Krishnaswamy, G, Dykes, R, Reynolds, S, & Berk, S. (1997). Clinical manifestations of IgE hypogammaglobulinemia. Ann Allergy Asthma Immunol.Mar;78(3):313-8.

Suñol, C. (2009) Use of Gene Expression of Neural Markers in Cultured Neural Cells to Identify Developmental Neurotoxicants, *Toxicological Sciences*, 113, 1-3.

Surolia, I.; Pirnie, S., Chellappa, V, Taylor, K, Cariappa, A, Moya, J, Liu, H, Bell, D, Driscoll, D, Diederichs, S, Haider, K, Netravali, I, Le, S, Elia, R, Dow, E, Lee, A, Freudenberg, J, De Jager, P, Chretien, Y, Varki, A, & et al.(2010) Functionally defective germline variants of sialic acid acetylesterase in autoimmunity. *Nature* 466:243-7.

Takeuchi, K.; Turley, S, Tan, E., Pollard, L. (1995) Analysis of the autoantibody response to fibrillarin in human disease and murine models of autoimmunity. *J. Immunol. 154,* 961-969

Theofilopoulos, A, & Dixon, F (1985). Murine models of systemic lupus erythematosus. *Adv Immunol* 37:269-379.

Tsao, B. (2003). The genetics of human systemic lupus erythematosus. Trends Immunol 24:595-602.

Van Vliet, E.; Uhrberg, M, Stein, C, & Gleichmann, E. (1993). MHC control of IL-4-dependent enhancement of B cell Ia expression and Ig class switching in mice treated with mercuric chloride. Int Arch Allergy Immunol. 1993;101(4):392-401.PMID:8102566 [PubMed - indexed for MEDLINE]

Vereecke, L.; Beyaert, R, van Loo, G.(2009) The ubiquitin-editing enzyme A20 (TNFAIP3) is a central regulator of immune pathology. Trends Immunol 30:383-91.

Vermeire, K.; Heremans, H, Vandeputte, M, Huang, S, Billiau, A, Matthys, P. (1997). Accelerated collagen-induced arthritis in IFN-γ receptor-deficient mice. J Immunol 158:5507-5513.

Wandstrat, A, Nguyen, C, Limaye, N, Chan, A, Subramanian, S, Tian, X, Yim, Y, Pertsemlidis, A, Garner, H, Morel, L, & Wakeland, E. (2004). Association of extensive polymorphisms in the SLAM/CD2 gene cluster with muri- nelupus. *Immunity* 21:769-80.

Waters, S.; McDuffie, M, Bagavant, H, Deshmukh, U, Gaskin, F, Jiang, C, Tung, K, & Fu, S. (2004). Breaking tolerance to double stranded DNA, nucleosome, and other nuclear antigens is not required for the pathogenesis of lupus glome -rulonephritis. *J Exp Med* 199:255-64, 2004.

Weiss, S. (2002) Eat dirt — The hygiene hypothesis and allergic diseases. *N Engl J Med*. 2002; 347: 930-931.

WHO, World Health Organization Geneva, (1990) Methylmercury.Environmental healthcriteria;101

Whitekus, M.; Santini, R, Rosenspire, A, McCabe, M, Jr. (1999). Protection Against CD95-Mediated Apoptosis by Inorganic Mercury in Jurkat T Cells. *The J Immunol* 162:7162-7170.

Wilson, R.; Goyal, L, Ditzel, M, Zachariou, A, Baker, D, Agapite, J, Steller, H, Meier,P, (2002). The DIAP1 RING finger mediates ubiquitination of Dronc and is indispensable for regulating apoptosis. *Nat. Cell Biol. 4(6); 445-450. (Export to RIS)* 12021771

Wollenberger, L. (March 2005). *Toxicity tests with crustaceans for detecting sublethal effects of potential endocrine disrupting chemicals.* Ph.D. thesis. Lyngby, Denmark: Environment and Resources, Technical University of Denmark. Available: http://www2.er.dtu.dk/publications/fulltext/2005/MR2005-012.pdf.

Wu, H.; Boackle, S, Hanvivadhanakul, P, Ulgiati, D, Grossman, J, Lee, Y, Shen, N, Abraham, L, Mercer, T, Park, E, Hebert, L, Rovin, B, Birmingham, D, Chang, D, Chen, C, McCurdy, D, Badsha, H, Thong, B, Chung, H, Arnett F, & et al. (2007). Association of a common complement receptor 2 haplotype with increased risk of systemic lupus erythematosus. *Proc Natl Acad Sci U S A* 104:3961-6.

Wu, W, Samoszuk, M , Comhair S. & et al (2000). Eosinophils generate brominating oxidants in allergen-induced asthma. *J Clin Invest.* 105: 1455-1463.

www.nhlbi.nih.gov/guidelines/asthma/epr3/index.htm

Xia, T.; Korge, P. Weiss, J, Li, N, Venkatesen, M, Sioutas, C, & Nel, A, (2004) Quinones and aromatic chemical compounds in particulate matter induce mitochondrial dysfunction: implications for ultrafine particle toxicity. Environ Health Perspect. Oct;112 (14):1347-58.

Xiu, Y.; Nakamura, K, Abe, M, Li, N, Wen, X, Jiang, Y, Zhang, D, Tsurui, H, Matsuoka, S, Hamano, Y, Fujii, H, Ono, M, Takaj, T, Shimokawa, T, Ra, C, Shirai, T,& Hirose, S. (2002) Transcriptional regulation of Fcgr2b gene by polymorphic promoter region and its contribution to humoral immune responses. *J Immunol*169:4340-6.

Xu, Z, Duan, B, Croker, B, & Morel L. (2006) STAT4 deficiency reduces autoantibody production and glomerulonephritis in a mouse model of lupus. *Clin Immunol* 120:189-98.

2

HLA and Citrullinated Peptides in Rheumatoid Arthritis

Iñaki Álvarez
Immunology Unit. Department of Cell Biology,
Physiology and Immunology. Institut de Biotecnologia i Biomedicina,
Universitat Autònoma de Barcelona,
Spain

1. Introduction

Rheumatoid arthritis (RA) is a chronic systemic inflammatory disease that mostly attacks synovial joints, although other tissues and organs can be affected. The final effect is usually the destruction of articular cartilage and ankylosis of the joints, with a prevalence of the wrist and small joints of the hand. Diagnostic criteria have recently been revised (Aletaha et al., 2010; Neogi et al., 2010). The prevalence of RA is about 1% in the total population, being women more affected than men in a ratio of approximately 2-3:1 (Alamanos & Drosos, 2005).

RA is considered an autoimmune disorder, although the etiology and pathogenesis of the disease remain unclear. A complex set of factors are involved in the onset of the disease, including genetic and environmental. The strongest genetic association is with the genes encoding major histocompatibility complex (MHC, HLA in human) class II molecules (Gregersen et al., 1987; Stastny, 1978), although other genes have been associated with RA, including *PTPN22, STAT4, TRAF1/C5*, and others.

Antibodies against the Fc fraction of IgG are found in the serum of about 80% of patients with RA. These autoantibodies are called rheumatoid factor (RF), and the consideration of RA as an autoimmune disease has largely been based on the presence of RF in the serum of patients. Nevertheless, the presence of RF is not exclusive of RA and that, together with the absence of definitive data demonstrating an arthritogenic effect of RF, suggest that these antibodies are produced as a consequence of the immune response rather than being the cause of it (Nemazee, 1985; Tarkowski et al., 1985). However, the adaptive immune response seems to play an important role in the disease as suggested by the strong association of RA with the presence of some HLA class II alleles. Autoantibodies against citrullinated proteins (ACPAs) have been described in the serum of about 50-70% of RA patients in comparison with about 2% of the healthy population (Avouac et al., 2006; Kroot et al., 2000; Nishimura et al., 2007; Schellekens et al., 2000; van Gaalen et al., 2004; Vincent et al., 2002). The presence of ACPAs is very stable during the course of the disease and is quite specific for RA. These antibodies can be detected several years before of symptomatic disease, making the presence of ACPAs a good clinical marker for RA. Patients containing ACPAs in the serum usually have a more severe disease. The presence of these antibodies correlates very well with the presence of some of the HLA-DR alleles containing the "shared epitope" (see below). All of these data have led to the postulation that there actually are two different disorders (Klareskog et al., 2008). However, the cause of the specificity of the generation of ACPAs in RA and whether the antibodies are pathogenic or secondary to the joint inflammation remain unanswered.

Many reports have been published in the last years describing some of the features of the antibodies that recognize citrullinated proteins and showing some of the proteins that are target of these autoantibodies. The generation of an effective B cell response requires the recognition by specific CD4+ T cells of peptides derived of the antigen in the context of MHC class II molecules. In this chapter some of the data indicating the importance of anti-citrulline responses will be reviewed and concretely emphasize on reviewing the last reports dealing with MHC presentation and T cell responses to citrullinated peptides will be done.

2. HLA and rheumatoid arthritis

The strongest genetic association of RA susceptibility is with some specific HLA class II alleles. In Northern Europe, the strongest association is with the serotype HLA-DR4 (Jaraquemada et al., 1986; Stastny, 1978). The association is with some allelic variants of HLA-DR4, including DRB1*0401, *0404, *0405 and *0408. However, other HLA-DR4 subtypes do not confer predisposition to RA. In Southern Europe and other populations the susceptibility to RA is associated to alleles other than DR4. Thus, DRB1*0101, *0102, *1402 and *1001 have been reported with predisposition to RA (Cutbush et al., 1993; de Juan et al., 1994; Gonzalez-Escribano et al., 1999; Hameed et al., 1997; Lacki et al., 2000; Mody & Hammond, 1994; Poor et al., 2007; Salvarani et al., 1999; Sanchez et al., 1990; Yelamos et al., 1993). A major feature shared by the alleles that confer susceptibility to RA is the presence of some residues at position 67 and 70-74 of the third hypervariable region of DRB1 (Table 1). Thus, the presence of specific residues in these positions (L...(Q/R)(K/R)RAA) led to the proposal of the "shared epitope" hypothesis (Gregersen et al., 1987), in which the molecular basis for the association of some alleles with RA was restricted to this critical region in the β chain of HLA-DR molecules. The P4 residue of the peptide core directly interacts with some of the residues that are part of the shared epitope (SE). Other residues are exposed to outside the binding groove. Thus, the side chains of these amino acids could be involved in the pathogenesis of the disease by defining the peptide preference or directly interacting with the T cell receptor (TCR), influencing the T cell repertoire selection, and specific T cell activation. Alternatively, molecular mimicry of this HLA-DR region and proteins from pathogenic agents might contribute to the disease process. Other mechanisms have been proposed to explain the role that the SE plays in the disease, including direct triggering by the five-amino acid SE sequence leading to NO production (Ling et al., 2007), ability to bind to heat shock proteins (Auger et al., 1996), and the ability to present citrullinated peptides (Hill et al., 2003). A putative "protective epitope" has also been defined for the same region, with the sequence DERAA, corresponding to DRB1*0402, *1102, *1301, *1302, and *1304, and is associated with a less severe disease (van der Helm-van Mil et al., 2005).

HLA genes show strong linkage disequilibrium, so they segregate as haplotypes with a low recombination rate, specially between HLA-DR and HLA-DQ. Different data indicate that some HLA-DQ alleles that segregate with given HLA-DR alleles play an important role in RA, although these data are not totally understood. The combination of the presence of the SE-containing HLA-DR alleles and specific HLA-DQ alleles opened the possibility that peptides containing the SE can be presented to T cells in the context of specific HLA-DQ, shaping the T-cell repertoire (Salvat et al., 1994).

HLA-DRB1 allele	Amino acid residue					
	67	70	71	72	73	74
High risk						
*04:01	L	Q	K	R	A	A
*01:01	-	-	R	-	-	-
*01:02	-	-	R	-	-	-
*04:04	-	-	R	-	-	-
*04:05	-	-	R	-	-	-
*04:08	-	-	R	-	-	-
*10:01	-	R	R	-	-	-
Protection or low risk						
*04:02	I	D	E	-	-	-
*07:01	I	D	R	-	G	Q
*11:02	I	D	E	-	-	-
*13:01	I	D	E	-	-	-
*13:02	I	D	E	-	-	-
*13:04	I	D	E	-	-	-
*15:01	I	-	A	-	-	-

Table 1. Residues in the shared epitope positions in HLA-DR molecules differentially associated to RA

3. Citrullination

Citrullination is a post-translational protein modification that consists in the deimination of the positive charged amino acid arginine, generating the neutral amino acid citrulline (Figure 1). The process requires high concentrations of Ca^{2+} and is produced in inflammatory environments (Baeten et al., 2001; Chavanas et al., 2004; Vossenaar et al., 2003). Other mechanism that triggers arginine deimination is apoptosis (Baeten et al., 2001). Environmental insults such as smoking increases the expression of PAD2 and induces citrullination in the mouse (Makrygiannakis et al., 2008).

The conversion of arginine to citrulline is carried out by a family of enzymes known as peptidyl arginine deiminases (PADs) (Vossenaar et al., 2003). Five members of this family of enzymes have been described in human (PAD1, PAD2, PAD3, PAD4 and PAD6). The members or this family are differentially expressed in many cell types (including neutrophils, monocytes, and macrophages) and tissues (Migliorini et al., 2005; Nijenhuis et al., 2004; van Venrooij & Pruijn, 2000; Vossenaar et al., 2003; Wysocka et al., 2006). Thus, PAD2 and PAD4 are expressed in the synovium of patients with RA, but PAD1, PAD3 and PAD6 are not (Foulquier et al., 2007). At least some functional haplotypes of PAD4 are associated with RA (Suzuki et al., 2003). Interestingly, PAD4 is capable of self-citrullination, which can regulate its activity and control the citrullination of other proteins (Andrade et al., 2010).

Citrullinated proteins have been detected in several inflamed tissues: arthritic joins (Vossenaar et al., 2004a), brain (Nicholas & Whitaker, 2002), muscle and lymphoid organs (Makrygiannakis et al., 2006) and lungs (Bongartz et al., 2007; Klareskog et al., 2006). In addition, some proteins from the epidermis and central nervous system are constitutively citrullinated (Kubilus et al., 1979; Nicholas et al., 2003).

The function of citrullination is not totally understood, although it is important in some physiological processes such as apoptosis (Asaga et al., 1998) and cell differentiation (Senshu et al., 1996). The loss of a positive charge can produce changes in some relevant protein features. Thus, electrostatic interactions are usually important in generating and maintaining protein structures. A citrullinated protein modifies some of the interactions that stabilize the native conformation, and decreases its isoelectric point, affecting the secondary and tertiary structure, which can result in a different protein folding that may modify the function of the protein (Gyorgy et al., 2006). Regarding the specific protein functions affected by citrullination it has been reported that arginine deimination influences protein–protein interaction (Tarcsa et al., 1996), and can modulate signalling potency (Proost et al., 2008). In addition, citrullinated proteins often change their sensitivity to degradation by proteolytic enzymes (Pritzker et al., 2000).

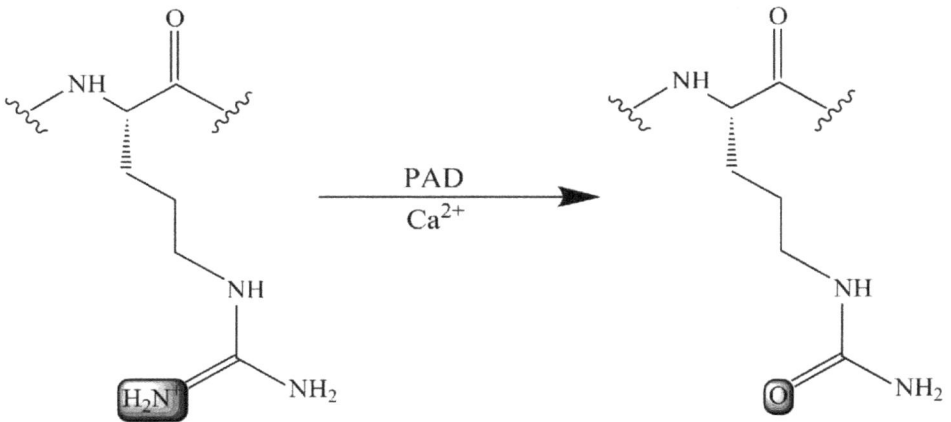

Fig. 1. **Conversion of arginine to citrulline**. The protein posttranslational modification known as citrullination consists in a deimination of arginine to citrulline. The reaction is carried out by an enzyme of the family of peptidyl arginine deiminases (PAD), and requires high concentration of Ca^{2+}. This reaction results in the loss of a positive charge in the protein.

4. Citrulline and rheumatoid arthritis

As mentioned above, the presence of citrullinated proteins is detected in the joints of patients with RA (Baeten et al., 2001), although it is not exclusive for rheumatoid synovial tissue (Vossenaar et al., 2004a). The specificity of citrullination has not been solved and several proteins have been found to be citrullinated in the synovium, including vimentin (Bang et al., 2007; Vossenaar et al., 2004b), fibrinogen (Masson-Bessiere et al., 2001), and collagen type II (Klareskog et al., 2008). The role of these modified proteins in the joints remains unknown, although some of these proteins are known targets of the autoimmune response. Thus, specific antibodies have been detected in RA patients that recognize citrullinated filaggrin (Nijenhuis et al., 2004; Schellekens et al., 1998; Sebbag et al., 1995; Simon et al., 1993), fibrinogen (Bang et al., 2007), vimentin (Burkhardt et al., 2005; Despres et al., 1994; Hayem et al., 1999; Hueber et al., 1999) and collagen type II (Burkhardt et al., 2005).

A relevant feature of ACPAs is that their presence is RA specific. Thus, in contrast with RF, patients with inflammatory diseases other than RA rarely carry ACPAs in serum. It still remains unclear why ACPAs are present in the serum of most RA patients but absent in the serum of other systemic autoinflammatory diseases.

As with RF, the generation of ACPAs in the serum of RA patients can occur several years before the onset of the disease (Aho et al., 2000; Kurki et al., 1992; Nielen et al., 2004; Rantapaa-Dahlqvist et al., 2003). The detection of these ACPAs can be used as clinical tests to predict the clinical course of the disease (Kastbom et al., 2004; Ronnelid et al., 2005). There are some clinical and genetic differences between ACPA+ and ACPA- RA patients. Clinically, ACPA+ RA patients have a more severe disease course than patients without detectable ACPAs (Forslind et al., 2004; Kastbom et al., 2004; Kroot et al., 2000; Ronnelid et al., 2005). Genetically, the detection of ACPAs in the serum of RA patients correlates very well with the presence of HLA-DR alleles containing the SE, which does not happen with RF. Some reports have shown that the presence of HLA-DRB1 alleles containing the SE is directly related and restricted to the ACPA+ subset of RA (Huizinga et al., 2005; van der Helm-van Mil et al., 2006) and SE alleles influence both the magnitude and the specificity of this RA-specific antibody response (Verpoort et al., 2007). Other HLA-DRB1-independent genetic associations in the HLA region to ACPA positivity have been reported (Okada et al., 2009). In contrast, ACPA- RA is not related with the SE-carrying HLA-DRB1 alleles and it has been associated with HLA-DRB1*03 (Irigoyen et al., 2005), an DRB1 allele that does not contain the SE. Taking together, it seems clear that ACPA+ and ACPA- RA do not present the same genetic background or clinical course and evidence strongly suggest that these are two different RA subsets, so they should be considered as different entities when treated.

Since ACPAs are developed before the onset of the disease and their presence predicts a more severe clinical course, this seems to indicate that the immune response against citrullinated proteins contribute to the pathogenesis of this form of RA.

5. Citrullinated peptides and HLA

The SE contains residues 70-74 of the DRβ chain, and is located in one α-helix of the binding groove. These residues are located in a position such that some of them can interact with the peptide bound to the HLA-DR molecule. Concretely, the crystal structures of HLA-DR1 and HLA-DR4 with different peptides have shown that the residues Lys71 in DRB1*0401 and Arg71 in DRB1*0101 directly interact with the amino acid located in position 4 (P4) of the peptide core bound to the binding groove of HLA-DR molecules (Dessen et al., 1997; Rosloniec et al., 2006). The binding motifs of the peptides associated to HLA-DR1 and HLA-DR4 were described years ago. More recently, our group reported an exhaustive analysis of the peptide pool associated to HLA-DR10 by mass spectrometry and identified the anchor motif of the peptide repertoire bound to this RA-associated allele (Alvarez et al., 2008). This motif was consistent with a more recent report by Kwok´s group using an approach based on binding assays (James et al., 2010). An important structural information extracted from these data is that HLA-DR molecules containing the SE do not bind peptides with basic residues in P4 position. This is due to the presence of basic residues at position 71 of the HLA-DR β chain (table 1).

Conversion of the basic amino acid arginine to the neutral citrulline produces the loss of a net positive charge on the protein or peptide that suffer this post-translational modification. Thus, citrulline is a neutral, polar, large amino acid with structural features similar to glutamine. Interestingly, peptides with arginine in P4 are poorly tolerated for the HLA-DR molecules that comprise the SE alleles (Fremont et al., 1996; Friede et al., 1996), while peptides with glutamine in P4 of the binding core have been described for DRB1*0101, DRB1*0401 and DRB1*1001 (Alvarez et al., 2008; Dengjel et al., 2005; Muntasell et al., 2004; Stern et al., 1994; Verreck et al., 1996). Basic residues, such as arginine or lysine, in P4 position of the peptide core produce electrostatic repulsion with the basic residues in position 71 of the β chain in the HLA-DR molecules that contain the SE. However, glutamine can accommodate well in the pocket and can be stabilized by hydrogen bonds with Arg71 or Lys71 in the HLA-DR β chain. Thus, positively charged amino acids (e.g., arginine) in P4 inhibit peptide binding to RA-related HLA-DR molecules containing the SE, whereas peptides with uncharged polarity (e.g., glutamine) are bound to these molecules with high affinity (Hammer et al., 1994; Hammer et al., 1995). Peptides with citrullin in P4 would interact favourably at the P4 anchoring pocket of SE-containing HLA-DR molecules. This was confirmed both for DRB1*0101, DRB1*0401 (Hill et al., 2003) and DRB1*1001 (James et al., 2010). Concretely, modified peptides derived from joint associated proteins were able to bind to RA-associated MHC molecules: the peptide spanning residues 65-77 from vimentin, vimentin (65-77) to DRB1*0101 and DRB1*0401 (Hill et al., 2003), and peptides vimentin (58-72), Fib A (737-751), Fib B (68-82) and cartilage intermediate layer protein CILP (982-996) to DRB1*1001 (James et al., 2010). These data open the possibility that in the inflamed joint, some arginines may be deiminated by activated PAD2 or PAD4 and, after protein catabolism, citrulline-containing peptides would be bound to SE HLA-DR molecules.

The peptide repertoires associated to many MHC molecules have been described, both for MHC class I and for MHC class II. However, up to now, no peptide with citrulline in P4 has been reported to be a natural ligand of any HLA-DR molecule. Some reasons make the identification of citrullinated peptides from the peptide repertoire bound to HLA-DR molecules very difficult. First, the conditions to obtain high level of protein citrullination are not totally controlled, although some protocols have been reported, as increasing intracellular calcium by the addition of ionomicine to the cell culture (Vossenaar et al., 2004c). Second and more important, after deimination induction, most of the peptides will remain containing arginine instead of citrulline, and probably, the amount of citrullinated peptides in the peptide pool will be low. Mass spectrometry analysis give information of the most abundant peptides in the MHC-associated peptide pools making complicated to find a low-abundance citrullinated peptide. An approach that could be used to solve these problems would be to enrich citrullinated peptides in the sample. Antibodies specific for citrullinated peptides can not be used because they can recognize some peptides but not others. A technique for the specific enrichment of citrulline-containing peptides has been described, based on the immobilization of a glyoxal derivative that reacts exclusively with the ureido group of the citrulline residue al low pH (Tutturen et al., 2010). The ureido group can be chemically modified by diacetyl monoxime and antipyrine (Senshu et al., 1992). The chemically modified citrulline can be detected, using a specific antibody, by Western blotting and immunohistochemistry (Makrygiannakis et al., 2008). Peptides or proteins containing the modified citrulline can also be detected by mass spectrometry (Stensland et al., 2009).

6. T cell responses to HLA-restricted citrullinated peptides

The induction of a typical humoral response that results in a production of classes of antibodies others than IgM requires the help of CD4 T cells. T cells recognize complexes formed by MHC molecules and peptides derived from antigenic proteins. In the case of ACPAs, the targets of the immune response are modified self proteins, as vimentin, fillagrin, fibrinogen and collagen type II. CD4 T cells that help in the generation of an anti-citrullinated proteins B cell response do not necessarily recognize citrullinated peptides. However, a role of T cell responses in RA is well known, which makes the identification of T cell responses against citrullinated peptides presented in the context of RA-related HLA-DR of great interest. These peptides could be citrullinated outside the binding core, in the core positions other than P4, or in P4, as discussed above.

In the last years, T cell responses to citrulline-containing peptides have been studied. First, using DR4-IE transgenic mice (expressing the chimeric molecule DR4-IE, that contains the DR4 binding groove and part of the murine class II molecule), Hill and collaborators demonstrated that deimination of arginine to citrulline significantly increased the peptide-MHC affinity when arginine was in P4 position. In addition, activated CD4$^+$ T cells were detected in these transgenic mice against a peptide spanning residues 65 to 77 of vimentin, vimentin (65-77), which had a citrulline in position 70 instead of the arginine of the unmodified protein. These results revealed that HLA-DRB1 alleles with the SE could initiate an specific autoimmune response to citrullinated self-antigens in DR4-transgenic mice (Hill et al., 2003). In this animal model, citrullinated fibrinogen induced arthritis. The disease induced in these mice was characterized by synovial hyperplasia followed by ankylosis, but lacked a large leukocyte infiltrate. Specific humoral and cellular responses to citrullinated components were observed, which were absent in wild-type mice immunized with citrullinated or unmodified fibrinogen and in transgenic mice immunized with unmodified fibrinogen (Hill et al., 2008). HLA-DRB1*0401–restricted T cell reactivity to fibrinogen (371-383) was clearly seen in transgenic mice after immunization with either citrullinated fibrinogen or unmodified fibrinogen, whereas no specific response to this peptide was detected in wild-type mice. Ten peptides derived from α, β or γ chains of human fibrinogen containing an aliphatic or aromatic residue in P1 position of the binding core and arginine or citrulline at P4 were tested to generate T cell responses. Only one citrullinated peptide, Fibα$_{R84Cit}$, induced a consistent T cell response, whereas no response was seen against the corresponding arginine-containing peptide Fibα$_{79-91}$. Therefore, these data confirm that a citrullinated protein can be arthritogenic when RA-associated alleles are expressed, and specific T cell responses to citrullinated peptides are part of the immune response. Citrullinated peptides-specific T cell activation plays an important role in the development and progression of arthritis in this animal model. Thus, when given prior to disease onset, treatment with CTLA-4Ig, an agent that blocks T cell costimulation, prevented T cell activation induced by citrullinated human fibrinogen. This effect was not seen with non-specific IgG1 (Yue et al.).

Other approach using the mouse model detected that a response against citrullinated peptides could be generated even when the antigen was administrated in unmodified form. Concretely, HEL was used as a model antigen, and T cells specifically reactive to citrullinated epitopes were detected among the responding repertoire to immunization with an unmodified HEL protein. In addition, antigen presenting cells (APCs), including dendritic cells and peritoneal macrophages, were able to present citrullinated peptides when provided an intact, unmodified HEL *ex vivo* (Ireland et al., 2006). Therefore, APCs were capable to capture and process the antigen, to deiminate some specific arginine residues and to present some citrullin-containing peptides to T cells in a correct way to induce an specific response against citrullinated peptides.

More than 90% of patients positive for citrullinated vimentin-specific ACPAs carry SE-containing HLA-DRB1 alleles. In a DR4-transgenic mouse model, animals were immunized with 33 citrulline-containing peptides (all possible citrullinated peptides of human vimentin) and tested for T cell reactivity. T cell responses were generated against some of these peptides restricted by HLA-DRB1*0401 (vimentin (26-44) and vimentin (415-433). Antigen presenting cells were able to generate these peptides from entire vimentin. In addition, T cell reactivity against these citrullinated peptides derived from vimentin were observed when PBMCs from ACPAs-positive, HLA-DR4-positive patients with RA were used (Feitsma et al.). These data strongly suggest the presence of HLA-DRB1*0401-restricted T cell responses against citrullinated vimentin-derived peptides in RA patients. The data do not exclude T cell responses against non-citrullinated peptides restricted by this or other HLA-DRB1 alleles, that also could facilitate a humoral response against citrullinated epitopes.

The generation of T cell responses against citrullinated peptides has also been confirmed for other autoantigens. Thus, a proliferative response was observed in more than 60% RA patients after stimulation with citrullinated aggrecan-derived peptide, aggrecan (84-103) (von Delwig et al., 2010). This response was absent in PBMCs from healthy controls, and there was no response to the unmodified aggrecan analog peptide, indicating that citrulline residue is required for T cell recognition. In addition, cytokine production was analyzed by ELISA and intracellular cytokine analysis. High levels of the proinflammatory cytokine interleukin-17 (IL-17) was produced by PBMCs from RA patients in response to stimulation with citrullinated aggrecan. This IL-17 production was absent when PBMCs from RA patients and healthy controls were stimulated with the unmodified aggrecan-derived peptide. Therefore, citrullinated aggrecan-specific T cells may play a role in the pathogenesis of RA and in the inflammatory process.

Most of the T cell responses to citrullinated peptides have been generated in models that express HLA-DRB1*0401. In addition, responses against citrullinated peptides restricted by the RA-associated, SE-containing HLA-DRB1*1001 molecule have been obtained (James et al., 2010). Authors demonstrated that HLA-DRB1*1001 can accommodate citrulline in three anchor positions, and three of the modified peptides that were evaluated developed specific CD4+ T cell responses. These peptides derived from fibrinogen α, fibrinogen β and cartilage intermediate-layer protein, and these data suggest a role for these three proteins as relevant antigens in RA in HLA-DRB1*1001+ patients. In addition, T cell clones specific for these sequences proliferated only in response to citrullinated peptides. One more time, these data suggest that deimination of arginine can have as a consequence the generation of new HLA-DR ligands that can be recognized by T cells as neoepitopes, and may play an important role in the initiation or progression of RA. As described recently, T cell responses to other post-translational modifications may play a similar role in generating inflammatory responses. One of this could be carbamylation of lysine to homocitrulline. Thus, mice were immunized with carbamylated peptides, which induced chemotaxis, and T and B cell responses. Mice immunized with carbamylated peptides developed erosive arthritis when citrullinated peptides were injected intra-articularly. In addition, T and B cells induced arthritis after adoptive transfer into normal recipients (Mydel et al., 2010). Therefore, the T cell response to homocitrulline-derived peptides, as well as the subsequent production of anti-homocitrulline Abs, was critical for the induction of autoimmune responses against citrulline-derived peptides which may provide a novel mechanism for the pathogenesis of arthritis.

Constitutive protein citrullination occurs in some tissues in absence of inflammation, which imply the existence of tolerance against these modified proteins. The thymus is the organ where the immunocompetent T cell repertoire is generated. During selection processes to generate central T cell tolerance, about 95-97% of the thymocytes die by apoptosis, which is an inductor of citrullination. Thus, PAD activity and arginine deimination may be active in this organ. Citrullinated peptides that bind to HLA-DR molecules in the thymus should not be able to induce an immune response in periphery. Differences in the machinery of antigen processing have been reported between thymic cells and other presenting cells. Thus, the identification and analysis of HLA-DR-associated citrullinated peptides in the thymus could reveal which peptides can generate central tolerance.

7. Conclusions

The finding that the sera of most RA patients contain antibodies specifc for citrullinated proteins opened the possibility of a new mechanism in the etiology of the disease. These antibodies are specific for RA, can be detected years before the development of the disease, and correlate with the presence of SE-containing alleles. In the last years, relevant advances on the identification of the citrullination process in the inflamed joints by PADs´activity, the presentation by RA-associated HLA-DR molecules that contain the SE, and T cell responses against citrullinated proteins have been made. Nevertheless, it remains to be defined which citrullinated peptides are really involved in the development of the disease in humans and if any of them can efficiently be presented in the context of various SE-containing HLA-DR molecules.

8. Acknowledgments

The author thanks Dr. Dolores Jaraquemada for her critical review of the manuscript.

9. References

Aho, K.;Palosuo, T.;Heliovaara, M., et al. (2000). Antifilaggrin antibodies within "normal" range predict rheumatoid arthritis in a linear fashion. *J Rheumatol,*Vol. 27 No. (12) (Dec 2000), pp. 2743-2746.

Alamanos, Y.& Drosos, A. A. (2005). Epidemiology of adult rheumatoid arthritis. *Autoimmun Rev,*Vol. 4 No. (3) (Mar 2005), pp. 130-136.

Aletaha, D.;Neogi, T.;Silman, A. J., et al. (2010). 2010 Rheumatoid arthritis classification criteria: an American College of Rheumatology/European League Against Rheumatism collaborative initiative. *Arthritis Rheum,*Vol. 62 No. (9) (Sep 2010), pp. 2569-2581.

Alvarez, I.;Collado, J.;Daura, X., et al. (2008). The rheumatoid arthritis-associated allele HLA-DR10 (DRB1*1001) shares part of its repertoire with HLA-DR1 (DRB1*0101) and HLA-DR4 (DRB*0401). *Arthritis Rheum,*Vol. 58 No. (6) (Jun 2008), pp. 1630-1639.

Andrade, F.;Darrah, E.;Gucek, M., et al. (2010). Autocitrullination of human peptidyl arginine deiminase type 4 regulates protein citrullination during cell activation. *Arthritis Rheum,*Vol. 62 No. (6) (Jan 2010), pp. 1630-1640.

Asaga, H.;Yamada, M.& Senshu, T. (1998). Selective deimination of vimentin in calcium ionophore-induced apoptosis of mouse peritoneal macrophages. *Biochem Biophys Res Commun,*Vol. 243 No. (3) (Feb 24 1998), pp. 641-646.

Auger, I.;Escola, J. M.;Gorvel, J. P., et al. (1996). HLA-DR4 and HLA-DR10 motifs that carry susceptibility to rheumatoid arthritis bind 70-kD heat shock proteins. *Nat Med,*Vol. 2 No. (3) (Mar 1996), pp. 306-310.

Avouac, J.;Gossec, L.& Dougados, M. (2006). Diagnostic and predictive value of anti-cyclic citrullinated protein antibodies in rheumatoid arthritis: a systematic literature review. *Ann Rheum Dis,*Vol. 65 No. (7) (Jul 2006), pp. 845-851.

Baeten, D.;Peene, I.;Union, A., et al. (2001). Specific presence of intracellular citrullinated proteins in rheumatoid arthritis synovium: relevance to antifilaggrin autoantibodies. *Arthritis Rheum,*Vol. 44 No. (10) (Oct 2001), pp. 2255-2262.

Bang, H.;Egerer, K.;Gauliard, A., et al. (2007). Mutation and citrullination modifies vimentin to a novel autoantigen for rheumatoid arthritis. *Arthritis Rheum,*Vol. 56 No. (8) (Aug 2007), pp. 2503-2511.

Bongartz, T.;Cantaert, T.;Atkins, S. R., et al. (2007). Citrullination in extra-articular manifestations of rheumatoid arthritis. *Rheumatology (Oxford),*Vol. 46 No. (1) (Jan 2007), pp. 70-75.

Burkhardt, H.;Sehnert, B.;Bockermann, R., et al. (2005). Humoral immune response to citrullinated collagen type II determinants in early rheumatoid arthritis. *Eur J Immunol,*Vol. 35 No. (5) (May 2005), pp. 1643-1652.

Cutbush, S.;Chikanza, I. C.;Biro, P. A., et al. (1993). Sequence-specific oligonucleotide typing in Shona patients with rheumatoid arthritis and healthy controls from Zimbabwe. *Tissue Antigens,*Vol. 41 No. (4) (Apr 1993), pp. 169-172.

Chavanas, S.;Mechin, M. C.;Takahara, H., et al. (2004). Comparative analysis of the mouse and human peptidylarginine deiminase gene clusters reveals highly conserved non-coding segments and a new human gene, PADI6. *Gene,*Vol. 330 No. (Apr 14 2004), pp. 19-27.

de Juan, M. D.;Belmonte, I.;Barado, J., et al. (1994). Differential associations of HLA-DR antigens with rheumatoid arthritis (RA) in Basques: high frequency of DR1 and DR10 and lack of association with HLA-DR4 or any of its subtypes. *Tissue Antigens,*Vol. 43 No. (5) (May 1994), pp. 320-323.

Dengjel, J.;Schoor, O.;Fischer, R., et al. (2005). Autophagy promotes MHC class II presentation of peptides from intracellular source proteins. *Proc Natl Acad Sci U S A,*Vol. 102 No. (22) (May 31 2005), pp. 7922-7927.

Despres, N.;Boire, G.;Lopez-Longo, F. J., et al. (1994). The Sa system: a novel antigen-antibody system specific for rheumatoid arthritis. *J Rheumatol,*Vol. 21 No. (6) (Jun 1994), pp. 1027-1033.

Dessen, A.;Lawrence, C. M.;Cupo, S., et al. (1997). X-ray crystal structure of HLA-DR4 (DRA*0101, DRB1*0401) complexed with a peptide from human collagen II. *Immunity,*Vol. 7 No. (4) (Oct 1997), pp. 473-481.

Feitsma, A. L.;van der Voort, E. I.;Franken, K. L., et al. Identification of citrullinated vimentin peptides as T cell epitopes in HLA-DR4-positive patients with rheumatoid arthritis. *Arthritis Rheum,*Vol. 62 No. (1) (Jan pp. 117-125.

Forslind, K.;Ahlmen, M.;Eberhardt, K., et al. (2004). Prediction of radiological outcome in early rheumatoid arthritis in clinical practice: role of antibodies to citrullinated peptides (anti-CCP). *Ann Rheum Dis,*Vol. 63 No. (9) (Sep 2004), pp. 1090-1095.

Foulquier, C.;Sebbag, M.;Clavel, C., et al. (2007). Peptidyl arginine deiminase type 2 (PAD-2) and PAD-4 but not PAD-1, PAD-3, and PAD-6 are expressed in rheumatoid arthritis synovium in close association with tissue inflammation. *Arthritis Rheum,*Vol. 56 No. (11) (Nov 2007), pp. 3541-3553.

Fremont, D. H.;Hendrickson, W. A.;Marrack, P., et al. (1996). Structures of an MHC class II molecule with covalently bound single peptides. *Science,*Vol. 272 No. (5264) (May 17 1996), pp. 1001-1004.

Friede, T.;Gnau, V.;Jung, G., et al. (1996). Natural ligand motifs of closely related HLA-DR4 molecules predict features of rheumatoid arthritis associated peptides. *Biochim Biophys Acta,*Vol. 1316 No. (2) (Jun 7 1996), pp. 85-101.

Gonzalez-Escribano, M. F.;Rodriguez, R.;Valenzuela, A., et al. (1999). Complex associations between HLA-DRB1 genes and female rheumatoid arthritis: results from a prospective study. *Hum Immunol,*Vol. 60 No. (12) (Dec 1999), pp. 1259-1265.

Gregersen, P. K.;Silver, J.& Winchester, R. J. (1987). The shared epitope hypothesis. An approach to understanding the molecular genetics of susceptibility to rheumatoid arthritis. *Arthritis Rheum,*Vol. 30 No. (11) (Nov 1987), pp. 1205-1213.

Gyorgy, B.;Toth, E.;Tarcsa, E., et al. (2006). Citrullination: a posttranslational modification in health and disease. *Int J Biochem Cell Biol,*Vol. 38 No. (10) 2006), pp. 1662-1677.

Hameed, K.;Bowman, S.;Kondeatis, E., et al. (1997). The association of HLA-DRB genes and the shared epitope with rheumatoid arthritis in Pakistan. *Br J Rheumatol,*Vol. 36 No. (11) (Nov 1997), pp. 1184-1188.

Hammer, J.;Bono, E.;Gallazzi, F., et al. (1994). Precise prediction of major histocompatibility complex class II-peptide interaction based on peptide side chain scanning. *J Exp Med,*Vol. 180 No. (6) (Dec 1 1994), pp. 2353-2358.

Hammer, J.;Gallazzi, F.;Bono, E., et al. (1995). Peptide binding specificity of HLA-DR4 molecules: correlation with rheumatoid arthritis association. *J Exp Med,*Vol. 181 No. (5) (May 1 1995), pp. 1847-1855.

Hayem, G.;Chazerain, P.;Combe, B., et al. (1999). Anti-Sa antibody is an accurate diagnostic and prognostic marker in adult rheumatoid arthritis. *J Rheumatol,*Vol. 26 No. (1) (Jan 1999), pp. 7-13.

Hill, J. A.;Southwood, S.;Sette, A., et al. (2003). Cutting edge: the conversion of arginine to citrulline allows for a high-affinity peptide interaction with the rheumatoid arthritis-associated HLA-DRB1*0401 MHC class II molecule. *J Immunol,*Vol. 171 No. (2) (Jul 15 2003), pp. 538-541.

Hill, J. A.;Bell, D. A.;Brintnell, W., et al. (2008). Arthritis induced by posttranslationally modified (citrullinated) fibrinogen in DR4-IE transgenic mice. *J Exp Med,*Vol. 205 No. (4) (Apr 14 2008), pp. 967-979.

Hueber, W.;Hassfeld, W.;Smolen, J. S., et al. (1999). Sensitivity and specificity of anti-Sa autoantibodies for rheumatoid arthritis. *Rheumatology (Oxford),*Vol. 38 No. (2) (Feb 1999), pp. 155-159.

Huizinga, T. W.;Amos, C. I.;van der Helm-van Mil, A. H., et al. (2005). Refining the complex rheumatoid arthritis phenotype based on specificity of the HLA-DRB1 shared epitope for antibodies to citrullinated proteins. *Arthritis Rheum,*Vol. 52 No. (11) (Nov 2005), pp. 3433-3438.

Ireland, J.;Herzog, J.& Unanue, E. R. (2006). Cutting edge: unique T cells that recognize citrullinated peptides are a feature of protein immunization. *J Immunol,*Vol. 177 No. (3) (Aug 1 2006), pp. 1421-1425.

Irigoyen, P.;Lee, A. T.;Wener, M. H., et al. (2005). Regulation of anti-cyclic citrullinated peptide antibodies in rheumatoid arthritis: contrasting effects of HLA-DR3 and the shared epitope alleles. *Arthritis Rheum,*Vol. 52 No. (12) (Dec 2005), pp. 3813-3818.

James, E. A.;Moustakas, A. K.;Bui, J., et al. (2010). HLA-DR1001 presents "altered-self" peptides derived from joint-associated proteins by accepting citrulline in three of its binding pockets. *Arthritis Rheum,*Vol. 62 No. (10) (Oct 2010), pp. 2909-2918.

Jaraquemada, D.;Ollier, W.;Awad, J., et al. (1986). HLA and rheumatoid arthritis: a combined analysis of 440 British patients. *Ann Rheum Dis,*Vol. 45 No. (8) (Aug 1986), pp. 627-636.

Kastbom, A.;Strandberg, G.;Lindroos, A., et al. (2004). Anti-CCP antibody test predicts the disease course during 3 years in early rheumatoid arthritis (the Swedish TIRA project). *Ann Rheum Dis,*Vol. 63 No. (9) (Sep 2004), pp. 1085-1089.

Klareskog, L.;Ronnelid, J.;Lundberg, K., et al. (2008). Immunity to citrullinated proteins in rheumatoid arthritis. *Annu Rev Immunol,*Vol. 26 No. 2008), pp. 651-675.

Klareskog, L.;Stolt, P.;Lundberg, K., et al. (2006). A new model for an etiology of rheumatoid arthritis: smoking may trigger HLA-DR (shared epitope)-restricted immune reactions to autoantigens modified by citrullination. *Arthritis Rheum,*Vol. 54 No. (1) (Jan 2006), pp. 38-46.

Kroot, E. J.;de Jong, B. A.;van Leeuwen, M. A., et al. (2000). The prognostic value of anti-cyclic citrullinated peptide antibody in patients with recent-onset rheumatoid arthritis. *Arthritis Rheum,*Vol. 43 No. (8) (Aug 2000), pp. 1831-1835.

Kubilus, J.;Waitkus, R. W.& Baden, H. P. (1979). The presence of citrulline in epidermal proteins. *Biochim Biophys Acta,*Vol. 581 No. (1) (Nov 23 1979), pp. 114-121.

Kurki, P.;Aho, K.;Palosuo, T., et al. (1992). Immunopathology of rheumatoid arthritis. Antikeratin antibodies precede the clinical disease. *Arthritis Rheum,*Vol. 35 No. (8) (Aug 1992), pp. 914-917.

Lacki, J. K.;Wassmuth, R.;Korczowska, I., et al. (2000). Does the presence of HLA-DR B1 shared motif affect progression of the disease in rheumatoid arthritis patients? *Int J Immunopathol Pharmacol,*Vol. 13 No. (2) (May-Aug 2000), pp. 83-89.

Ling, S.;Li, Z.;Borschukova, O., et al. (2007). The rheumatoid arthritis shared epitope increases cellular susceptibility to oxidative stress by antagonizing an adenosine-mediated anti-oxidative pathway. *Arthritis Res Ther,*Vol. 9 No. (1) 2007), pp. R5.

Makrygiannakis, D.;af Klint, E.;Lundberg, I. E., et al. (2006). Citrullination is an inflammation-dependent process. *Ann Rheum Dis,*Vol. 65 No. (9) (Sep 2006), pp. 1219-1222.

Makrygiannakis, D.;Hermansson, M.;Ulfgren, A. K., et al. (2008). Smoking increases peptidylarginine deiminase 2 enzyme expression in human lungs and increases citrullination in BAL cells. *Ann Rheum Dis,*Vol. 67 No. (10) (Oct 2008), pp. 1488-1492.

Masson-Bessiere, C.;Sebbag, M.;Girbal-Neuhauser, E., et al. (2001). The major synovial targets of the rheumatoid arthritis-specific antifilaggrin autoantibodies are deiminated forms of the alpha- and beta-chains of fibrin. *J Immunol*,Vol. 166 No. (6) (Mar 15 2001), pp. 4177-4184.

Migliorini, P.;Pratesi, F.;Tommasi, C., et al. (2005). The immune response to citrullinated antigens in autoimmune diseases. *Autoimmun Rev*,Vol. 4 No. (8) (Nov 2005), pp. 561-564.

Mody, G. M.& Hammond, M. G. (1994). Differences in HLA-DR association with rheumatoid arthritis among migrant Indian communities in South Africa. *Br J Rheumatol*,Vol. 33 No. (5) (May 1994), pp. 425-427.

Muntasell, A.;Carrascal, M.;Alvarez, I., et al. (2004). Dissection of the HLA-DR4 peptide repertoire in endocrine epithelial cells: strong influence of invariant chain and HLA-DM expression on the nature of ligands. *J Immunol*,Vol. 173 No. (2) (Jul 15 2004), pp. 1085-1093.

Mydel, P.;Wang, Z.;Brisslert, M., et al. (2010). Carbamylation-dependent activation of T cells: a novel mechanism in the pathogenesis of autoimmune arthritis. *J Immunol*,Vol. 184 No. (12) (Jun 15 2010), pp. 6882-6890.

Nemazee, D. A. (1985). Immune complexes can trigger specific, T cell-dependent, autoanti-IgG antibody production in mice. *J Exp Med*,Vol. 161 No. (1) (Jan 1 1985), pp. 242-256.

Neogi, T.;Aletaha, D.;Silman, A. J., et al. (2010). The 2010 American College of Rheumatology/European League Against Rheumatism classification criteria for rheumatoid arthritis: Phase 2 methodological report. *Arthritis Rheum*,Vol. 62 No. (9) (Sep 2010), pp. 2582-2591.

Nicholas, A. P.& Whitaker, J. N. (2002). Preparation of a monoclonal antibody to citrullinated epitopes: its characterization and some applications to immunohistochemistry in human brain. *Glia*,Vol. 37 No. (4) (Mar 15 2002), pp. 328-336.

Nicholas, A. P.;King, J. L.;Sambandam, T., et al. (2003). Immunohistochemical localization of citrullinated proteins in adult rat brain. *J Comp Neurol*,Vol. 459 No. (3) (May 5 2003), pp. 251-266.

Nielen, M. M.;van Schaardenburg, D.;Reesink, H. W., et al. (2004). Specific autoantibodies precede the symptoms of rheumatoid arthritis: a study of serial measurements in blood donors. *Arthritis Rheum*,Vol. 50 No. (2) (Feb 2004), pp. 380-386.

Nijenhuis, S.;Zendman, A. J.;Vossenaar, E. R., et al. (2004). Autoantibodies to citrullinated proteins in rheumatoid arthritis: clinical performance and biochemical aspects of an RA-specific marker. *Clin Chim Acta*,Vol. 350 No. (1-2) (Dec 2004), pp. 17-34.

Nishimura, K.;Sugiyama, D.;Kogata, Y., et al. (2007). Meta-analysis: diagnostic accuracy of anti-cyclic citrullinated peptide antibody and rheumatoid factor for rheumatoid arthritis. *Ann Intern Med*,Vol. 146 No. (11) (Jun 5 2007), pp. 797-808.

Okada, Y.;Yamada, R.;Suzuki, A., et al. (2009). Contribution of a haplotype in the HLA region to anti-cyclic citrullinated peptide antibody positivity in rheumatoid arthritis, independently of HLA-DRB1. *Arthritis Rheum*,Vol. 60 No. (12) (Dec 2009), pp. 3582-3590.

Poor, G.;Nagy, Z. B.;Schmidt, Z., et al. (2007). Genetic background of anticyclic citrullinated peptide autoantibody production in Hungarian patients with rheumatoid arthritis. *Ann N Y Acad Sci*,Vol. 1110 No. (Sep 2007), pp. 23-32.

Pritzker, L. B.;Joshi, S.;Gowan, J. J., et al. (2000). Deimination of myelin basic protein. 1. Effect of deimination of arginyl residues of myelin basic protein on its structure and susceptibility to digestion by cathepsin D. *Biochemistry,*Vol. 39 No. (18) (May 9 2000), pp. 5374-5381.

Proost, P.;Loos, T.;Mortier, A., et al. (2008). Citrullination of CXCL8 by peptidylarginine deiminase alters receptor usage, prevents proteolysis, and dampens tissue inflammation. *J Exp Med,*Vol. 205 No. (9) (Sep 1 2008), pp. 2085-2097.

Rantapaa-Dahlqvist, S.;de Jong, B. A.;Berglin, E., et al. (2003). Antibodies against cyclic citrullinated peptide and IgA rheumatoid factor predict the development of rheumatoid arthritis. *Arthritis Rheum,*Vol. 48 No. (10) (Oct 2003), pp. 2741-2749.

Ronnelid, J.;Wick, M. C.;Lampa, J., et al. (2005). Longitudinal analysis of citrullinated protein/peptide antibodies (anti-CP) during 5 year follow up in early rheumatoid arthritis: anti-CP status predicts worse disease activity and greater radiological progression. *Ann Rheum Dis,*Vol. 64 No. (12) (Dec 2005), pp. 1744-1749.

Rosloniec, E. F.;Ivey, R. A., 3rd;Whittington, K. B., et al. (2006). Crystallographic structure of a rheumatoid arthritis MHC susceptibility allele, HLA-DR1 (DRB1*0101), complexed with the immunodominant determinant of human type II collagen. *J Immunol,*Vol. 177 No. (6) (Sep 15 2006), pp. 3884-3892.

Salvarani, C.;Boiardi, L.;Mantovani, V., et al. (1999). HLA-DRB1 alleles associated with polymyalgia rheumatica in northern Italy: correlation with disease severity. *Ann Rheum Dis,*Vol. 58 No. (5) (May 1999), pp. 303-308.

Salvat, S.;Auger, I.;Rochelle, L., et al. (1994). Tolerance to a self-peptide from the third hypervariable region of HLA DRB1*0401 in rheumatoid arthritis patients and normal subjects. *J Immunol,*Vol. 153 No. (11) (Dec 1 1994), pp. 5321-5329.

Sanchez, B.;Moreno, I.;Magarino, R., et al. (1990). HLA-DRw10 confers the highest susceptibility to rheumatoid arthritis in a Spanish population. *Tissue Antigens,*Vol. 36 No. (4) (Oct 1990), pp. 174-176.

Schellekens, G. A.;de Jong, B. A.;van den Hoogen, F. H., et al. (1998). Citrulline is an essential constituent of antigenic determinants recognized by rheumatoid arthritis-specific autoantibodies. *J Clin Invest,*Vol. 101 No. (1) (Jan 1 1998), pp. 273-281.

Schellekens, G. A.;Visser, H.;de Jong, B. A., et al. (2000). The diagnostic properties of rheumatoid arthritis antibodies recognizing a cyclic citrullinated peptide. *Arthritis Rheum,*Vol. 43 No. (1) (Jan 2000), pp. 155-163.

Sebbag, M.;Simon, M.;Vincent, C., et al. (1995). The antiperinuclear factor and the so-called antikeratin antibodies are the same rheumatoid arthritis-specific autoantibodies. *J Clin Invest,*Vol. 95 No. (6) (Jun 1995), pp. 2672-2679.

Senshu, T.;Sato, T.;Inoue, T., et al. (1992). Detection of citrulline residues in deiminated proteins on polyvinylidene difluoride membrane. *Anal Biochem,*Vol. 203 No. (1) (May 15 1992), pp. 94-100.

Senshu, T.;Kan, S.;Ogawa, H., et al. (1996). Preferential deimination of keratin K1 and filaggrin during the terminal differentiation of human epidermis. *Biochem Biophys Res Commun,*Vol. 225 No. (3) (Aug 23 1996), pp. 712-719.

Simon, M.;Girbal, E.;Sebbag, M., et al. (1993). The cytokeratin filament-aggregating protein filaggrin is the target of the so-called "antikeratin antibodies," autoantibodies specific for rheumatoid arthritis. *J Clin Invest,*Vol. 92 No. (3) (Sep 1993), pp. 1387-1393.

Stastny, P. (1978). Association of the B-cell alloantigen DRw4 with rheumatoid arthritis. *N Engl J Med,*Vol. 298 No. (16) (Apr 20 1978), pp. 869-871.

Stensland, M.;Holm, A.;Kiehne, A., et al. (2009). Targeted analysis of protein citrullination using chemical modification and tandem mass spectrometry. *Rapid Commun Mass Spectrom,*Vol. 23 No. (17) (Sep 2009), pp. 2754-2762.

Stern, L. J.;Brown, J. H.;Jardetzky, T. S., et al. (1994). Crystal structure of the human class II MHC protein HLA-DR1 complexed with an influenza virus peptide. *Nature,*Vol. 368 No. (6468) (Mar 17 1994), pp. 215-221.

Suzuki, A.;Yamada, R.;Chang, X., et al. (2003). Functional haplotypes of PADI4, encoding citrullinating enzyme peptidylarginine deiminase 4, are associated with rheumatoid arthritis. *Nat Genet,*Vol. 34 No. (4) (Aug 2003), pp. 395-402.

Tarcsa, E.;Marekov, L. N.;Mei, G., et al. (1996). Protein unfolding by peptidylarginine deiminase. Substrate specificity and structural relationships of the natural substrates trichohyalin and filaggrin. *J Biol Chem,*Vol. 271 No. (48) (Nov 29 1996), pp. 30709-30716.

Tarkowski, A.;Czerkinsky, C.& Nilsson, L. A. (1985). Simultaneous induction of rheumatoid factor- and antigen-specific antibody-secreting cells during the secondary immune response in man. *Clin Exp Immunol,*Vol. 61 No. (2) (Aug 1985), pp. 379-387.

Tutturen, A. E.;Holm, A.;Jorgensen, M., et al. (2010). A technique for the specific enrichment of citrulline-containing peptides. *Anal Biochem,*Vol. 403 No. (1-2) (Aug 2010), pp. 43-51.

van der Helm-van Mil, A. H.;Huizinga, T. W.;Schreuder, G. M., et al. (2005). An independent role of protective HLA class II alleles in rheumatoid arthritis severity and susceptibility. *Arthritis Rheum,*Vol. 52 No. (9) (Sep 2005), pp. 2637-2644.

van der Helm-van Mil, A. H.;Verpoort, K. N.;Breedveld, F. C., et al. (2006). The HLA-DRB1 shared epitope alleles are primarily a risk factor for anti-cyclic citrullinated peptide antibodies and are not an independent risk factor for development of rheumatoid arthritis. *Arthritis Rheum,*Vol. 54 No. (4) (Apr 2006), pp. 1117-1121.

van Gaalen, F. A.;Linn-Rasker, S. P.;van Venrooij, W. J., et al. (2004). Autoantibodies to cyclic citrullinated peptides predict progression to rheumatoid arthritis in patients with undifferentiated arthritis: a prospective cohort study. *Arthritis Rheum,*Vol. 50 No. (3) (Mar 2004), pp. 709-715.

van Venrooij, W. J.& Pruijn, G. J. (2000). Citrullination: a small change for a protein with great consequences for rheumatoid arthritis. *Arthritis Res,*Vol. 2 No. (4) 2000), pp. 249-251.

Verpoort, K. N.;Cheung, K.;Ioan-Facsinay, A., et al. (2007). Fine specificity of the anti-citrullinated protein antibody response is influenced by the shared epitope alleles. *Arthritis Rheum,*Vol. 56 No. (12) (Dec 2007), pp. 3949-3952.

Verreck, F. A.;van de Poel, A.;Drijfhout, J. W., et al. (1996). Natural peptides isolated from Gly86/Val86-containing variants of HLA-DR1, -DR11, -DR13, and -DR52. *Immunogenetics,*Vol. 43 No. (6) 1996), pp. 392-397.

Vincent, C.;Nogueira, L.;Sebbag, M., et al. (2002). Detection of antibodies to deiminated recombinant rat filaggrin by enzyme-linked immunosorbent assay: a highly effective test for the diagnosis of rheumatoid arthritis. *Arthritis Rheum,*Vol. 46 No. (8) (Aug 2002), pp. 2051-2058.

von Delwig, A.;Locke, J.;Robinson, J. H., et al. (2010). Response of Th17 cells to a citrullinated arthritogenic aggrecan peptide in patients with rheumatoid arthritis. *Arthritis Rheum,*Vol. 62 No. (1) (Jan 2010), pp. 143-149.

Vossenaar, E. R.;Zendman, A. J.;van Venrooij, W. J., et al. (2003). PAD, a growing family of citrullinating enzymes: genes, features and involvement in disease. *Bioessays,*Vol. 25 No. (11) (Nov 2003), pp. 1106-1118.

Vossenaar, E. R.;Smeets, T. J.;Kraan, M. C., et al. (2004a). The presence of citrullinated proteins is not specific for rheumatoid synovial tissue. *Arthritis Rheum,*Vol. 50 No. (11) (Nov 2004a), pp. 3485-3494.

Vossenaar, E. R.;Despres, N.;Lapointe, E., et al. (2004b). Rheumatoid arthritis specific anti-Sa antibodies target citrullinated vimentin. *Arthritis Res Ther,*Vol. 6 No. (2) 2004b), pp. R142-150.

Vossenaar, E. R.;Radstake, T. R.;van der Heijden, A., et al. (2004c). Expression and activity of citrullinating peptidylarginine deiminase enzymes in monocytes and macrophages. *Ann Rheum Dis,*Vol. 63 No. (4) (Apr 2004c), pp. 373-381.

Wysocka, J.;Allis, C. D.& Coonrod, S. (2006). Histone arginine methylation and its dynamic regulation. *Front Biosci,*Vol. 11 No. 2006), pp. 344-355.

Yelamos, J.;Garcia-Lozano, J. R.;Moreno, I., et al. (1993). Association of HLA-DR4-Dw15 (DRB1*0405) and DR10 with rheumatoid arthritis in a Spanish population. *Arthritis Rheum,*Vol. 36 No. (6) (Jun 1993), pp. 811-814.

Yue, D.;Brintnell, W.;Mannik, L. A., et al. CTLA-4Ig blocks the development and progression of citrullinated fibrinogen-induced arthritis in DR4-transgenic mice. *Arthritis Rheum,*Vol. 62 No. (10) (Oct pp. 2941-2952.

3

IRF-5 - A New Link to Autoimmune Diseases

Sujayita Roy and Paula M. Pitha

Krieger School of Arts & Sciences, Department of Biology, Johns Hopkins University
Department of Oncology, Johns Hopkins School of Medicine
United States of America

1. Introduction

Transcription factors of the interferon regulatory factor (IRF) family have a critical role in the activation of interferon (IFN) genes. All cellular IRFs share a region of homology in the amino terminus encompassing a highly conserved DNA binding motif characterized by five tryptophan repeats, but show variability in the carboxy (C-) terminal part of the IRF polypeptides. While some of these IRFs like IRF-3 and IRF-7 have a critical role in the antiviral response, the others like IRF-1, IRF-4 and IRF-8 have basic roles in the development and function of lymphoid cells. Recently, the importance of IRF-5 in the antiviral and inflammatory response *in vivo* has been clearly established, but it was also shown that this IRF has a basic function in apoptosis and B cells and macrophage differentiation. More interestingly, the role of IRF-5 pathogenicity in autoimmune diseases has been also established, as IRF-5 has been identified as one of the primary risk factors associated with Systemic Lupus Erythematosus (SLE) and other autoimmune diseases. This chapter will review the current knowledge of the mechanisms of IRF-5 activation by the TLR7 pathway and the genetic modifications of IRF-5 that may contribute to the dysregulation of the innate and adaptive immune response associated with the autoimmune disease. Furthermore we will summarize the contribution of the SLE mouse models to our understanding of the role of IRF-5 and TLR7 in the induction of the autoimmune diseases.

2. Type I IFN and SLE

Autoimmune diseases are characterized by a dysregulated expression of Type I IFN, hyper-reactivity of B cells and the production of auto-antibodies. Leukocytes from patients with different autoimmune disorders such as SLE, psoriasis, dermatomyositis and rheumatic arthritis all show overexpression of interferon-induced genes. Furthermore, clinical use of IFNα leads to development of autoimmune syndromes like type I diabetes, psoriasis and inflammatory arthritis (Gota and Calabrese 2003). Till date, it has not been determined whether the uncontrolled production of Type I IFN is a consequence of dysregulated function of the immune system or due to genetic variations of the factors involved in IFN induction or IFN signalling pathway. Type I IFNs are produced by all leucocytes in response to TLR7 or TLR9 activation and the plasmacytoid dendritic cells (pDC) are the most active producer of IFNα. pDCs represent only about 1% of the PBMCs, but they can secrete up to 10^9 IFNα molecules per cell within 12 hours (Fitzgerald-Bocarsly *et al.*, 2008).

SLE is a classical systemic autoimmune disease. The link between SLE and Type I IFN is indisputable, reviewed in (Crow 2009). The elevation of type I IFNs is the hallmark of autoimmune diseases. In SLE, there is a correlation between IFN levels and the presence of anti-ds (double-stranded) DNA antibodies and disease progression. Interferon-stimulated genes (ISG) signature is a marker for severity of the disease (Baechler et al., 2003). Also the high levels of IFNα are a heritable risk for SLE (Niewold et al., 2007).

Clinical findings show that elevated pDC populations along with higher IFN mRNA levels present in dermal lesions of SLE patients contribute to elevated IFN levels. (Blomberg et al., 2001). pDCs also accumulate in active lupus nephritis and migrate to the glomeruli (Silvestris et al., 2003). Immune complexes containing nucleic acid found in the serum from lupus patients are known to trigger a type I IFN response in pDCs (Bengtsson et al., 2000). The IgG RNA/DNA complexes are internalized via receptors [fragment crystallizable gamma receptor IIa (FcγRIIa)] expressed on pDCs, and stimulate endosomic TLR7 or TLR9 followed by activation of IRF-5 and IRF-7 and IFNα production. Both TLR7 and TLR9 are expressed in pDCs. RNA-containing immune complexes signalling through TLR7 are especially efficient in inducing IFNα and there is a direct correlation between serum levels of IFNα and the presence of autoantibodies to RNA-protein complexes (Vollmer et al., 2005). Autoantibodies reactive against RNA-containing autoantigens are detected in the cerebrospinal fluid of patients with cerebral lupus (Santer et al., 2009). An indirect evidence for the role of IFNα in autoimmune disease is the observation showing that patients receiving anti-IFN therapy for other diseases (such as HCV-related hepatitis treated with IFNα) develop autoantibodies and SLE-like syndrome (Ho et al., 2008). Another indirect observation is the induction of anti-dsDNA antibodies and full-blown SLE during a clinical anti-TNFα therapy in patients with rheumatoid arthritis (RA) (De Rycke et al., 2005). In vitro, TNFα suppresses IFNα expression and thus suppression of TNFα in patients with arthritis, with the antibody treatment, may result in enhancement of IFNα production.

3. Induction of innate antiviral response

Almost all nucleated cells respond to viral infections by producing Type I IFNs. Type I IFNs (IFNα and IFNβ) are an essential part of the antiviral response; however, their unregulated production is associated with pathology. Virus mediated Type I IFN induction is a classical example of transcriptional regulation. Virus infection induces activation of two families of transcriptional factors, NFκB and IRF family. The IRF proteins possess a common DNA binding domain at the N terminus characterized by a helix-turn-helix motif. The motif is rich in tryptophan residues and binds the GAAA and AANNGAAA domains in the virus responsive element (VRE) of Type I IFN promoters. The C-terminal regions of IRFs are distinct and contain IRF-associated domains (IADs) which are required for protein-protein interactions: either with other IRFs or other transcriptional factors. Two members of the IRF family, IRF-3 and IRF-7 are the major players in the induction of Type I IFN (Au et al., 1998; Au et al., 1995; Marie et al., 1998; Ronco et al., 1998). In the uninfected cell, they are localized to the cytoplasm, but in response to a viral infection, they are phosphorylated and translocate to the nucleus where they associate with the co-activator CREB-binding protein and stimulate transcription of IfnA and IfnB genes. While IRF-3 alone is sufficient for induction of IfnB gene, IRF-7 expression is essential for expression of the entire battery of IfnA genes, reviewed in (Pitha and Kunzi 2007). Both IRFs can be activated by a signalling pathway that initiates upon binding of viral dsRNA to membrane Toll-like Receptors, TLR3 and TL4, or cytoplasmic receptors, Retinoic acid-Inducible Gene (RIG)-I or Melanoma Differentiation-Associated gene (MDA)-5. Recent data, however, shows that IRF-3 can be also activated by binding of the viral DNA to the cytoplasmic receptor, Absent In Melanoma (AIM)-2 (Ishikawa and Barber 2011).

4. Role of IRF-5 in the induction of an antiviral response

Another IRF, IRF-5 also stimulates Type I IFN production in infected cells. IRF-5 differs from IRF-3 and IRF-7 in activation and function. While IRF-3 and IRF-7 are induced by TLR3, TLR4 or RIG-I/MDA5 pathways, IRF-5 is activated only by TLR7 and TLR9 in a Myeloid Differentiation factor 88 (MyD88)-dependent pathway and consequently, only certain viral infections (Newcastle disease virus, NDV; VSV; and HSV) can activate IRF-5 (Barnes *et al.*, 2001). The activation of IRF-5 results in the transcription of nine differently alternatively spliced IRF-5 mRNAs, these isoforms are cell-type specific and have distinct functions (Mancl *et al.*, 2005).

Ectopic expression of IRF-5 induces several IFNα subtypes; however, the subtypes induced by IRF-5 and IRF-7 are distinct, *e.g.* IRF-7 induces mostly *IfnA1* while the major subtype induced by IRF-5 is *IfnA8* (Barnes *et al.*, 2001).

5. Downstream effectors of IFNs

The Type I IFN system is well characterized and well-studied. Type I IFNs mediate their action by engaging the ubiquitously expressed IFNα receptor (IFNAR) complex which has two units, IFNAR1 and IFNAR2, reviewed in (Uze *et al.*, 2007). On binding to their respective receptors, IFNs exert their multiple effects through receptor-mediated signalling pathways, resulting in the induction of IFN-stimulated genes (ISGs). The major signalling pathway is the JAK-STAT pathway; beginning from the Janus kinases (JAK1 and Tyk2) and followed by tyrosine phosphorylation of pre-existing signal transducer and activator of transcription (STAT). On phosphorylation, STAT1 and STAT2 assemble together, associate with interferon regulatory factor 9 (IRF-9) and form a multimeric complex (ISGF3) that translocates to the nucleus, where it interacts with interferon-responsive elements (ISRE) present in the 5′ flanking region of ISG (Improta *et al.*, 1994; Levy and Darnell 2002). While ISGF3 seems to be the main transcription factor regulating transcription of ISGs, Type I IFN also stimulates formation of STAT1 homodimers that bind to a slightly different DNA domain, the IFNγ activated site (GAS), present in the promoters of ISG that can be induced both by Type I IFN and IFNγ. The signalling by Type I IFN is not limited to the JAK–STAT pathway as this receptor can also activate both the Mitogen-Activated Protein kinase (MAPK) and Phosphoinositide 3-kinase (PI3K) pathways (Platanias 2005). Activation of IFNs through the IFNARs followed by amplification of the signal via downstream pathways results in activation of more than 300 ISGs. The function of the majority of ISGs has yet to be determined; however, the antiviral function of several of the ISG have been recently characterized, and the proteins described (Samuel 2001; Schoggins *et al.*, 2011).

Among these, ISG15 is one of the very early induced ISGs that influence a panoply of cellular functions; ISG15 is a ubiquitin homologue which is covalently attached to lysine residues (ISGylation) of the targeted proteins. Recent evidence indicates the existence of cross-talk between ubiquitinylation and ISGylation. Since ubiquitinylation is a component of many cellular and stress induced signalling pathway, ISGylation can effectively interfere with these pathways. Activation of ISGylation proceeds by similar enzymatic pathways as used for ubiquitinylation, and interestingly, all enzymes required for ISGylation are induced by IFN. Similar to ubiquitinylation, the ISGylation process is reversible and de-ISGYlating enzymes provide an additional level of control over the entire process. More than a hundred ISG15 targets have been identified, and some of these genes such as RIG-I, JAK1, Protein Kinase R (PKR) and STAT-1 are part of the IFN response system while others have different cellular functions. However, unlike the degradation-driven ubiquitinylation, ISGylation in many cases inhibits ubiquitinylation, reviewed in (Skaug and Chen 2010).

Another IFN induced gene with multiple functions is a constitutively expressed dsRNA dependent PKR whose expression is enhanced by Type I IFN. The inactive monomers of PKR are activated by viral RNA, PKR is phosphorylated and forms active dimers. Activated PKR catalyzes phosphorylation of several substrates including the α subunit of the initiation factor eIF-2 (eIF-2α) (Samuel 1993), as well as the transcription factor inhibitor IκB (Kumar et al., 1994). Thus PKR affects both viral replication and many cellular functions, reviewed in (Pindel and Sadler 2011).

Other ISGs such as cytidine deaminases of the APOBEC family and adenosine deaminase ADAR1 have been recently characterized but their cellular functions are yet to be determined (Chiu and Greene 2008; George et al., 2011; Schoggins et al., 2011). Also interesting is a recent finding from the Rice group (Schoggins et al., 2011) which shows that IRF-1, induced by both IFNγ and Type I IFN has antiviral activity against a large group of distinct viruses and that this antiviral activity is not IFN-mediated. This group also identified large number of novel antiviral ISGs and showed that a number of these proteins function at the translational level.

In addition, there are reports of host-produced antiviral micro-RNAs (miRNAs) in response to IFNs (Hansen et al., 2010; Lagos et al., 2010; O'Connell et al., 2007; Pedersen et al., 2007). Even though first identified in fishes and invertebrates, it was assumed that miRNAs were not elicited as a first line of defence in mammals. However, microarray analysis of general IFNα/β response identified a few candidate miRNAs which are increased or attenuated in response to IFNα/β. Some of these target IFNB mRNA and thus serve as negative regulators of the IFN system, while others are induced during the innate antiviral response. Therefore it seems that IFN-induced cellular miRNAs may represent fine-tuning of the IFN system.

6. Role of IRF-5 in the innate immune response

The transcription factor IRF-5 plays a key role in the innate antiviral and inflammatory response. In vitro studies had initially indicated that IRF-5 may be involved in the antiviral response (Barnes et al., 2001), and when genetically modified Irf-5-/- mice became available, the importance of IRF-5 in the antiviral and inflammatory response in vivo was also demonstrated (Paun et al., 2008; Takaoka et al., 2005). Irf-5-/- mice exhibit high susceptibility to viral infection and show reductions in serum levels of Type I IFN as well as inflammatory cytokines such as IL-6 and TNFα. IRF-5 shows a cell type specific expression in B cells, DC, monocytes and macrophages. In contrast to IRF-3 and IRF-7, IRF-5 is activated only by TLR7 and TLR9 MyD88 dependent pathway and unlike IRF-3 and IRF-7, not by TLR3 or RIG I pathways (Schoenemeyer et al., 2005). The MyD88 mediated activation of IRF-5 involves the formation of a tertiary complex consisting of MyD88 and tetramers of IRAK1, IRAK4, TRAF6 and IRF-5 and IRF-7. It was shown that both K63 ubiquitinylation by TRAF6 and phosphorylation are necessary for activation and translocation of IRF-5 to the nucleus, but the kinase that activates IRF-5 has not yet been identified (Balkhi *et al.*, 2008). Activated IRF-5 forms homodimers and heterodimers with IRF-3 and IRF-7, but while the IRF-5 synergizes with IRF-3 activation, it inhibits the transcriptional activity of IRF-7 (Barnes *et al.*, 2004). In addition to its role in the early inflammatory response, IRF-5 also has pro-apoptotic functions.

The observations discussed above show an important role for IRF-5 in the regulation of early inflammatory cytokines and chemokines' expression, as well as Type I IFN genes. The function of IRF-5 was also examined *in vivo* using the genetically modified *Irf-5⁻/⁻* mouse model. These mice exhibit an increased susceptibility to viral infection and reductions in serum levels of type I IFNs as well as inflammatory cytokines such as interleukin-6 and tumor necrosis factor alpha (TNFα) (Paun *et al.*, 2008; Takaoka *et al.*, 2005). Examination of the cells type in which expression of inflammatory cytokines and IFN depends on IRF-5 show that IRF-5 is required for the TLR9 mediated induction of IFN β in DC, but not in peritoneal macrophages, while the stimulation of inflammatory cytokines expression was dependent on IRF-5 in both cell types. These data indicate that the function of IRF-5 may be cell type specific.

Unexpectedly, approximately 80% of *Irf-5⁻/⁻* mice, (94% C57BL/6) developed an age-related splenomegaly, associated with a dramatic accumulation of CD19⁺B220⁻ B cells (Lien *et al.*, 2010). The age-related splenomegaly was dependent on genotype, and developed in mice with the mixture of 129 and C57BL/6 genotype, but did not occur in mice that were 98% of C57BL/6 background (unpublished data). Interestingly, the *Irf-5⁻/⁻* C57BL6 mice have attenuated responses to T-cell dependent (TD) and T-cell independent (TI) antigens (unpublished data), with a marked down-regulation of serum levels of antigen specific IgG2a and IgG2c. The Taniguchi group (Savitsky *et al.*, 2010) has shown that the down-regulation of IgG2a production occurred also in *in vitro* cultured IRF-5 knockout DC cells stimulated with CpG oligodeoxynucleotides. The synthesis of IL-6 and TNFα was also down-regulated in IRF-5 knockout B cell stimulated with TLR 9 ligand, indicating that the function of these cells is impaired (Lien *et al.*, 2010).

7. Role of IRF-5 in autoimmune diseases

The demonstration that IRF-5 is important not only for the induction of Type I IFN genes, but also for the inflammatory cytokines gave new insights into the regulation of the innate inflammatory response. However, there is also accumulating evidence that IRF-5 may play an important role in the dysregulation of the immune system leading to autoimmune diseases. Several distinctly spliced human IRF-5 isoforms (designated variants 1-10), which show cell type-specific expression and distinct cellular localization, were identified (Mancl *et al.*, 2005). The most common variations are insertions or deletions in exon 6. The majority of IRF-5 isotypes do not differ in their DNA binding sites, but differ in the interaction domain. The transcription of IRF-5 is started at one of the three different promoters. Transcript initiated at exon 1A and 1B are expressed constitutively in B cells and pDC, while transcript 1c is induced by IFN. It should be however noted that spliced variants of IRF-5 were identified only in human cells, while in inbred strains of mice, *IRF-5* encodes for a dominant unspliced transcript.

It has been known for a long time that the autoimmune disease SLE exhibits genetic predisposition, which was later mapped to a specific region on human chromosome 6. When the sequence of the human genome became available, it was found that the genomic region associated with predisposition to SLE showed the presence of several genes associated with the Type I IFN induction and signalling pathway. One of these genes is IRF-5 and a common SNP haplotype in IRF-5 (rs 2004640T) was identified in Scandinavian cohorts as a risk factor for SLE. Interestingly, the same SNP haplotype of IRF-5 has been shown later to be associated with numerous other autoimmune disorders, such as rheumatoid arthritis (RA) (Sigurdsson *et al.*, 2007) and others (Kozyrev and Alarcon-Riquelme 2007). Three specific functional alleles of IRF-5 were identified that define risk factors for SLE (Graham et al., 2006). The rs 2004640 G allele expresses isotypes initiated from exon 1A and 1C, while the rs 2004640T allele expresses transcripts from exon 1B, which provides a stronger promoter and increases the expression of IRF-5. The second SNP is the in-frame insertion- of 30 bp in exon 6 that alters the proline, glutamic acid and serine rich regions and encodes a protein that is similar to unspliced isotype IRF-5v5. The third SNP introduces a variation in the poly A termination site that makes the 3'UTR shorter which leads to an increased stability of IRF-5 mRNA (Graham *et al.*, 2006). All together, these modifications in the *IRF-5* gene result in elevated levels of IRF-5 protein which is larger than the proteins encoded by the spliced IRF- transcripts. Many additional SNPs in IRF-5 have been later identified and are reviewed in (Kozyrev and Alarcon-Riquelme 2007). The high levels of lupus associated IRF-5 expression have been detected in PBMCs of Lupus patients (Feng *et al.*, 2010). Dysregulated expression of Type I IFN is associated with SLE pathogenesis (Niewold *et al.*, 2007) and gene array analysis of PMBCs from SLE patients has revealed elevated expression of IFN-stimulated genes (Crow *et al.*, 2003). Thus, the connection between expression of specific IRF-5 haplotypes and dysregulated production of Type I IFN has been emerging. Interestingly neither IRF-3 or IRF-7 or other members of IRF family were found to be associated with predisposition to autoimmune disease. Thus IRF-5 is possibly the most important factor in the predisposition to the inflammatory diseases.

8. IRF-5 functions in uninfected cells

Another unique feature of IRF-5 is that it is also induced upon DNA damage by p53 (Mori *et al.*, 2002). This establishes the connection between IRF-5 and p53-apoptotic pathways and identifies its possible role in tumor suppression. However, IRF-5 induces apoptosis in p53 independent manner (Barnes *et al.*, 2003). *Irf-5−/−* Mouse Embryonic Fibroblasts (MEFs) expressing c-Ras do not undergo apoptosis even under DNA damage and can efficiently form tumors in mice. These MEFs are also resistant to viral induced apoptosis even though their IFN and cytokine profiles are normal (Yanai *et al.*, 2007). However, there are several indications that IRF-5 and p53 pro-apoptotic function are independent. Several p53 targets are activated in *Irf-5−/−* cells and overexpression of IRF-5 can stop the growth of B cell tumor lymphoma in the absence of p53 (Barnes *et al.*, 2003). Ectopic expression of IRF-5 induces DNA damage-induced apoptosis in p53-deficient colon cancer cells (Hu *et al.*, 2005). IRF-5 is also involved in Fas/CD95-induced apoptosis, a p53 independent phenomenon (Couzinet *et al.*, 2008). IRF-5 stimulates the cyclin-dependent kinase inhibitor p21, but it also stimulates the expression of the pro-apoptotic genes *Bak1*, *Bax*, caspase 8, and DAP kinase 2, thus indicating its ability to promote cell cycle arrest and apoptosis independently of p53 (Barnes *et al.*, 2003).

Udalova and colleagues have also identified IRF-5 as a lineage-defining factor for macrophages (Krausgruber *et al.*, 2011). Their work shows, for the first time, that IRF-5 can be both a transcription activator and repressor. Macrophages differentiate into two functionally opposite types depending on the differentiation stimulus. When bone marrow macrophages are grown with granulocyte–macrophage colony stimulating factor (GM-CSF), they differentiate into M1 type, classical pro-inflammatory macrophages which secrete cytokines like IL-12. However, when they are differentiated with M-CSF, they differentiate to the M2 type, which secretes anti-inflammatory cytokines like IL-10. The authors show that differentiation to M1 macrophages is accompanied by an increase in IRF-5 levels. Overexpression of IRF-5 in M2 macrophages forces them to express a pro-inflammatory profile of cytokines and lowers IL-10 levels, basically making the M2 macrophages functionally similar to M1. Conversely, knockdown of IRF-5 levels in M1 macrophages converts M1 macrophages to the M2 expression profile, producing high levels of IL-10 and low levels of proinflammatory cytokines. Thus IRF-5 is a determinant of macrophage plasticity. The authors also demonstrate that in macrophages, IRF-5 functions as a negative regulator of IL-10. These results open the field to many other questions such as possible cell type specificity of the suppression of IL-10 transcription, or how many other genes are negatively regulated by IRF-5. The analysis of the IRF-5 signature profile in human B cell line BJAB identifies large number of both up-regulated and down regulated genes (Barnes *et al.*, 2004).

9. Activation of IRF-5 by the TLR7 pathway

TLR7 and TLR9 recognize viral ss (single stranded)-RNA or a B form of dsDNA respectively. The recognition is dependent on endosomal internalization and acidification. The TLR7/9 signalling pathway is mediated by an adaptor molecule MyD88 (Kawai *et al.*, 1999; Muzio *et al.*, 1997). MyD88 has two domains: a C-terminal Toll/IL-1 Receptor (TIR) domain that is required for the interaction with the TLRs and an amino terminal death domain (DD) that interacts with members of the IL-1 receptor associated kinase (IRAK) family (Martin and Wesche 2002). This association between IRAK1 and MyD88 results in self-phosphorylation of IRAK-1, as well as phosphorylation by the related kinase, IRAK-4 (Cao *et al.*, 1996; Li *et al.*, 2002). After phosphorylation, IRAK1 dissociates from MyD88 and now binds to TRAF6 (TNF receptor-associated factor 6) (Burns *et al.*, 2000). TRAF6-mediated K63-linked ubiquitinylation is required for IRF-5 nuclear translocation in TLR7/9-MyD88-dependent signalling (Balkhi *et al.*, 2008). IRF-5 homo-dimerizes upon phosphorylation of serine/ threonine residues at the C-terminal end by a still undefined kinase and translocates to the nucleus (Chen *et al.*, 2008). Thus, both ubiquitinylation and phosphorylation of IRF-5 are required for nuclear translocation. IRF-5 also associates with Ikkα kinase, but that results in degradation of IRF-5-rather than activation (Balkhi *et al.*, 2010). It should be noted that TLR 7 and TL9 are the only know pathways that lead to the activation of IRF-5. Unlike IRF-3 or IRF-7, IRF-5 is not activated by TLR3 or TLR 4 via TIR-domain-containing adapter-inducing IFNβ (Trif) pathways or by the RIG-I/MAV IPS-1 pathways.

Several ligands can activate TLR7. TLR7 recognizes viral ssRNA , but IFN production can be also induced in response to imiquimod and resiquimod (Hemmi *et al.*, 2002). In addition, several other guanine nucleoside analogs are recognized exclusively via TLR7 (Lee and Kim 2007). Of physiological ligands, guanosine and uridine-rich ssRNA oligonucleotides derived from HIV-1, stimulate DCs and macrophages to secrete IFNα and other pro-inflammatory cytokines via murine TLR7 (Heil *et al.*, 2004). TLR7 also responds to ssRNA (polyU) or ssRNA derived from wild-type influenza virus (Diebold *et al.*, 2004). Since these sequences can originate from viral as well as endogenous RNA, TLR7 may be unable to discriminate between self and non-self RNA and see the self RNA as sensors of endogenous danger signals. Accordingly, small nuclear ribonucleoproteins (snRNPs), a major component of the immune complexes associated with SLE can activate human pDCs by TLR7 induced signaling pathway and stimulate production of Type I IFNs and other proinflammatory cytokines. Interestingly, the TLR7 pathway can also be activated by nuclear ribonucleoprotein complexes (Savarese et al., 2006).

10. Mouse models of SLE

The mouse model of SLE provides additional information on the mechanism of SLE pathogenicity. NZB mice develop spontaneous lupus, produce autoantibodies and develop glomerulonephritis. Duplication of TLR7 and transposition of the TLR7 gene as seen in the *Yaa* mutation promotes the SLE like symptoms. The B cells of murine lupus model also show an accelerated class switching, which is controlled by the genotype (Vyse et al., 1996). Our results showed that in addition to a decreased production of Type I IFN and inflammatory cytokines, *Irf-5$^{-/-}$* mice exhibit an alteration of the B cells phenotype, associated with age related expansion of CD19$^+$B220$^-$ group of B cells, decrease in plasma cells and splenomegaly (Lien et al., 2010). However, the mechanism by which IRF-5 controls B cells differentiation to plasma cells is not known. *Irf-5$^{-/-}$* mice have also decreased levels of natural antibodies and T cells dependent antigenic stimulation leads to profound decrease in serum IgG2a (Savitsky et al., 2010). Finally the requirement of IRF-5 for the development of lupus like disease was demonstrated in *FcγRIIB$^{-/-}$* mice, where IRF-5 deficiency profoundly decreased the manifestation of the disease (Richez et al., 2010). Two other IRFs, IRF-4 and IRF-8 have critical functions in the B cell differentiation program. B cells development is blocked at the pre-B cells stage in IRF-4 and IRF-8 compound null mice (Lu et al., 2003). IRF-4 also functions in late B cells development regulating IgG class switching and plasma cell development (Sciammas et al., 2006). IRF-8 has a role in germinal centre transcription program (Lee et al., 2006). Altogether, these data indicate that several members of the IRF family can affect B-cell development, however the strong genetic association between IRF-5 and autoimmune disease point out to a unique functions of IRF-5 in the immune system.

11. Induction of autoimmunity by IFNs

How the IFNs contribute to SLE and its progress remains to be fully explained. The presence of immunogenic complexes leads to dendritic cell activation and thus there is a greater antigen presentation and more IFNs are secreted. IFNα increases the expression of autoantigens such as Ro52 and also induces apoptosis via translocation of Ro52 to the nucleus (Baechler et al., 2004; Bennett et al., 2003). Type I IFNs also induce the maturation and activation of dendritic cells, along with upregulation of MHC Class I and II molecules (Baccala et al., 2007). This promotes the development of helper T cells (Th1). In addition, Type I IFNs also enhance antibody production and class switching, decrease the selectivity of B cells for CpG-rich DNA, and permit stimulation by even non-CpG DNA and thereby promote an autoimmune response (Jego et al., 2003; Le Bon et al., 2006). How does IRF-5 contribute to this picture?

12. Genetic association studies and SLE

Genetic and population association studies provide a more comprehensive picture of the role of IFNs in SLE, reviewed in (Delgado-Vega et al., 2010). Of the entire battery of genes identified by genome wide association studies, most of the genes are involved in innate and adaptive immune responses. These can be divided into the following groups: (1) genes implicated in processing and presentation of immune complexes, (2) genes involved in the IFN-inducing pathways, and (3) genes involved in the Type I IFN signalling pathway. Of the first group, the MHC region shows up as a prime candidate in correlation studies, but is challenging to study since the region has hundreds of potential candidate genes (Deng and Tsao 2010; Sestak *et al.*, 2011). In the IFN-inducing pathways, transcription factor IRF-5 was the first identified gene directly to be associated with increased risk of lupus (Graham *et al.*, 2006; Sigurdsson *et al.*, 2005). IRF-5 allele variants with the highest probability of being causal were identified and shown to affect IRF-5 expression. Patients with a risk haplotype of IRF-5 show higher serum IFN activity, when compared to patients lacking this risk genotype. Finally, in the IFN signalling pathway, STAT4, a downstream interacting protein of IFNAR, is also strongly associated with lupus (Kariuki *et al.*, 2009). STAT4 is associated with increased sensitivity to IFNα and the presence of anti-dsDNA autoantibodies. In addition, polymorphisms in the Janus kinase tyrosine kinase 2 (TYK2), which binds to IFNAR, and is part of the initiation of the JAK-STAT pathway, was also found to be associated with lupus and strengthen the link between IFNα expression and SLE. Several other gene products that are part of the IFN signalling pathway, such as TNFAIP3, TYK2, and TREX1, have been also associated with susceptibility to SLE (Adrianto *et al.*, 2011; Fan *et al.*, 2011; Hellquist *et al.*, 2009). Recently identified SNPs in IRF7 also seem to be associated with SLE. (Fu *et al.*, 2011). It is unlikely that the alteration of the function of a single master gene will be responsible for the pathogenesis of SLE; rather it may be combination of malfunction of several genes. Without doubt there is still the potential of finding new genes that contribute to the development of SLE.

13. IRF-5 polymorphisms and association with SLE

IRF-5 was identified as a risk factor for SLE in two very important association studies. Sigurdsson *et al.* looked at sets of lupus patients from Sweden, Finland and Iceland and analyzed 4 SNPs of IRF-5 (Sigurdsson *et al.*, 2005). Graham *et al.* (Graham *et al.*, 2007) describe two functional SNPs within the IRF-5 gene which are a risk haplotype for SLE. One SNP, rs2004640, creates a donor splice site in intron 1 of IRF-5 and the isoform expresses an alternative of untranslated exon 1B. A second SNP is located about 5 kb downstream of IRF-5 and could not be tied to functional importance but is used as a haplotype tag (Graham *et al.*, 2007). Later, several groups identified a second polymorphism that has more easily identifiable functional roles. rs10954213 alters the polyadenylation site of IRF-5 and the resultant mRNA cal be correlated to higher levels of IRF-5 seen in SLE (Sigurdsson *et al.*, 2008). The A allele of this SNP leads to a shorter and more stable mRNA. Finally, an insertion- deletion is found in the 6th exon of IRF-5 that can potentially change the protein isoforms expressed IRF-5 by 10 amino acids (Kozyrev *et al.*, 2007). The deletion results in expression of the isoforms V1 and V4, while the insertion give rise to isoforms V5 and V6. The lupus risk haplotype, TCA, includes the insertion TCA and thus individuals with lupus are expected to express the corresponding isoforms (V5 and V6). The sequence added by the insertion/deletion gives rise to a proline-rich region which can be potentially recruited for additional protein –protein interactions and/or protein stability by altering the degradation rate of the resulting protein.

Even though the genetic association of lupus and IRF-5 has been consistent, the initial studies dealt with an overwhelmingly European population and there are some suggestions that the association factors might be population specific. Studies in Asian populations have identified new susceptibility genes for lupus, while some of the previously known ones have been discounted (Kawasaki et al., 2008; Li et al., 2011; Shimane et al., 2009; Shin et al., 2008; Siu et al., 2008), reviewed in (Kim et al., 2009). Given that the majority of lupus patients are women, genetic imprinting remains yet an unexplored topic. However very interesting is a recent finding showing that IRF-5 is expressed at higher levels in female than in male mice and that the IRF-5 promoter is under hormonal regulation (Shen et al., 2010).

14. Conclusions and future perspectives

Identification of the IRF-5 gene as a genetic risk factor for SLE helps to dissect its role in the IFNα pathway in pathogenesis of SLE. The SNP, rs10954213, that affects the levels of IRF-5 expression through increasing the stability of its mRNA, has a great impact on function and expression of protein, but has not found to be strongly associated as a risk haplotype. Thus many questions remain. Higher levels of IRF-5 might result not only in continued production of type I IFN but also of the proinflammatory cytokines. Are these cytokines responsible for the activation of the immune cells such as B cells? Hyper activation of B cells is one of the markers of SLE and the results in mice indicate that IRF-5 has an important role in cell differentiation and induction of IgG2a subtype, which is an important subtype for the induction of autoimmunity. In humans, the IgG2a isotype corresponds to IgG1, which is the dominant subclass of serum autoantibodies in SLE (Manolova et al., 2002). The biological role of IRF-5 isoforms remains to be determined. Presently we do not know whether TCA haplotype IRF-5 has a distinct function from the other IRF-5 variants or whether it induces different group of the inflammatory genes or IFN A variants. It would be of great interest to learn about the roles of the IRF-5 induced genes and their variation in SLE patients. Now

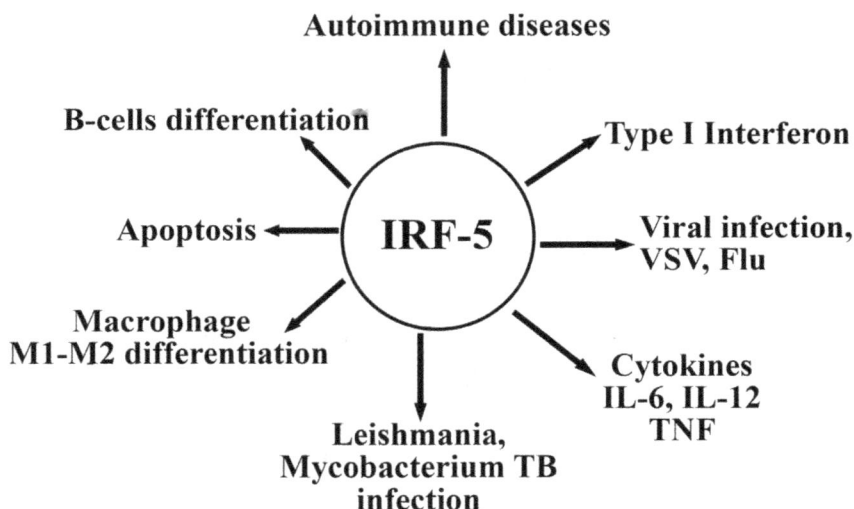

Fig. 1. Various roles of IRF-5 in immunity and autoimmune diseases.

that IRF-5 has been identified as an important factor in induction of type IFN in lupus, it will be important to determine which of the other IRF-5 regulated genes contribute to the pathogenicity of the disease. A recent observation that EBV might also be implicated in the activation of Type I IFN in SLE patients (Yadav *et al.*, 2011) might be an important link in dissecting the cross-talk between genetic predisposition or risk factors and environmental stimuli. Is there any cross talk between IRF-5 and some of the other gene products that were also identified to be associated with Lupus disease? Many of these questions remain yet to be explored to understand the impact of IRF-5 in SLE biology (Figure 1).

15. Acknowledgement

This work was supported by the NIAID grant R01 AI067632-05 to PMP.

16. References

Adrianto I, Wen F, Templeton A, Wiley G, King JB, Lessard CJ, Bates JS, Hu Y, Kelly JA, Kaufman KM, Guthridge JM, Alarcon-Riquelme ME, Anaya JM, Bae SC, Bang SY, Boackle SA, Brown EE, Petri MA, Gallant C, Ramsey-Goldman R, Reveille JD, Vila LM, Criswell LA, Edberg JC, Freedman BI, Gregersen PK, Gilkeson GS, Jacob CO, James JA, Kamen DL, Kimberly RP, Martin J, Merrill JT, Niewold TB, Park SY, Pons-Estel BA, Scofield RH, Stevens AM, Tsao BP, Vyse TJ, Langefeld CD, Harley JB, Moser KL, Webb CF, Humphrey MB, Montgomery CG, Gaffney PM. 2011. Association of a functional variant downstream of TNFAIP3 with systemic lupus erythematosus. *Nat Genet* 43(3):253-8.

Au WC, Moore PA, LaFleur DW, Tombal B, Pitha PM. 1998. Characterization of the interferon regulatory factor-7 and its potential role in the transcription activation of interferon A genes. *J Biol Chem* 273(44):29210-7.

Au WC, Moore PA, Lowther W, Juang YT, Pitha PM. 1995. Identification of a member of the interferon regulatory factor family that binds to the interferon-stimulated response element and activates expression of interferon-induced genes. *Proc Natl Acad Sci U S A* 92(25):11657-61.

Baccala R, Hoebe K, Kono DH, Beutler B, Theofilopoulos AN. 2007. TLR-dependent and TLR-independent pathways of type I interferon induction in systemic autoimmunity. *Nat Med* 13(5):543-51.

Baechler EC, Batliwalla FM, Karypis G, Gaffney PM, Moser K, Ortmann WA, Espe KJ, Balasubramanian S, Hughes KM, Chan JP, Begovich A, Chang SY, Gregersen PK, Behrens TW. 2004. Expression levels for many genes in human peripheral blood cells are highly sensitive to ex vivo incubation. *Genes Immun* 5(5):347-53.

Baechler EC, Batliwalla FM, Karypis G, Gaffney PM, Ortmann WA, Espe KJ, Shark KB, Grande WJ, Hughes KM, Kapur V, Gregersen PK, Behrens TW. 2003. Interferon-inducible gene expression signature in peripheral blood cells of patients with severe lupus. *Proc Natl Acad Sci U S A* 100(5):2610-5.

Balkhi MY, Fitzgerald KA, Pitha PM. 2008. Functional regulation of MyD88-activated interferon regulatory factor 5 by K63-linked polyubiquitination. *Mol Cell Biol* 28(24):7296-308.

Balkhi MY, Fitzgerald KA, Pitha PM. 2010. IKKalpha negatively regulates IRF-5 function in a MyD88-TRAF6 pathway. *Cell Signal* 22(1):117-27.

Barnes BJ, Kellum MJ, Pinder KE, Frisancho JA, Pitha PM. 2003. Interferon regulatory factor 5, a novel mediator of cell cycle arrest and cell death. *Cancer Res* 63(19):6424-31.

Barnes BJ, Moore PA, Pitha PM. 2001. Virus-specific activation of a novel interferon regulatory factor, IRF-5, results in the induction of distinct interferon alpha genes. *J Biol Chem* 276(26):23382-90.

Barnes BJ, Richards J, Mancl M, Hanash S, Beretta L, Pitha PM. 2004. Global and distinct targets of IRF-5 and IRF-7 during innate response to viral infection. *J Biol Chem* 279(43):45194-207.

Bengtsson AA, Sturfelt G, Truedsson L, Blomberg J, Alm G, Vallin H, Ronnblom L. 2000. Activation of type I interferon system in systemic lupus erythematosus correlates with disease activity but not with antiretroviral antibodies. *Lupus* 9(9):664-71.

Bennett L, Palucka AK, Arce E, Cantrell V, Borvak J, Banchereau J, Pascual V. 2003. Interferon and granulopoiesis signatures in systemic lupus erythematosus blood. *J Exp Med* 197(6):711-23.

Blomberg S, Eloranta ML, Cederblad B, Nordlin K, Alm GV, Ronnblom L. 2001. Presence of cutaneous interferon-alpha producing cells in patients with systemic lupus erythematosus. *Lupus* 10(7):484-90.

Burns K, Clatworthy J, Martin L, Martinon F, Plumpton C, Maschera B, Lewis A, Ray K, Tschopp J, Volpe F. 2000. Tollip, a new component of the IL-1RI pathway, links IRAK to the IL-1 receptor. *Nat Cell Biol* 2(6):346-51.

Cao Z, Henzel WJ, Gao X. 1996. IRAK: a kinase associated with the interleukin-1 receptor. *Science* 271(5252):1128-31.

Chen W, Lam SS, Srinath H, Jiang Z, Correia JJ, Schiffer CA, Fitzgerald KA, Lin K, Royer WE, Jr. 2008. Insights into interferon regulatory factor activation from the crystal structure of dimeric IRF5. *Nat Struct Mol Biol* 15(11):1213-20.

Chiu YL, Greene WC. 2008. The APOBEC3 cytidine deaminases: an innate defensive network opposing exogenous retroviruses and endogenous retroelements. *Annu Rev Immunol* 26:317-53.

Couzinet A, Tamura K, Chen HM, Nishimura K, Wang Z, Morishita Y, Takeda K, Yagita H, Yanai H, Taniguchi T, Tamura T. 2008. A cell-type-specific requirement for IFN regulatory factor 5 (IRF5) in Fas-induced apoptosis. *Proc Natl Acad Sci U S A* 105(7):2556-61.

Crow MK. 2009. Developments in the clinical understanding of lupus. *Arthritis Res Ther* 11(5):245.

Crow MK, Kirou KA, Wohlgemuth J. 2003. Microarray analysis of interferon-regulated genes in SLE. *Autoimmunity* 36(8):481-90.

De Rycke L, Baeten D, Kruithof E, Van den Bosch F, Veys EM, De Keyser F. 2005. The effect of TNFalpha blockade on the antinuclear antibody profile in patients with chronic arthritis: biological and clinical implications. *Lupus* 14(12):931-7.

Delgado-Vega AM, Alarcon-Riquelme ME, Kozyrev SV. 2010. Genetic associations in type I interferon related pathways with autoimmunity. *Arthritis Res Ther* 12 Suppl 1:S2.

Deng Y, Tsao BP. 2010. Genetic susceptibility to systemic lupus erythematosus in the genomic era. *Nat Rev Rheumatol* 6(12):683-92.

Diebold SS, Kaisho T, Hemmi H, Akira S, Reis e Sousa C. 2004. Innate antiviral responses by means of TLR7-mediated recognition of single-stranded RNA. *Science* 303(5663):1529-31.

Feng D, Stone RC, Eloranta ML, Sangster-Guity N, Nordmark G, Sigurdsson S, Wang C, Alm G, Syvanen AC, Ronnblom L, Barnes BJ. 2010. Genetic variants and disease-associated factors contribute to enhanced interferon regulatory factor 5 expression in blood cells of patients with systemic lupus erythematosus. *Arthritis Rheum* 62(2):562-73.

Fitzgerald-Bocarsly P, Dai J, Singh S. 2008. Plasmacytoid dendritic cells and type I IFN: 50 years of convergent history. *Cytokine Growth Factor Rev* 19(1):3-19.

Fu Q, Zhao J, Qian X, Wong JL, Kaufman KM, Yu CY, Mok MY, Harley JB, Guthridge JM, Song YW, Cho SK, Bae SC, Grossman JM, Hahn BH, Arnett FC, Shen N, Tsao BP. 2011. Association of a functional IRF7 variant with systemic lupus erythematosus. *Arthritis Rheum* 63(3):749-54.

George CX, Gan Z, Liu Y, Samuel CE. 2011. Adenosine deaminases acting on RNA, RNA editing, and interferon action. *J Interferon Cytokine Res* 31(1):99-117.

Gota C, Calabrese L. 2003. Induction of clinical autoimmune disease by therapeutic interferon-alpha. *Autoimmunity* 36(8):511-8.

Graham RR, Kozyrev SV, Baechler EC, Reddy MV, Plenge RM, Bauer JW, Ortmann WA, Koeuth T, Gonzalez Escribano MF, Pons-Estel B, Petri M, Daly M, Gregersen PK, Martin J, Altshuler D, Behrens TW, Alarcon-Riquelme ME. 2006. A common haplotype of interferon regulatory factor 5 (IRF5) regulates splicing and expression and is associated with increased risk of systemic lupus erythematosus. *Nat Genet* 38(5):550-5.

Graham RR, Kyogoku C, Sigurdsson S, Vlasova IA, Davies LR, Baechler EC, Plenge RM, Koeuth T, Ortmann WA, Hom G, Bauer JW, Gillett C, Burtt N, Cunninghame Graham DS, Onofrio R, Petri M, Gunnarsson I, Svenungsson E, Ronnblom L, Nordmark G, Gregersen PK, Moser K, Gaffney PM, Criswell LA, Vyse TJ, Syvanen AC, Bohjanen PR, Daly MJ, Behrens TW, Altshuler D. 2007. Three functional variants of IFN regulatory factor 5 (IRF5) define risk and protective haplotypes for human lupus. *Proc Natl Acad Sci U S A* 104(16):6758-63.

Hansen A, Henderson S, Lagos D, Nikitenko L, Coulter E, Roberts S, Gratrix F, Plaisance K, Renne R, Bower M, Kellam P, Boshoff C. 2010. KSHV-encoded miRNAs target MAF to induce endothelial cell reprogramming. *Genes Dev* 24(2):195-205.

Heil F, Hemmi H, Hochrein H, Ampenberger F, Kirschning C, Akira S, Lipford G, Wagner H, Bauer S. 2004. Species-specific recognition of single-stranded RNA via toll-like receptor 7 and 8. *Science* 303(5663):1526-9.

Hellquist A, Jarvinen TM, Koskenmies S, Zucchelli M, Orsmark-Pietras C, Berglind L, Panelius J, Hasan T, Julkunen H, D'Amato M, Saarialho-Kere U, Kere J. 2009. Evidence for genetic association and interaction between the TYK2 and IRF5 genes in systemic lupus erythematosus. *J Rheumatol* 36(8):1631-8.

Hemmi H, Kaisho T, Takeuchi O, Sato S, Sanjo H, Hoshino K, Horiuchi T, Tomizawa H, Takeda K, Akira S. 2002. Small anti-viral compounds activate immune cells via the TLR7 MyD88-dependent signaling pathway. *Nat Immunol* 3(2):196-200.

Ho V, McLean A, Terry S. 2008. Severe systemic lupus erythematosus induced by antiviral treatment for hepatitis C. *J Clin Rheumatol* 14(3):166-8.

Hu G, Mancl ME, Barnes BJ. 2005. Signaling through IFN regulatory factor-5 sensitizes p53-deficient tumors to DNA damage-induced apoptosis and cell death. *Cancer Res* 65(16):7403-12.

Improta T, Schindler C, Horvath CM, Kerr IM, Stark GR, Darnell JE, Jr. 1994. Transcription factor ISGF-3 formation requires phosphorylated Stat91 protein, but Stat113 protein is phosphorylated independently of Stat91 protein. *Proc Natl Acad Sci U S A* 91(11):4776-80.

Ishikawa H, Barber GN. 2011. The STING pathway and regulation of innate immune signaling in response to DNA pathogens. *Cell Mol Life Sci* 68(7):1157-65.

Jego G, Palucka AK, Blanck JP, Chalouni C, Pascual V, Banchereau J. 2003. Plasmacytoid dendritic cells induce plasma cell differentiation through type I interferon and interleukin 6. *Immunity* 19(2):225-34.

Kariuki SN, Kirou KA, MacDermott EJ, Barillas-Arias L, Crow MK, Niewold TB. 2009. Cutting edge: autoimmune disease risk variant of STAT4 confers increased sensitivity to IFN-alpha in lupus patients in vivo. *J Immunol* 182(1):34-8.

Kawai T, Adachi O, Ogawa T, Takeda K, Akira S. 1999. Unresponsiveness of MyD88-deficient mice to endotoxin. *Immunity* 11(1):115-22.

Kawasaki A, Kyogoku C, Ohashi J, Miyashita R, Hikami K, Kusaoi M, Tokunaga K, Takasaki Y, Hashimoto H, Behrens TW, Tsuchiya N. 2008. Association of IRF5 polymorphisms with systemic lupus erythematosus in a Japanese population: support for a crucial role of intron 1 polymorphisms. *Arthritis Rheum* 58(3):826-34.

Kim I, Kim YJ, Kim K, Kang C, Choi CB, Sung YK, Lee HS, Bae SC. 2009. Genetic studies of systemic lupus erythematosus in Asia: where are we now? *Genes Immun* 10(5):421-32.

Kozyrev SV, Alarcon-Riquelme ME. 2007. The genetics and biology of Irf5-mediated signaling in lupus. *Autoimmunity* 40(8):591-601.

Kozyrev SV, Lewen S, Reddy PM, Pons-Estel B, Witte T, Junker P, Laustrup H, Gutierrez C, Suarez A, Francisca Gonzalez-Escribano M, Martin J, Alarcon-Riquelme ME. 2007. Structural insertion/deletion variation in IRF5 is associated with a risk haplotype and defines the precise IRF5 isoforms expressed in systemic lupus erythematosus. *Arthritis Rheum* 56(4):1234-41.

Krausgruber T, Blazek K, Smallie T, Alzabin S, Lockstone H, Sahgal N, Hussell T, Feldmann M, Udalova IA. 2011. IRF5 promotes inflammatory macrophage polarization and TH1-TH17 responses. *Nat Immunol* 12(3):231-8.

Kumar A, Haque J, Lacoste J, Hiscott J, Williams BR. 1994. Double-stranded RNA-dependent protein kinase activates transcription factor NF-kappa B by phosphorylating I kappa B. *Proc Natl Acad Sci U S A* 91(14):6288-92.

Lagos D, Pollara G, Henderson S, Gratrix F, Fabani M, Milne RS, Gotch F, Boshoff C. 2010. miR-132 regulates antiviral innate immunity through suppression of the p300 transcriptional co-activator. *Nat Cell Biol* 12(5):513-9.

Le Bon A, Thompson C, Kamphuis E, Durand V, Rossmann C, Kalinke U, Tough DF. 2006. Cutting edge: enhancement of antibody responses through direct stimulation of B and T cells by type I IFN. *J Immunol* 176(4):2074-8.

Lee CH, Melchers M, Wang H, Torrey TA, Slota R, Qi CF, Kim JY, Lugar P, Kong HJ, Farrington L, van der Zouwen B, Zhou JX, Lougaris V, Lipsky PE, Grammer AC, Morse HC, 3rd. 2006. Regulation of the germinal center gene program by interferon (IFN) regulatory factor 8/IFN consensus sequence-binding protein. *J Exp Med* 203(1):63-72.

Lee MS, Kim YJ. 2007. Signaling pathways downstream of pattern-recognition receptors and their cross talk. *Annu Rev Biochem* 76:447-80.

Levy DE, Darnell JE, Jr. 2002. Stats: transcriptional control and biological impact. *Nat Rev Mol Cell Biol* 3(9):651-62.

Li P, Chang YK, Shek KW, Lau YL. 2011. Lack of association of TYK2 gene polymorphisms in chinese patients with systemic lupus erythematosus. *J Rheumatol* 38(1):177-8.

Li S, Strelow A, Fontana EJ, Wesche H. 2002. IRAK-4: a novel member of the IRAK family with the properties of an IRAK-kinase. *Proc Natl Acad Sci U S A* 99(8):5567-72.

Lien C, Fang CM, Huso D, Livak F, Lu R, Pitha PM. 2010. Critical role of IRF-5 in regulation of B-cell differentiation. *Proc Natl Acad Sci U S A* 107(10):4664-8.

Lu R, Medina KL, Lancki DW, Singh H. 2003. IRF-4,8 orchestrate the pre-B-to-B transition in lymphocyte development. *Genes Dev* 17(14):1703-8.

Mancl ME, Hu G, Sangster-Guity N, Olshalsky SL, Hoops K, Fitzgerald-Bocarsly P, Pitha PM, Pinder K, Barnes BJ. 2005. Two discrete promoters regulate the alternatively spliced human interferon regulatory factor-5 isoforms. Multiple isoforms with distinct cell type-specific expression, localization, regulation, and function. *J Biol Chem* 280(22):21078-90.

Manolova I, Dancheva M, Halacheva K. 2002. Predominance of IgG1 and IgG3 subclasses of autoantibodies to neutrophil cytoplasmic antigens in patients with systemic lupus erythematosus. *Rheumatol Int* 21(6):227-33.

Marie I, Durbin JE, Levy DEs. 1998. Differential viral induction of distinct interferon-alpha genes by positive feedback through interferon regulatory factor-7. *EMBO J.* 17(22):6660-9.

Martin MU, Wesche H. 2002. Summary and comparison of the signaling mechanisms of the Toll/interleukin-1 receptor family. *Biochim Biophys Acta* 1592(3):265-80.

Mori T, Anazawa Y, Iiizumi M, Fukuda S, Nakamura Y, Arakawa H. 2002. Identification of the interferon regulatory factor 5 gene (IRF-5) as a direct target for p53. *Oncogene* 21(18):2914-8.

Muzio M, Ni J, Feng P, Dixit VM. 1997. IRAK (Pelle) family member IRAK-2 and MyD88 as proximal mediators of IL-1 signaling. *Science* 278(5343):1612-5.

Niewold TB, Hua J, Lehman TJ, Harley JB, Crow MK. 2007. High serum IFN-alpha activity is a heritable risk factor for systemic lupus erythematosus. *Genes Immun* 8(6):492-502.

O'Connell RM, Taganov KD, Boldin MP, Cheng G, Baltimore D. 2007. MicroRNA-155 is induced during the macrophage inflammatory response. *Proc Natl Acad Sci U S A* 104(5):1604-9.

Paun A, Reinert JT, Jiang Z, Medin C, Balkhi MY, Fitzgerald KA, Pitha PM. 2008. Functional characterization of murine interferon regulatory factor 5 (IRF-5) and its role in the innate antiviral response. *J Biol Chem* 283(21):14295-308.

Pedersen IM, Cheng G, Wieland S, Volinia S, Croce CM, Chisari FV, David M. 2007. Interferon modulation of cellular microRNAs as an antiviral mechanism. *Nature* 449(7164):919-22.

Pindel A, Sadler A. 2011. The role of protein kinase R in the interferon response. *J Interferon Cytokine Res* 31(1):59-70.

Pitha PM, Kunzi MS. 2007. Type I interferon: the ever unfolding story. *Curr Top Microbiol Immunol* 316:41-70.

Platanias LC. 2005. Introduction: interferon signals: what is classical and what is nonclassical? *J Interferon Cytokine Res* 25(12):732.

Richez C, Yasuda K, Bonegio RG, Watkins AA, Aprahamian T, Busto P, Richards RJ, Liu CL, Cheung R, Utz PJ, Marshak-Rothstein A, Rifkin IR. 2010. IFN regulatory factor 5 is required for disease development in the FcgammaRIIB-/-Yaa and FcgammaRIIB-/- mouse models of systemic lupus erythematosus. *J Immunol* 184(2):796-806.

Ronco LV, Karpova AY, Vidal M, Howley PM. 1998. Human papillomavirus 16 E6 oncoprotein binds to interferon regulatory factor-3 and inhibits its transcriptional activity. *Genes Dev* 12(13):2061-72.

Samuel CE. 1993. The eIF-2 alpha protein kinases, regulators of translation in eukaryotes from yeasts to humans. *J Biol Chem* 268(11):7603-6.

Samuel CE. 2001. Antiviral actions of interferons. *Clin Microbiol Rev* 14(4):778-809, table of contents.

Santer DM, Yoshio T, Minota S, Moller T, Elkon KB. 2009. Potent induction of IFN-alpha and chemokines by autoantibodies in the cerebrospinal fluid of patients with neuropsychiatric lupus. *J Immunol* 182(2):1192-201.

Savarese E, Chae OW, Trowitzsch S, Weber G, Kastner B, Akira S, Wagner H, Schmid RM, Bauer S, Krug A. 2006. U1 small nuclear ribonucleoprotein immune complexes induce type I interferon in plasmacytoid dendritic cells through TLR7. *Blood* 107(8):3229-34.

Savitsky DA, Yanai H, Tamura T, Taniguchi T, Honda K. 2010. Contribution of IRF5 in B cells to the development of murine SLE-like disease through its transcriptional control of the IgG2a locus. *Proc Natl Acad Sci U S A* 107(22):10154-9.

Schoenemeyer A, Barnes BJ, Mancl ME, Latz E, Goutagny N, Pitha PM, Fitzgerald KA, Golenbock DT. 2005. The interferon regulatory factor, IRF5, is a central mediator of toll-like receptor 7 signaling. *J Biol Chem* 280(17):17005-12.

Schoggins JW, Wilson SJ, Panis M, Murphy MY, Jones CT, Bieniasz P, Rice CM. 2011. A diverse range of gene products are effectors of the type I interferon antiviral response. *Nature*.

Sciammas R, Shaffer AL, Schatz JH, Zhao H, Staudt LM, Singh H. 2006. Graded expression of interferon regulatory factor-4 coordinates isotype switching with plasma cell differentiation. *Immunity* 25(2):225-36.

Sestak AL, Furnrohr BG, Harley JB, Merrill JT, Namjou B. 2011. The genetics of systemic lupus erythematosus and implications for targeted therapy. *Ann Rheum Dis* 70 Suppl 1:i37-43.

Shen H, Panchanathan R, Rajavelu P, Duan X, Gould KA, Choubey D. 2010. Gender-dependent expression of murine Irf5 gene: implications for sex bias in autoimmunity. *J Mol Cell Biol* 2(5):284-90.

Shimane K, Kochi Y, Yamada R, Okada Y, Suzuki A, Miyatake A, Kubo M, Nakamura Y, Yamamoto K. 2009. A single nucleotide polymorphism in the IRF5 promoter region is associated with susceptibility to rheumatoid arthritis in the Japanese population. *Ann Rheum Dis* 68(3):377-83.

Shin HD, Kim I, Choi CB, Lee SO, Lee HW, Bae SC. 2008. Different genetic effects of interferon regulatory factor 5 (IRF5) polymorphisms on systemic lupus erythematosus in a Korean population. *J Rheumatol* 35(11):2148-51.

Sigurdsson S, Goring HH, Kristjansdottir G, Milani L, Nordmark G, Sandling JK, Eloranta ML, Feng D, Sangster-Guity N, Gunnarsson I, Svenungsson E, Sturfelt G, Jonsen A, Truedsson L, Barnes BJ, Alm G, Ronnblom L, Syvanen AC. 2008. Comprehensive evaluation of the genetic variants of interferon regulatory factor 5 (IRF5) reveals a novel 5 bp length polymorphism as strong risk factor for systemic lupus erythematosus. *Hum Mol Genet* 17(6):872-81.

Sigurdsson S, Nordmark G, Goring HH, Lindroos K, Wiman AC, Sturfelt G, Jonsen A, Rantapaa-Dahlqvist S, Moller B, Kere J, Koskenmies S, Widen E, Eloranta ML, Julkunen H, Kristjansdottir H, Steinsson K, Alm G, Ronnblom L, Syvanen AC. 2005. Polymorphisms in the tyrosine kinase 2 and interferon regulatory factor 5 genes are associated with systemic lupus erythematosus. *Am J Hum Genet* 76(3):528-37.

Sigurdsson S, Padyukov L, Kurreeman FA, Liljedahl U, Wiman AC, Alfredsson L, Toes R, Ronnelid J, Klareskog L, Huizinga TW, Alm G, Syvanen AC, Ronnblom L. 2007. Association of a haplotype in the promoter region of the interferon regulatory factor 5 gene with rheumatoid arthritis. *Arthritis Rheum* 56(7):2202-10.

Silvestris F, Tucci M, Quatraro C, Dammacco F. 2003. Recent advances in understanding the pathogenesis of anemia in multiple myeloma. *Int J Hematol* 78(2):121-5.

Siu HO, Yang W, Lau CS, Chan TM, Wong RW, Wong WH, Lau YL, Alarcon-Riquelme ME. 2008. Association of a haplotype of IRF5 gene with systemic lupus erythematosus in Chinese. *J Rheumatol* 35(2):360-2.

Skaug B, Chen ZJ. 2010. Emerging role of ISG15 in antiviral immunity. *Cell* 143(2):187-90.

Takaoka A, Yanai H, Kondo S, Duncan G, Negishi H, Mizutani T, Kano S, Honda K, Ohba Y, Mak TW, Taniguchi T. 2005. Integral role of IRF-5 in the gene induction programme activated by Toll-like receptors. *Nature* 434(7030):243-9.

Uze G, Schreiber G, Piehler J, Pellegrini S. 2007. The receptor of the type I interferon family. *Curr Top Microbiol Immunol* 316:71-95.

Vollmer J, Tluk S, Schmitz C, Hamm S, Jurk M, Forsbach A, Akira S, Kelly KM, Reeves WH, Bauer S, Krieg AM. 2005. Immune stimulation mediated by autoantigen binding sites within small nuclear RNAs involves Toll-like receptors 7 and 8. *J Exp Med* 202(11):1575-85.

Vyse TJ, Morel L, Tanner FJ, Wakeland EK, Kotzin BL. 1996. Backcross analysis of genes linked to autoantibody production in New Zealand White mice. *J Immunol* 157(6):2719-27.

Yadav P, Tran H, Ebegbe R, Gottlieb P, Wei H, Lewis RH, Mumbey-Wafula A, Kaplan A, Kholdarova E, Spatz L. 2011. Antibodies elicited in response to EBNA-1 may cross-react with dsDNA. *PLoS One* 6(1):e14488.

Yanai H, Chen HM, Inuzuka T, Kondo S, Mak TW, Takaoka A, Honda K, Taniguchi T. 2007.
    Role of IFN regulatory factor 5 transcription factor in antiviral immunity and tumor
    suppression. *Proc Natl Acad Sci U S A* 104(9):3402-7.

4

Cell Surface Glycans at SLE – Changes During Cells Death, Utilization for Disease Detection and Molecular Mechanism Underlying Their Modification

Bilyy Rostyslav[1,2], Tomin Andriy[1], Yaroslav Tolstyak[2],
Havrylyuk Anna[2], Chopyak Valentina[2],
Kit Yuriy[1] and Stoika Rostyslav[1]
[1]Institute of Cell Biology, National Academy of Sciences of Ukraine, Lviv,
[2]Danylo Halytsky Lviv National Medical University, Lviv,
Ukraine

1. Introduction

Autoimmune diseases develop when the immune system starts producing antibodies and T cells that are targeting components of the body. Such state occurs when the ability to recognition of self is disturbed and the immune cells attack healthy cells. The autoimmune diseases are frequently accompanied by self-destruction which is realized via apoptosis. There are two signaling pathways how the immune cells induce apoptosis in the target cells: 1) receptor-mediated; 2) receptor-independent. In the first mechanism, so called "death receptors" that are located on plasma membrane of the target cell are involved, while their "death ligands" are either located on the surface of the immune cell, or released by these cells and acting in free form. The corresponding ligand-receptor interactions cause activation of "death receptors" which use special "death domains" for contacting with specific intracellular signaling proteins and formation of death-inducing signaling complex (DISC). It is considered that this complex is capable of interacting with procaspase 8 and activating this initiator caspase. It is also probable that from this moment (activation of caspase 8), cascade of the apoptotic events gains irreversible character (Ashkenazi & Dixit, 1998). The receptor-independent mechanisms of apoptosis induction in which the immune cells take part, differ significantly (Vermijlen et al., 2001). These mechanisms are based on the ability of cytotoxic T cells to induce formation of special pores in plasma membrane of the target cells. Through these pores, calcium cations and protein granzyme B penetrates the target cells where they directly activate apoptotic enzymes – the caspases.

Fas-receptor that belongs to a family of tumor necrosis factor (TNF) receptors (Orlinick & Chao, 1998) is a typical "death receptor". It is known that TNF is produced by activated macrophages and T cells as a host response to infection (Tartaglia & Goeddel, 1992). Its interaction with specific plasma membrane receptors induces production of transcription factors NF-kB and AP-1 which take part in the activation of specific genes whose products are involved in the inflammation and immunomodulation (Tartaglia & Goeddel, 1992).

After association with the adaptor protein TRADD, TNF receptor can interact with the procaspase 8, and this occurs during the TNF-induced apoptosis.

Apo2L or TRAIL is another TNF-like ligand that can induce apoptosis in various cell lines including tumor ones (Pradhan, Krahling, Williamson, & Schlegel, 1997). Since the population of mature T cells gains sensitivity to the TRAIL-induced apoptosis after their stimulation with the interleukin 2, it is considered that TRAIL takes part in elimination of the peripheral T lymphocytes.

The receptor-independent apoptosis is the main mechanism by which the cytotoxic lymphocytes destroy virus-infected cells, as well as tumor cells (Ploegh, 1998). This mechanism is based on exocytosis of special dense granules which interact with plasma membrane of the target cells. These granules contain cytolytic substances which can polymerize in the presence of calcium cations and form macromolecular channels in the plasma membrane of the target cells. These channels are used for penetration of the granzyme B – serine protease that is capable of activating various caspases, for example the procaspase 3 (Goping et al., 2003). An elevated expression of the antiapoptotic mitochondrial protein Bcl-2 blocks such activation of the caspase 3, while the granzyme B blocks functioning of the Bcl-2. Thus, granzyme B is critical agent in the induction of apoptosis caused by the cytotoxic T cells.

1.1 SLE

Systemic Lupus Erythematosus (SLE) is a chronic, usually life-long, potentially fatal autoimmune disease characterized by unpredictable exacerbations and remissions with variable clinical manifestations. In SLE patients, there is a high probability for clinical involvement of the joints, skin, kidney, brain, lung, heart, serosa and gastrointestinal tract. Women and minorities are disproportionately affected, and Lupus SLE is most common in women of child-bearing age. A recent study identified a prevalence in the Unites States of 500 per 100,000 (1:200) in women (Belmont, 2010). SLE is a multifactorial disease involving genetic, environmental and hormonal factors. Its precise pathogenesis is unclear. There is growing evidence in favor of clearance deficiency of apoptotic cells as a core mechanism in SLE pathogenesis.

1.2 Clearance and SLE

Defective clearance of apoptotic cells causes secondary necrosis with a release of intracellular content and inflammatory mediators. This occurrence is considered as an intrinsic defect that can cause permanent presence of cellular debris responsible for the initiation of systemic autoimmunity in such diseases as SLE (for details see the review (Munoz, Lauber, Schiller, Manfredi, & Herrmann, 2010)). Macrophages respond and present self-antigens to T and B cells. Pathogenic autoantibodies are the primary cause of tissue damage in patients with lupus. The production of these antibodies arises by means of complex mechanisms involving every key facet of the immune system. Thus, restoring organism's ability to remove dying cells and impaired macromolecules (improving clearance efficiency) can serve as a perspective approach to treatment of autoimmune disorders and achieving clinical remission.

1.3 Ways to improve clearance

The apoptotic markers located in plasma membrane of the cell are very important, since they allow detecting apoptosis without violation of cell integrity. At present, phosphatidyl serine externalization is the most widely used apoptotic marker on PM (Fadok et al., 1992). It is detected by the annexin V binding test (Reutelingsperger & Christiaan Peter, 1998). Recently, we found that apoptosis is accompanied by not only the loss of plasma membrane asymmetry caused by phosphatidyl serine externalization, but also by changes in cell surface glycoconjugates described by us (R. Bilyy & Stoika, 2007; R. O. Bilyy, Antonyuk, & Stoika, 2004; R. O. Bilyy & Stoika, 2003). Similar results were obtained by the group headed by Prof. Martin Herrmann (Heyder et al., 2003). Further findings of our (R. Bilyy et al., 2005; R. O. Bilyy et al., 2004) and other groups (Batisse et al., 2004; Franz et al., 2006; Franz et al., 2007) allowed us to consider that an increase in the exposure levels of α-D-mannose- and β-D-galactose-rich GPs of the PM is a characteristic feature of the apoptotic cells. Their expression is substantially increased after apoptosis induction. Two independent mechanisms can lead to the appearance of altered surface glycoepitopes. One mechanism is the activation of surface sialidases resulting in exposure of desialylated (galactose-rich) surface glycoepitopes.

These glyconeoepitopes have been proposed for both the detection of apoptotic cells (R. O. Bilyy et al., 2004) and their isolation from the mixed populations (Stoika, Bilyy, & Antoniuk, 2006). Moreover, these glycoepitops can be directly involved in clearance of the apoptotic cells by the macrophages, serving as an "eat-me" signals of the apoptotic cells, as we have shown in (Meesmann et al., 2010). Our finding explains the previously known fact of surface glycopattern contribution to the clearance of dying and aged cells (Savill, Fadok, Henson, & Haslett, 1993). We effectively used changed apoptotic cell glycopattern for detection of dying cells in blood samples at the autoimmune disorders (R. Bilyy et al., 2009). We have proved that artificial desialylation of apoptotic and viable cells enhances their clearance by macrophages. This was confirmed in both cell lines and isolated human PMN and monocytes differentiated to macrophages (Meesmann et al., 2010).

Detection of both annexin V (van den Eijnde et al., 1997) and fluorescent conjugates of lectins (Heyder et al., 2003) usually requires using complex equipment like flow cytometer and/or fluorescent microscope. Evaluation of phosphatidyl serine externalization should be conducted as soon as possible after blood isolation, and cannot be done after the majority of available fixation procedure, since it would result in false-positive results; while the GPs are not affected by cell fixation or staining procedure. We have focused at the development of a test aimed to detect cell surface glycoconjugate changes during apoptotic cell death. We utilized the multivalency of lectin molecules for inducing agglutination of apoptotic cells, resulting from their altered surface GP content, and developed a specific test for apoptosis measurement (R. Bilyy & Stoika, 2007; Stoika et al., 2006).

2. Lymphocyte desialylation at SLE

Previously, we (R. Bilyy et al., 2009) demonstrated a significant increase in apoptosis incidence in the perypheral blood lymphocytes of RA patients comparing with lymphocytes of clinically healthy donors. That increase was detected by both flow cytometry and lectin-induced agglutination testing of apoptosis. We concluded that apoptosis-related changes in glycoconjugates of plasma membrane of the peripheral blood lymphocytes in RA patients can be used as a reliable and simple tool for apoptosis measurement during this and, probably, other autoimmune disorders. Detection of glycoconjugates via specific lectin binding is compatible with other available fixation/staining procedures, and can be recommended as an additional indicator in the multi-parameter automated detection systems.

Here we estimated changes in cell surface GP expression, namely changes in ß-D-containing glycans, in the peripheral blood lymphocytes of SLE patients and clinically healthy donors, and compared these changes with the level of apoptotic cells detected by the alternative methods. Detection of ß-D-containing glycans was performed by using VAA lectin staining, since this lectin binds to the surface of both early and late apoptotic cells, as can be seen at the confocal image on Fig. 1.

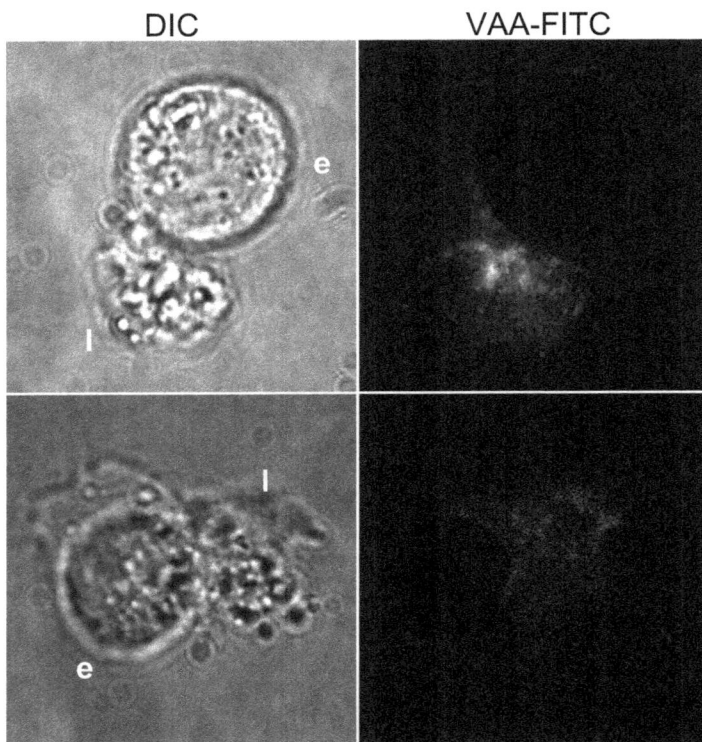

Fig. 1. Confocal microscopy of Jurkat T-cells at early (e) and late (l) stages of apoptosis progression, staining with VAA lectin. Lectin binds with cell surface, both cells are PI-negative.

Study of the peripheral blood lymphocytes of healthy donors revealed that their populations contained 0.707±0.121 % of cells with noticeable pre-G1 peak in cell cycle, with a range of 1.95% (minimal value - 0.14% and maximal value – 2.09), while the SLE patients were characterized by a markedly increased number of apoptotic cells (if judged by the appearance of G1 peak) – 4.47±0.50 %, with a wide range of 10.72% (minimal value – 0.86% and maximal value 11.62 %) (significance of the difference between two groups was P<0.001).

The lectin-induced agglutination test is based on the evaluation of minimal concentration of ß-D-galactose specific *Viscum album* lectin (VAA) used for cell agglutination. The principle of lectin-induced agglutination test is described in Fig. 2. Previously, it was proved that the level of these GPs was increased at apoptosis, and the concentration of lectin used for agglutination is in a reverse dependence upon the amount of cell surface GPs – the higher amount of the apoptotic like GPs is present on the cell surface - the less amount of lectin is needed for agglutination of these cells. Agglutination of lymphocytes of clinically healthy donors (0.32% and 0.12% of apoptotic cells), and of SLE patients (4.91% and 2.37% of apoptotic cells), as well as flow cytometry data on pre-G1 cell content are presented in Fig. 2.

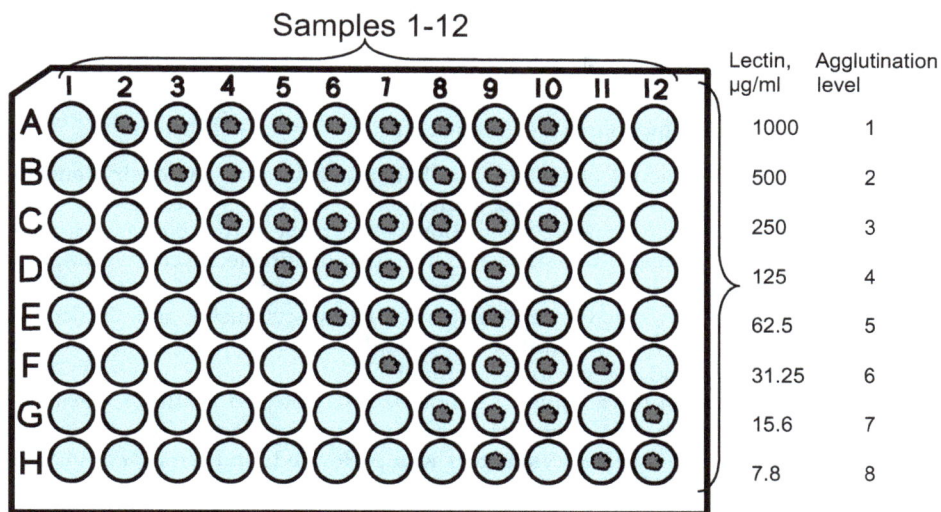

Fig. 2. Principle of lectin-stimulated agglutination test. Agglutination level corresponds to minimal lectin concentration, needed for cell agglutination. Notes: 1 – our data indicate that lectin concentration, 2000 µg/ml agglutinates almost all intact cells. 2,3,4 – this conditions indicates possible errors in sample preparation and needs to be re-tested.

In the group of healthy donors, the mean lectin concentration needed to agglutinate lymphocytes was $1,500 \pm 121.27$ µg/ml, while in the group of SLE patients, this indicator equaled 306.19 ± 128.17 (significance of the difference between two groups was $P < 0.001$) (Table 1). Thus, the ratio between the lectin concentrations in two studied groups constituted almost 4 times. This could be caused by two reasons: 1. increased basal (overall) lectin binding by cells in population; 2. increased number of cells that specifically bind the lectin. To clarify these mechanisms, smears of peripheral blood lymphocytes were subjected to lectin-cytochemical analysis based on using VAA lectin with subsequent microphotography and densitometric study. It revealed that basal staining in control group was 0.153 ± 0.013 a.u., while in the SLE patients it was 0.144 ± 0.01 a.u. There was no significant differences between two cell populations, while the number of cells that were intensively stained in both populations was significantly different (see Table 1). Thus, we suggested that difference in agglutination between lymphocytes of two groups is due to an increased percentage of cells exposing galactose-rich glycoconjugates on their surface.

	Healthy donors, n=18	SLE patients, n=23	p
% of apoptotic cells[1]	0.707 ± 0.121 %	4.471 ±0.502 %	p<0.001
Agglutination[2]	1,500 ± 121.27 µg/ml	306.19±128.17 µg/ml	p<0.001
Basal VAA staining[3]	0.153 ± 0.013 a.u.	0.144 ± 0.010 a.u.	0.061
% of VAA stained cells	4.783 ± 0.936 %	8.27 ± 1.30 %	p<0.05

1 – judged by content of pre-G1 cells, measured by flow cytometry;
2 – measured by lectin-induced agglutination;
3 – measured by lectin-cytochemical analysis.

Table 1. Number of apoptotic cells and changes in plasma membrane glycoconjugates of lymphocytes in clinically healthy donors and SLE patients.

Correlation analysis of the amount of apoptotic cells detected by flow cytometry, and of minimal lectin concentration, needed for cell agglutination detected by lectin-stimulated agglutination, revealed a strong negative correlation between these two parameters (R=-0,764, P<0.001, see Fig.4). As previously established, the agglutinating lectin concentration is reversely proportional to the amount of apoptotic cells. Thus, the amount of apoptotic cells established by both methods – pre-G1 cell detection by flow cytometry and the lectin-induced agglutination – is well correlated. It should be noted that lectin-induced agglutination is much easier and cheaper in performing.

The correlation study between the amount of apoptotic cells detected by the Annexin V-FITC labeling and by testing based on using mannose-specific lectin from *Narcissus pseudonarcissus* (both detected by flow cytometry) was performed, and strong correlation between both parameters (R=0.725) was demonstrated (Heyder et al., 2003). Thus, specific changes in cell surface glycoconjugate pattern can be effectively used for detection of apoptotic cells at SLE and, probably, other at other autoimmune disorders.

The study of peripheral blood lymphocytes of 23 SLE patients and that of 18 clinically healthy donors revealed a significantly increased incidence of apoptosis in the SLE patients. That was detected by both flow cytometry and lectin-induced agglutination testing. High correlation between these results obtained by using two different methods suggests that apoptosis-related changes in plasma membrane glycoconjugates of the peripheral blood lymphocytes at SLE can be used as a reliable and easy tool for apoptosis measurement during autoimmune disorders. Detection of glycoconjugates via specific lectin binding is compatible with other available fixation/staining procedures. It can be recommended as an additional indicator in the multi-parameter automated detection systems.

Thus, the obtained data demonstrated that SLE was accompanied by an appearance of apoptotic cells possessing desialylated glycoepitopes (rich in terminal ß-D-containing glycans). Taking into account the above described clauses that desialylated glycans are important for cell clearance and that SLE potentially results from insufficient cell clearance, an intriguing question appears– are there any desialylating agents in blood of SLE patients.

3. Desialylating abzymes at SLE

Mammalian sialidases (related enzymes including bacterial and viral are also referred as neuraminidases) are glycosidases responsible for the removal of sialic acids from the glycoproteins and glycolipids. They have been implicated to participate in many biological processes, particularly in lysosomal catabolism (Miyagi, Wada, Yamaguchi, Hata, &

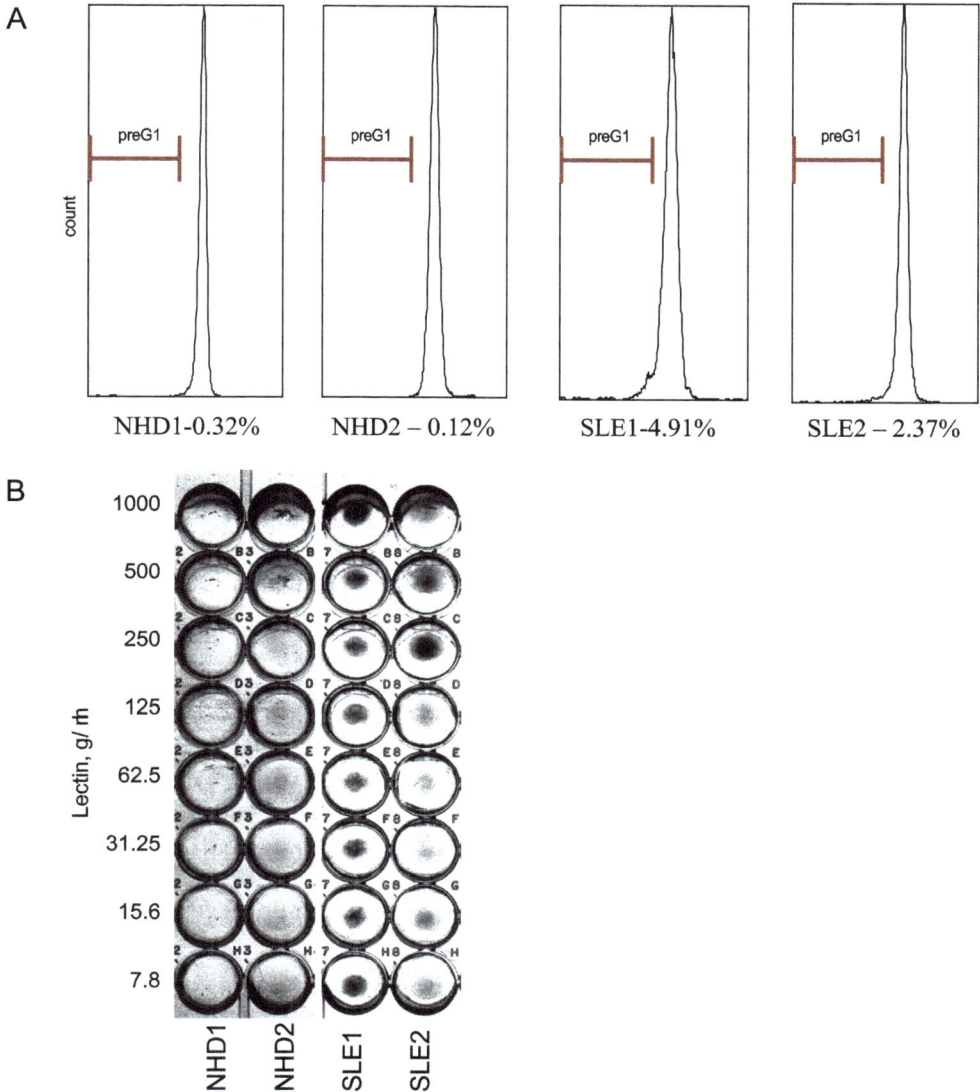

Fig. 3. Detection of apoptotic cells by measuring amount of pre-G1 cells using PI staining by
flow cytometry (A) and minimal concentration needed for lectin-induced agglutination (B)
of peripheral blood lymphocytes of two normal healthy donors and two SLE patients.

Shiozaki, 2008; Monti, Preti, Venerando, & Borsani, 2002). Altered sialylation of
glycoproteins and glycolipids is observed as a ubiquitous phenotype in cancer. It leads to an
appearance of tumor-associated antigens, aberrant adhesion and disturbance of
transmembrane signalling (Miyagi, Wada, & Yamaguchi, 2008; Miyagi, Wada, Yamaguchi,
& Hata, 2004). Aberrant sialylation is closely associated with the malignant phenotype of

cancer cells, including metastatic potential and invasiveness (Miyagi, Wada, & Yamaguchi, 2008; Miyagi et al., 2004; Miyagi, Wada, Yamaguchi, Shiozaki, et al., 2008). However, its biological significance and molecular mechanisms have not been fully elucidated.

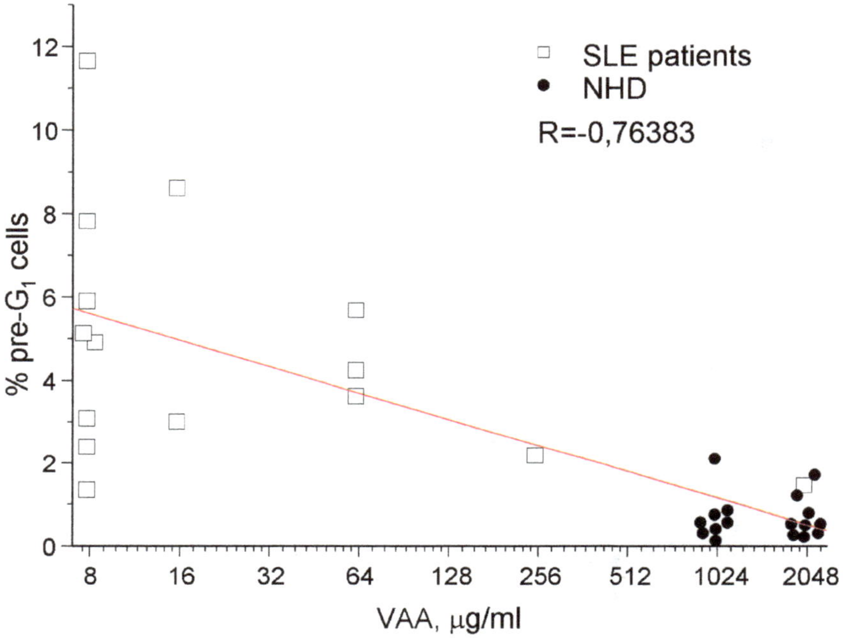

Fig. 4. Correlation analysis between specific lectin concentrations needed for lymphocyte agglutination and a percentage of the apoptotic cells. Lectin concentration needed for agglutination is reversely proportional to the amount of apoptotic cells.

Neuraminidases are abundant in prokaryotes and viruses, while only 4 sialidases are known in human (Miyagi, Wada, Yamaguchi, Shiozaki, et al., 2008). The last described one, Neu4, was reported only in 2003 (Comelli, Amado, Lustig, & Paulson, 2003). Neu 1 is a lysosomal sialidase, and Neu2 is localized in lysosomes and involved in digestion of N–glycans, and Neu3, known as ganglioside sialidase, is localized in plasma membrane and involved in ganglioside metabolism (Monti et al., 2000). Neu4 is localized in lysosomes (Seyrantepe et al., 2004) and can be translocated to mitochondria (Yamaguchi et al., 2005) and endoplasmic reticulum (Bigi et al.). However, none of known sialidases is active in the body fluids (blood or lymph). There is no evidence that plasma membrane sialidase Neu3 (or any other sialidase) can be shed from cell surface into the blood flow (Miyagi, Wada, Yamaguchi, Shiozaki, et al., 2008). While detecting increased neuraminidase activity on the surface of apoptotic cells (R. Bilyy, Tomin, & Stoika, 2010), we failed to detect any sialidase activity in culture media that could result from enzyme secretion/release during cell death.

We have focused our attention at the catalytic antibodies. These antibodies, now named as "abzymes", were first obtained in 1986 (Pollack, Jacobs, & Schultz, 1986; Tramontano, Janda, & Lerner, 1986), the first example of natural abzymes was IgG found in bronchial asthma

patients, cleaving intestinal vasoactive peptide (Paul et al., 1989). Abzyme's properties were
discussed in more detail in recent reviews (Belogurov, Kozyr, Ponomarenko, & Gabibov,
2009; Georgy A. Nevinsky & Buneva, 2005; Planque et al., 2008; Taguchi et al., 2008).
Abzymes were detected in human organism at a variety of autoimmune and non-
autoimmune pathologies (Gabibov, Ponomarenko, Tretyak, Paltsev, & Suchkov, 2006; G. A.
Nevinsky & Buneva, 2003), and various peptides, proteins, nucleic acids and
oligosaccharides can serve as substrates for the catalytically active antibodies in human and
other mammalians (Hanson, Nishiyama, & Paul, 2005; Lacroix-Desmazes et al., 2006). The
involvement of abzymes in pathogenesis of autoimmune disorders has been documented
(Gabibov et al., 2006; Hanson et al., 2005; Lacroix-Desmazes et al., 2006; G. A. Nevinsky &
Buneva, 2003). Catalytically active antibodies are typically found in patients with
autoimmune disorders, however, they have also been detected in cancer patients. DNA-
hydrolyzing activity of IgG auto-Ab from blood serum of patients with various types of
lymphoproliferative diseases was described (Kozyr et al., 1998; Kozyr et al., 1996). Testing of
the abzymes in patients with hematological tumors and SLE revealed a linkage of anti-DNA

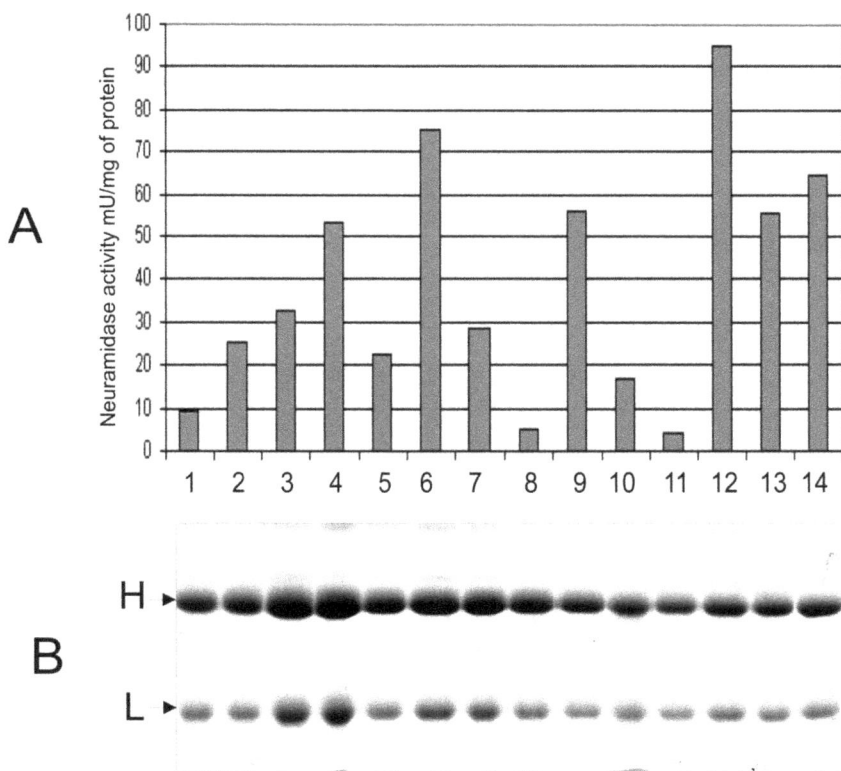

Fig. 5. Comparative analysis of sialidase activity of IgGs obtained by chromatography on
Protein G – Sepharose from blood serum of SLE patients (A) and SDS-PAG electrophoresis
of IgG-preparations (B), n = 14. The position on the gel of heavy (H) and light (L) chains of
IgGs molecules is indicated.

Ab catalysis with mature B-cell tumors, and an increased probability of DNA-abzymes formation at the autoimmune conditions (Gabibov et al., 2006). These data suggest a similarity between the mechanisms of abzyme formation at SLE and B-cell lymphomas. Peptide-hydrolyzing and DNA-hydrolyzing activities of Bence Jones proteins isolated from blood serum of myeloma patients are well studied (Paul et al., 1995; Sun, Gao, Kirnarskiy, Rees, & Paul, 1997). There are numerous data demonstrating that the catalytic activity of anti-DNA IgGs and Bence Jones proteins are associated with their cytotoxic activity and correlate with the disease pathogenesis (Gabibov, Kozyr, & Kolesnikov, 2000; Kozyr et al., 2002; Matsuura, Ohara, Munakata, Hifumi, & Uda, 2006; Sashchenko et al., 2001; Sinohara & Matsuura, 2000). Recently, we demonstrated that anti-histone H1 IgGs isolated from blood serum of multiple sclerosis patients, were capable of hydrolyzing histone H1 (Kit, Starykovych, Richter, & Stoika, 2008). IgGs with similar proteolytic activity were also found in blood serum of patients with SLE (Magorivska et al., 2010) and multiple myeloma (Magorivska et al., 2009). Recently, we have shown that in the blood serum of some multiple myeloma patients there are immunoglobulins IgG possessing sialidase activity (R. Bilyy, Tomin, Mahorivska, et al., 2010). These data suggest an important role of abzymes at the autoimmune and oncological diseases. However, further studies are needed for better understanding of humoral immunity functions under normal and pathological conditions.

Here we demonstrated for the first time that blood serum of SLE patients contains catalytically active IgGs possessing sialidase activity. Biological consequences of such phenomenon are discussed.

The reason for studying neuraminidase activity of Ab in SLE patients is based on data showing that Ig preparations obtained by precipitation with 50% saturated ammonium sulphate from blood serum of 14 SLE patients possessed a significant capability of hydrolyzing neuramidase substrate 4-MUNA (Fig. 5), while Ig preparations of 12 healthy

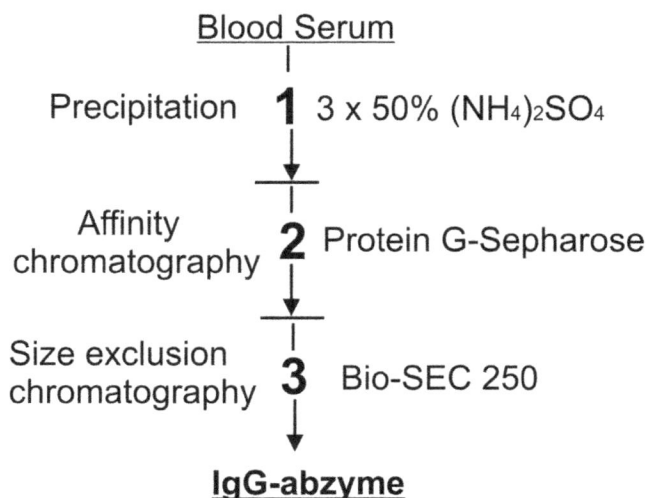

Blood Serum

Precipitation **1** 3 x 50% $(NH_4)_2SO_4$

Affinity chromatography **2** Protein G-Sepharose

Size exclusion chromatography **3** Bio-SEC 250

IgG-abzyme

Fig. 6. Purification of IgG-abzymes from blood serum of SLE patients. Step 1 - Three-fold Ab precipitation with ammonium sulfate. Step 2 - IgG isolation by affinity chromatography on protein G-Sepharose column. Step 3 - HPLC size exclusion chromatography at pH 2.6, favoring dissociation of the immune complexes on Bio-Sec 250 column.

donors, obtained in the similar manner, were devoid of significant level of sialidase activity. Thus, we suggested that at least a part of this catalytic activity could be linked to abzymes present in the Ig preparations. To verify this suggestion, the catalytically active Ig preparations obtained with ammonium sulphate precipitation were further purified by the chromatography on protein G-sepharose column (Fig. 6) and additionally purified by HPLC SEC at neutral and acidic conditions (Fig.7). Besides, we obtained (Fab)$_2$-fragments of this

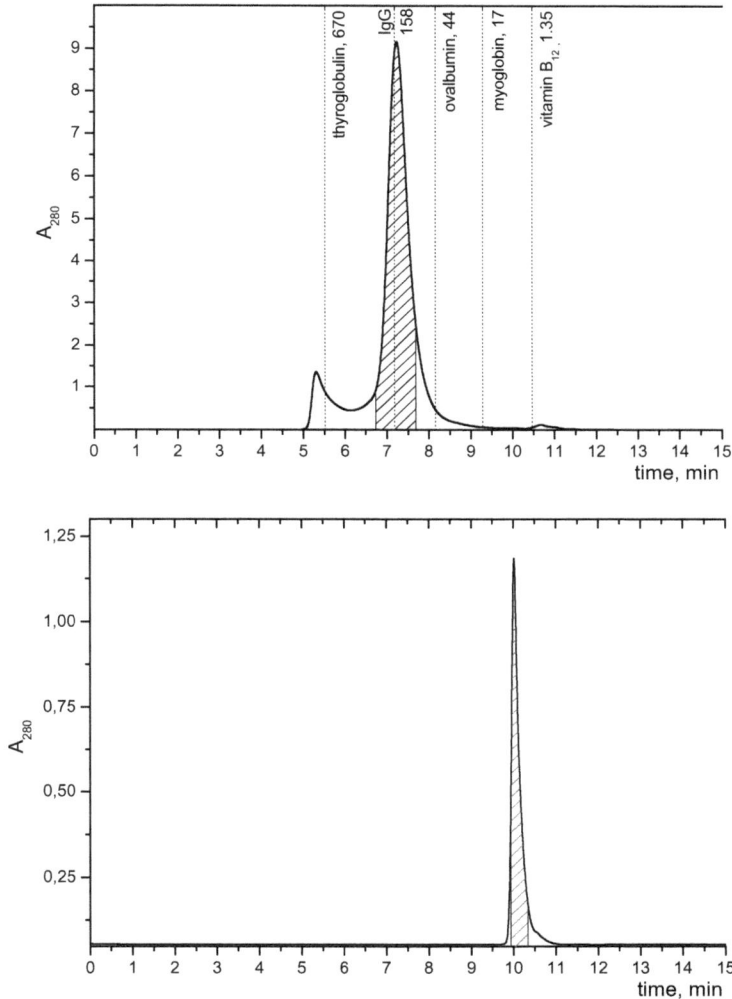

Fig. 7. Typical HPLC size exclusion chromatography on Bio-Sec 250 column (PBS, pH 6.8) elution profile of IgG preparation after purification by affinity chromatography on protein G-Sepharose (top) and additional size exclusion chromatography of this IgG sample at pH 2.6 (glycine*HCl), favoring dissociation of the immune complexes on Bio-Sec 250 column (bottom). Peaks indicated by shading were collected and used for further analysis.

IgG, and studied their sialidase activity. It was found that both IgG preparation and its (Fab)$_2$ fragments possessed sialidase activity towards 4-MUNA, but not galactosidase activity towards 4-MU-Gal (Fig. 8). Sialidase activity towards 4-MUNA was not inhibited in the presence of 10 mM 4-MU ($p<0.05$).

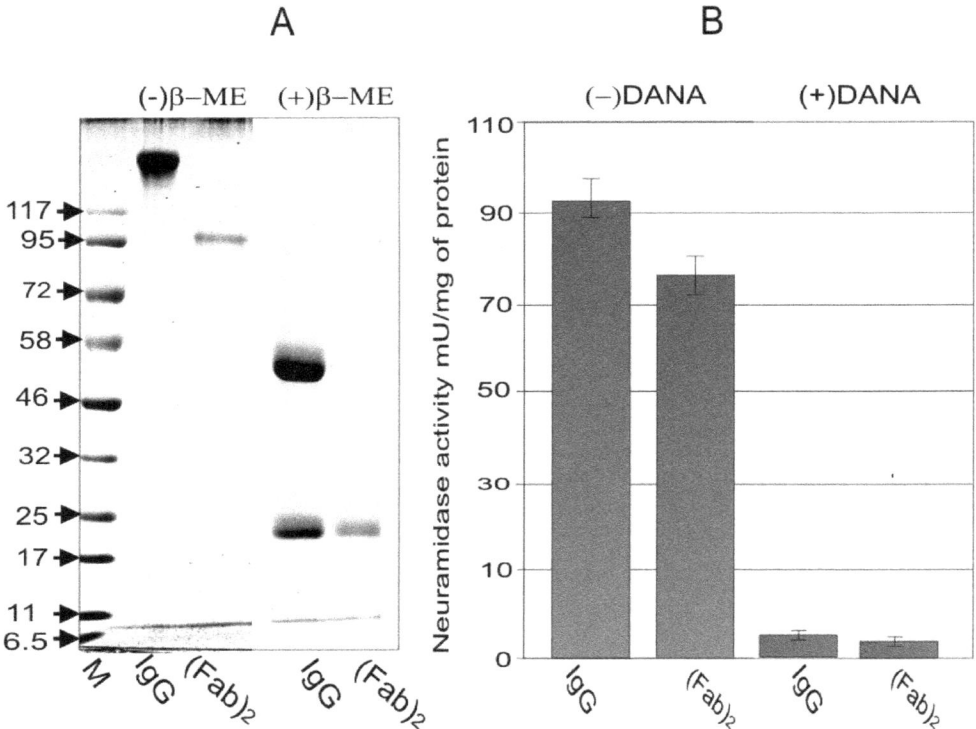

A – Homogeneity determination of IgGs and their (Fab)2 by SDS electrophoresis in gradient PAGE (5–16%) in the absence (-) or presence (+) of beta-mercaptoethanol (in non-reducing and reducing conditions, respectively). M: protein molecular mass markers (kDa).
B – Sialidase activity of IgGs and their (Fab)2 in the absence (-) or presence (+) of specific sialidase inhibitor DANA.

Fig. 8. Evidences that sialidase activity of IgG preparations purified by the affinity chromatography on protein G-sepharose from blood serum of SLE patient is an intrinsic properties of antibodies.

To prove that sialidase activity of IgG fractions isolated from the SLE patients is an intrinsic property of the abzymes and is not caused by the co-purified enzymes/impurities, we applied the same criteria to the purity of catalytic Ab which have been proposed earlier (G. A. Nevinsky & Buneva, 2003; Paul et al., 1989). To rule out possible enzymatic contamination tightly bound to IgG molecule, we performed HPLC-SEC chromatography at the acidic conditions (pH 2.6), that are known to guarantee dissociation of antibody-antigen complexes (Hanson et al., 2005; G. A. Nevinsky & Buneva, 2003) (Fig. 7). It was confirmed by the SDS-PAGE electrophoresis and Western-blot analysis using anti(human)-IgG Ab that

Cell Surface Glycans at SLE – Changes During Cells Death, Utilization for Disease Detection
and Molecular Mechanism Underlying Their Modification

81

the main chromatographic peak is an electrophoretically homogeneous IgG. Its sialidase activity was tested and shown to be attributable to IgG fraction. HPLC purification resulted in the retention of ~50% of original sialidase activity of protein-G purified IgG sample. Sialidase activity was significantly decreased when the reaction was performed in the presence of pan-neuraminidase inhibitor DANA that excludes a possibility of non-specific hydrolysis reaction. The mechanism of DANA action is connected with its resemblance of the unhydrolyzable transition-state analogue formed during sialic acid cleavage which is irreversibly bound by active centers of most neuraminidases (Chavas et al., 2005).

It is known, that the pH optimum of different sialidases is in range of pH 4–6.5. We have shown that isolated IgG is active under the physiological pH of blood serum. By using buffer systems in the pH range 3-9, we found that studied IgG samples revealed maximum speed reaction at pH range of 4.5÷6.0, nevertheless at pH 7.4 all samples retained from 27 to 52% of their maximal activity, measured at NaCl concentration equal to that of blood serum. This suggests its potential enzymatic effectiveness in blood serum.

In order to determine the speed of catalytic reaction of both IgG and corresponding (Fab)$_2$-fragments, we have calculated kinetic parameters (K_m, V_{max}, k_{cat}) for sialidase reaction at 0.1–100 µM concentrations of the substrate. Computer analysis demonstrated that the observed reaction belongs to a single substrate type, described by classical Michaelis-Menten equation. The calculated data for different studies sialyl abzymes were: Km=44.4÷1600 µM and kcat=0.045÷23.1 min-1 (Fig. 9). The catalysis mediated by an artificial abzymes is usually characterized by relatively low reaction rates: k_{cat} values are 10^2–10^6-fold lower than for the canonical enzymes (Georgy A. Nevinsky & Buneva, 2005). The known kcat values for natural abzymes vary in the range of 0.001–40 min^{-1}. The kcat values detected for MUNA hydrolysis (0.045÷23.1 depending on sample) are comparable with the typical k_{cat} values established for others abzymes. To validate the kinetics assay, we have used C. perfringens neuraminidase as standard for kinetic parameters measurement. According to the obtained results, C. perfringens Km equals to 89.2 µM for 4-MUNA, which is in a good accordance with the literature data of 120 µM (Li et al., 1994)(Inoue & Kitajima, 2006), while V_{max} was detected to be 2856 µmol/min/mg. The obtained Km value of IgG were of similar range, while V_{max} of IgG was significantly lower (k_{cat} significantly higher) than that of C. perfringens neuraminidase.

Principal question concerning a role of the discovered abzymes possessing sialidase activity is whether they can use as potential desialylation substrates also glycoproteins and glycolipids that are present in human's blood plasma and cells. Earlier, we have shown that sialyl-abzymes from multiple myeloma patients act towards human RBC by desialylating them and promoting agglutination with PNA lectins (R. Bilyy, Tomin, Mahorivska, et al., 2010). It is known that the peanut agglutinin (PNA) agglutinates human RBC after their sialidase treatment resulting in the exposure of sub-terminal Gal-residues (Nakano, Fontes Piazza, & Avila-Campos, 2006). Here, by incubating IgG preparation form SLE sera with RBC of NHD (blood group A(0)) and using subsequent agglutination test with different PNA lectin concentrations, we demonstrated an ability of IgG-abzyme obtained from blood serum of SLEs patient desialylate human RBCs directly. Agglutination was observed at PNA concentration 7 µg/ml, while when the IgG preparation from NHD was used, agglutination was achieved at 250 µg/ml; PBS served here as a negative control (no agglutination at 1,000 µg/ml, and Clostridium perfringens neuraminidase (10 mU) served as a positive control, agglutination at 7µg/ml of PNA. Thus treatment with sialyl abzymes from

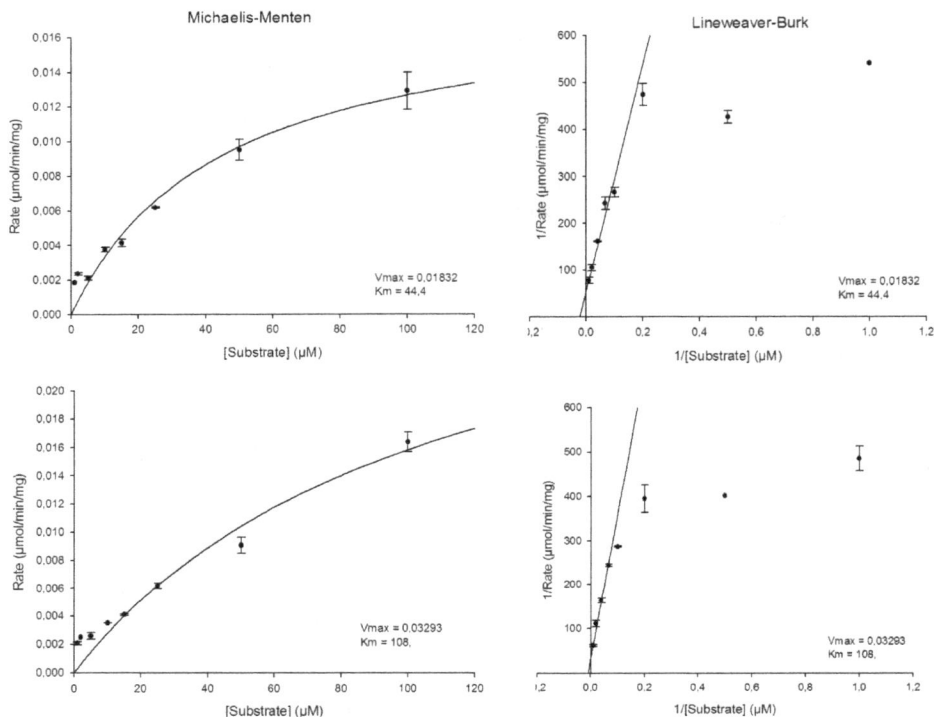

Fig. 9. Kinetic parameters (Michaelis-Menten and Lineweaver-Burk plots) of sialidase reaction catalyzed by the IgG (A) or its (Fab)₂-fragments (B). The incubation time for all samples was 180 min.

SLE patient have increased the amount of desialylated glycoepitopes for 250 µg /7 µg =35 times. We also used as substrates for sialyl abzymes: a) gangliodes of mouse brain and b) total surface glycans on eukaryotic (human T-leukemia Jurkat) cells. Ganglioside fraction was isolated from mouse brain and was incubated with sialil-abzyme and neuraminidase. Both sialil-abzyme and neuraminidase caused desialylation of GM3 and increase in the content of free sialic (neuraminic) acid (Fig.10). Treatment of human leukemia Jurkat cells with sialil-abzyme and neuraminidase caused a decrease in the level of a2,6-sialil-reach surface glycoconjugates (if judged by binding of FITC-labeled SNA lectin analyzed by flow cytometry) (Fig 11). Moreover, treatment of Jurkat cells with sialil-abzyme and neuraminidase also caused an increase in the level of desialylated glycoepitopes, if judged by binding of PNA lectin (biotynilated, treated with streptavidin-FITC and analyzed by flow cytometry) (Fig. 11).

Thus, isolated sialyl abzymes were desialylating both human RBC, gangliosides and total surface glycoepitopes of the eukaryotic cells and were active under pH and ion content values of human blood serum.

We have demonstrated previously unknown catalytic activity in the IgG antibodies of SLE patients – an intrinsic sialidase activity. Such activity was present in the IgG of blood serum

Cell Surface Glycans at SLE – Changes During Cells Death, Utilization for Disease Detection
and Molecular Mechanism Underlying Their Modification

83

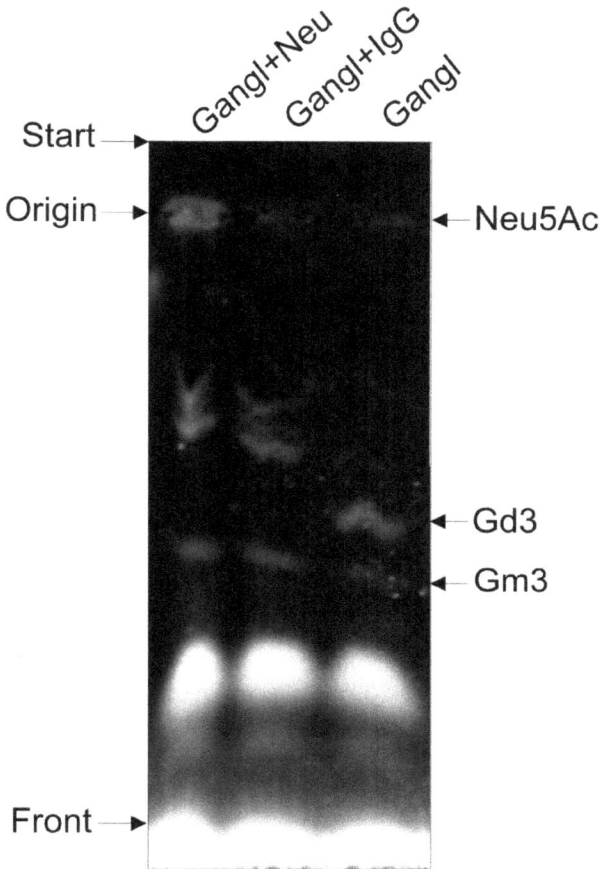

Fig. 10. Desialation of gangliosids by sialidase active IgGs obtained from blood serum of SLE patients possessing highest sialidase activity. Gangl+Neu – gangliosides incubated with neuramidase from *C. perphringers*; Gangl+IgG – gangliosides incubated with sialidase active IgGs; Gangl – gangliosides without incubation (control). The positions of free neuraninic acid (Neu5Ac), gangliosides GM3 and GD3 are shown by arrows on the right hand.

of SLE patients and absent in the IgG of NHD. Sialidase activity was detected under different conditions which exclude a possibility of contamination or artefacts. It was blocked by typical sialidase inhibitor (DANA), expressed under physiological pH, and corresponded to classical Michaelis-Menten kinetics. Since DANA is an unhydrolyzable transitional state analogue of hydrolysis reaction, one can assume that the mechanism of action of IgG with sialidase activity is similar to that of sialidase enzyme. Moreover, the described IgGs possessing sialidase activity were capable of direct desialylation of human RBCs, ganglyosides and T-lymphocytes. The reason for appearance of discovered sialidase activity is not fully understood. One of the possible suggestions is their anti-idiotypic antibody as the "internal image" of an active site of endo- or exogenic sialidases, as known for other abzymes (Friboulet, Izadyar, Avalle, Roseto, & Thomas, 1994).

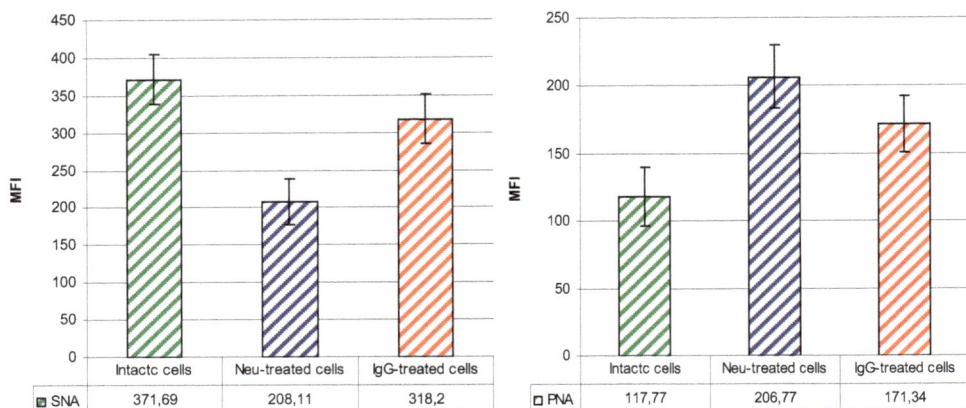

▨ SNA	371,69	208,11	318,2
Intactc cells	Neu-treated cells	IgG-treated cells	

▢ PNA	117,77	206,77	171,34
Intactc cells	Neu-treated cells	IgG-treated cells	

Jurkat cells were stained with FITC-labeled SNA (left), or biotinilated PNA lectin (right), stained with streptavidin-FITC. Cells were either treated with Neuraminidase, 10mU or sialil-abzyme, 10 uM for 3h at 37°C. Data represent normalized MFI of lectin binding. SNA lectin binds terminal a2,6-sialic acid residues, while PNA lectin binds desialylated glycoepitopes (Antonyuk, 2005).

Fig. 11. Analysis of lectin binding to human Jurkat T-cells.

The level of IgG molecule's sialylation was reported to be critical in defining their pro- or anti-inflamatory properties (Kaneko, Nimmerjahn, & Ravetch, 2006). Anti-inflamatory activity of immunoglobulins was tightly connected with the presence of a2,6-sialylated Asn^{297} in the IgG molecule (Anthony, Nimmerjahn, et al., 2008). Macrophages receptors responsible for binding sialylated IgG and modulating its anti-inflamatory action were also described (Anthony, Wermeling, Karlsson, & Ravetch, 2008). Agalactosylated and desialylated IgG antibodies' action *in vivo* depends on binding of cellular Fc receptors (Nimmerjahn, Anthony, & Ravetch, 2007). Specific glycoforms, if present in populations of immunoglobulin molecules, are connected with disease-associated alterations and can serve as diagnostic biomarkers at rheumatoid arthritis and other diseases (Arnold, Wormald, Sim, Rudd, & Dwek, 2007). Blood serum level of desialylylated form of IgG (IgG-G0) isolated from patients with rheumatoid arthritis, are more that 2 standard deviations above those levels in the age-matched healthy control (R. B. Parekh et al., 1985). They correlate with the disease activity and fall during remission periods (Rook et al., 1991). High levels of desialylylated IgG-G0 are also characteristic for other disorders: Crohn's disease, SLE complicated by Sjogren's syndrome, and tuberculosis (Bond et al., 1997; R. Parekh et al., 1989; R. B. Parekh et al., 1985). The enzyme EndoS from *Streptococcus pyogenes* that cleaves IgG glycan between two GlcNAc residues, was used for "making autoantibodies safe" (Scanlan, Burton, & Dwek, 2008). The action of EndoS truncated IgG glycans and IgG molecules lost the ability to initiate activating signals through C1q, FcγRs and MBL, while the ability to interact with inhibitory FcγRIIB was preserved (Collin, Shannon, & Bjorck, 2008).

4. Summary

In previous studies, we have shown that cell surface glycopattern is changed during apoptosis. This, in part, results from activation of surface sialidases, with desialylated glycoproteins being characteristic markers of apoptosis (R. Bilyy & Stoika, 2007). Such feature was successfully utilized for lymphocyte screening in the autoimmune patients (R. Bilyy et al., 2009). It is widely accepted that altered glycoepitopes (desialylaed) are important surface markers for clearance of apoptotic cells (R. Bilyy & Stoika, 2007). We have shown (Meesmann et al., 2010) that desialylation of cell surface epitopes in viable cells, caused by sialidase, acts as an "eat-me" signal for macrophages and is needed for elimination of late apoptotic cells along with phosphatydilserine exposure, needed for elimination of early apoptotic cells. Apoptotic cells possess an elevated neuraminidase activity on their surface, however, we failed to detect any sialidase activity in culture media that could result from enzyme secretion/release during cell death. As we have shown, SLE – a disease resulting from insufficient cell clearance (Munoz et al., 2010) - is accompanied by the appearance of desialylated lymphocytes in blood stream. At the same time, some of SLE patients possessed abzymes with sialydase activity in their blood. The exact role of sialyl abzymes at SLE is currently unclear, as well as their relation to apoptotic cell desialylation and clearance. The abzymes possessing sialidase activity can change surface sialylation level and, thus, alter the glycocalyx of SLE patients' cells and promote their clearance. They can also influence the immune response by acting towards blood serum IgG molecules.

5. Acknowledgements

The authors would like to acknowledge I. Kril' who greatly contributed to this work. The work was supported by the National Academy of Sciences of Ukraine, and grants awarded to R. Bilyy by the WUBMRC and the President of Ukraine.

6. Abbreviations

GP - glycoprotein, PI - propidium iodide, PM – plasma membrane, RA - rheumatoid arthritis, Ab – antibodies, DANA - 2,3-dehydro-2-deoxy-N-acetylneuraminic acid, SLE-multiple myeloma, 4-MUNA - 2'-(4-Methylumbelliferyl)-α-D-N-acetylneuralminic acid, 4-MU-Gal - 4-Methylumbelliferyl-β-D-galactopyranoside, NHD – normal healthy donors, RBC – red blood cells, SLE - systemic lupus erymatosus.

7. References

Anthony, R. M., Nimmerjahn, F., Ashline, D. J., Reinhold, V. N., Paulson, J. C. and Ravetch, J. V. (2008), Recapitulation of IVIG anti-inflammatory activity with a recombinant IgG Fc, *Science,* Vol. 320 No. 5874, pp. 373-376.
Anthony, R. M., Wermeling, F., Karlsson, M. C. and Ravetch, J. V. (2008), Identification of a receptor required for the anti-inflammatory activity of IVIG, *Proc Natl Acad Sci U S A,* Vol. 105 No. 50, pp. 19571-19578.
Antonyuk, V. O. (2005), *The lectins and their resources [in Ukrainian],* Quart, Lviv. 554 p.
Arnold, J. N., Wormald, M. R., Sim, R. B., Rudd, P. M. and Dwek, R. A. (2007), The impact of glycosylation on the biological function and structure of human immunoglobulins, *Annu Rev Immunol,* Vol. 25, pp. 21-50.
Ashkenazi, A. and Dixit, V. M. (1998), Death Receptors: Signaling and Modulation, *Science,* Vol. 281 No. 5381, pp. 1305-1308.
Batisse, C., Marquet, J., Greffard, A., Fleury-Feith, J., Jaurand, M. C. and Pilatte, Y. (2004), Lectin-based three-color flow cytometric approach for studying cell surface

glycosylation changes that occur during apoptosis, *Cytometry A*, Vol. 62 No. 2, pp. 81-88.

Belmont, M. (2010), Lupus Clinical Overview, http://cerebel.com/lupus/

Belogurov, A., Jr., Kozyr, A., Ponomarenko, N. and Gabibov, A. (2009), Catalytic antibodies: balancing between Dr. Jekyll and Mr. Hyde, *BioEssays*, Vol. 31 No. 11, pp. 1161-1171.

Bigi, A., Morosi, L., Pozzi, C., Forcella, M., Tettamanti, G., Venerando, B., Monti, E. and Fusi, P. (2010), Human sialidase NEU4 long and short are extrinsic proteins bound to outer mitochondrial membrane and the endoplasmic reticulum, respectively, *Glycobiology*, Vol. 20 No. 2, pp. 148-157.

Bilyy, R., Kit, Y., Hellman, U., Tryndyak, V., Kaminskyy, V. and Stoika, R. (2005), In vivo expression and characteristics of novel alpha-D-mannose-rich glycoprotein markers of apoptotic cells, *Cell Biol Int*, Vol. 29 No. 11, pp. 920-928.

Bilyy, R., Nemesh, L., Antonyuk, V., Kit, Y., Valchuk, I., Havryluk, A., Chopyak, V. and Stoika, R. (2009), Apoptosis-related changes in plasma membrane glycoconjugates of peripheral blood lymphocytes in rheumatoid arthritis, *Autoimmunity*, Vol. 42 No. 4, pp. 334 - 336.

Bilyy, R. and Stoika, R. (2007), Search for novel cell surface markers of apoptotic cells, *Autoimmunity*, Vol. 40 No. 4, pp. 249-253.

Bilyy, R., Tomin, A., Mahorivska, I., Shalay, O., Lohinskyy, V., Stoika, R. and Kit, Y. (2010), Antibody-Mediated Sialidase Activity in Blood Serum of Patients With Multiple Myeloma, *Journal of Molecular Recognition*, Vol. 23 No. 6, pp. DOI:10.1002/jmr.1071.

Bilyy, R., Tomin, A. and Stoika, R. (2010), Method of neuraminidase activity detection in cells and cellular compartments, in a201003168, U. (Ed.), *Bul.13, 12.07.2010*, UA.

Bilyy, R. O., Antonyuk, V. O. and Stoika, R. S. (2004), Cytochemical study of role of alpha-d-mannose- and beta-d-galactose-containing glycoproteins in apoptosis, *J Mol Histol*, Vol. 35 No. 8-9, pp. 829-838.

Bilyy, R. O. and Stoika, R. S. (2003), Lectinocytochemical detection of apoptotic murine leukemia L1210 cells, *Cytometry A*, Vol. 56 No. 2, pp. 89-95.

Bond, A., Alavi, A., Axford, J. S., Bourke, B. E., Bruckner, F. E., Kerr, M. A., Maxwell, J. D., Tweed, K. J., Weldon, M. J., Youinou, P. and Hay, F. C. (1997), A detailed lectin analysis of IgG glycosylation, demonstrating disease specific changes in terminal galactose and N-acetylglucosamine, *J Autoimmun*, Vol. 10 No. 1, pp. 77-85.

Chavas, L. M., Tringali, C., Fusi, P., Venerando, B., Tettamanti, G., Kato, R., Monti, E. and Wakatsuki, S. (2005), Crystal structure of the human cytosolic sialidase Neu2. Evidence for the dynamic nature of substrate recognition, *J Biol Chem*, Vol. 280 No. 1, pp. 469-475.

Collin, M., Shannon, O. and Bjorck, L. (2008), IgG glycan hydrolysis by a bacterial enzyme as a therapy against autoimmune conditions, *Proc Natl Acad Sci U S A*, Vol. 105 No. 11, pp. 4265-4270.

Comelli, E. M., Amado, M., Lustig, S. R. and Paulson, J. C. (2003), Identification and expression of Neu4, a novel murine sialidase, *Gene*, Vol. 321, pp. 155-161.

Fadok, V. A., Voelker, D. R., Campbell, P. A., Cohen, J. J., Bratton, D. L. and Henson, P. M. (1992), Exposure of phosphatidylserine on the surface of apoptotic lymphocytes triggers specific recognition and removal by macrophages, *J Immunol.*, Vol. 148 No. 7, pp. 2207-2216.

Franz, S., Frey, B., Sheriff, A., Gaipl, U. S., Beer, A., Voll, R. E., Kalden, J. R. and Herrmann, M. (2006), Lectins detect changes of the glycosylation status of plasma membrane constituents during late apoptosis, *Cytometry A*, Vol. 69 No. 4, pp. 230-239.

Franz, S., Herrmann, K., Fuhrnrohr, B., Sheriff, A., Frey, B., Gaipl, U. S., Voll, R. E., Kalden, J. R., Jack, H. M. and Herrmann, M. (2007), After shrinkage apoptotic cells expose internal membrane-derived epitopes on their plasma membranes, *Cell Death.Differ.*, Vol. 14 No. 4, pp. 733-742.

Friboulet, A., Izadyar, L., Avalle, B., Roseto, A. and Thomas, D. (1994), Abzyme generation using an anti-idiotypic antibody as the "internal image" of an enzyme active site, *Appl Biochem Biotechnol*, Vol. 47 No. 2-3, pp. 229-237; discussion 237-229.

Gabibov, A. G., Kozyr, A. V. and Kolesnikov, A. V. (2000), Disease association and cytotoxic effects of DNA-hydrolyzing autoantibodies, *Chem Immunol*, Vol. 77, pp. 130-156.

Gabibov, A. G., Ponomarenko, N. A., Tretyak, E. B., Paltsev, M. A. and Suchkov, S. V. (2006), Catalytic autoantibodies in clinical autoimmunity and modern medicine, *Autoimmun Rev*, Vol. 5 No. 5, pp. 324-330.

Goping, I. S., Barry, M., Liston, P., Sawchuk, T., Constantinescu, G., Michalak, K. M., Shostak, I., Roberts, D. L., Hunter, A. M., Korneluk, R. and Bleackley, R. C. (2003), Granzyme B-Induced Apoptosis Requires Both Direct Caspase Activation and Relief of Caspase Inhibition, *Immunity*, Vol. 18 No. 3, pp. 355-365.

Hanson, C. V., Nishiyama, Y. and Paul, S. (2005), Catalytic antibodies and their applications, *Curr Opin Biotechnol*, Vol. 16 No. 6, pp. 631-636.

Heyder, P., Gaipl, U. S., Beyer, T. D., Voll, R. E., Kern, P. M., Stach, C., Kalden, J. R. and Herrmann, M. (2003), Early detection of apoptosis by staining of acid-treated apoptotic cells with FITC-labeled lectin from Narcissus pseudonarcissus, *Cytometry*, Vol. 55A No. 2, pp. 86-93.

Inoue, S. and Kitajima, K. (2006), KDN (deaminated neuraminic acid): dreamful past and exciting future of the newest member of the sialic acid family, *Glycoconj J*, Vol. 23 No. 5-6, pp. 277-290.

Kaneko, Y., Nimmerjahn, F. and Ravetch, J. V. (2006), Anti-inflammatory activity of immunoglobulin G resulting from Fc sialylation, *Science*, Vol. 313 No. 5787, pp. 670-673.

Kit, Y. Y., Starykovych, M. A., Richter, V. A. and Stoika, R. S. (2008), Detection and characterization of IgG- and sIgA-Abzymes capable of hydrolyzing histone H1, *Biochemistry (Mosc)*, Vol. 73 No. 8, pp. 950-956.

Kozyr, A. V., Kolesnikov, A. V., Aleksandrova, E. S., Sashchenko, L. P., Gnuchev, N. V., Favorov, P. V., Kotelnikov, M. A., Iakhnina, E. I., Astsaturov, I. A., Prokaeva, T. B., Alekberova, Z. S., Suchkov, S. V. and Gabibov, A. G. (1998), Novel functional activities of anti-DNA autoantibodies from sera of patients with lymphoproliferative and autoimmune diseases, *Appl Biochem Biotechnol*, Vol. 75 No. 1, pp. 45-61.

Kozyr, A. V., Kolesnikov, A. V., Iakhnina, E. I., Astsaturov, I. A., Varlamova, E., Kirillov, E. V. and Gabibov, A. G. (1996), [DNA-hydrolyzing antibodies in lymphoproliferative disorders], *Biull Eksp Biol Med*, Vol. 121 No. 2, pp. 204-206.

Kozyr, A. V., Sashchenko, L. P., Kolesnikov, A. V., Zelenova, N. A., Khaidukov, S. V., Ignatova, A. N., Bobik, T. V., Gabibov, A. G., Alekberova, Z. S., Suchkov, S. V. and

Gnuchev, N. V. (2002), Anti-DNA autoantibodies reveal toxicity to tumor cell lines, *Immunol Lett,* Vol. 80 No. 1, pp. 41-47.

Lacroix-Desmazes, S., Wootla, B., Delignat, S., Dasgupta, S., Nagaraja, V., Kazatchkine, M. D. and Kaveri, S. V. (2006), Pathophysiology of catalytic antibodies, *Immunol Lett,* Vol. 103 No. 1, pp. 3-7.

Li, Y. T., Yuziuk, J. A., Li, S. C., Nematalla, A., Hasegawa, A., Kimura, M. and Nakagawa, H. (1994), A novel sialidase capable of cleaving 3-deoxy-D-glycero-D-galacto-2-nonulosonic acid (KDN), *Arch Biochem Biophys,* Vol. 310 No. 1, pp. 243-246.

Magorivska, I., Bilyy, R., Havryluk, A., Chop'yak, V., Stoika, R. and Kit, Y. (2010), Anti-histone H1 IgGs from blood serum of systemic lupus erythematosus patients are capable of hydrolyzing histone H1 and myelin basic protein, *Journal of Molecular Recognition,* Vol. 23, pp. DOI:10.1002/jmr.1033.

Magorivska, I., Bilyy, R., Shalay, O., Loginsky, V., Kit, Y. and Stoika, R. (2009), Blood serum immunoglobulins of patients with multiple myeloma are capable of hydrolysing histone H1, *Exp Oncol,* Vol. 31 No. 2, pp. 97-101.

Matsuura, K., Ohara, K., Munakata, H., Hifumi, E. and Uda, T. (2006), Pathogenicity of catalytic antibodies: catalytic activity of Bence Jones proteins from myeloma patients with renal impairment can elicit cytotoxic effects, *Biol Chem,* Vol. 387 No. 5, pp. 543-548.

Meesmann, H. M., Fehr, E.-M., Kierschke, S., Herrmann, M., Bilyy, R., Heyder, P., Blank, N., Krienke, S., Lorenz, H.-M. and Schiller, M. (2010), Decrease of sialic acid residues as an eat-me signal on the surface of apoptotic lymphocytes, *J Cell Sci,* Vol. 123 No. 19, pp. 3347-3356.

Miyagi, T., Wada, T. and Yamaguchi, K. (2008), Roles of plasma membrane-associated sialidase NEU3 in human cancers, *Biochim Biophys Acta,* Vol. 1780 No. 3, pp. 532-537.

Miyagi, T., Wada, T., Yamaguchi, K. and Hata, K. (2004), Sialidase and malignancy: a minireview, *Glycoconj J,* Vol. 20 No. 3, pp. 189-198.

Miyagi, T., Wada, T., Yamaguchi, K., Hata, K. and Shiozaki, K. (2008), Plasma membrane-associated sialidase as a crucial regulator of transmembrane signalling, *J Biochem,* Vol. 144 No. 3, pp. 279-285.

Miyagi, T., Wada, T., Yamaguchi, K., Shiozaki, K., Sato, I., Kakugawa, Y., Yamanami, H. and Fujiya, T. (2008), Human sialidase as a cancer marker, *Proteomics,* Vol. 8 No. 16, pp. 3303-3311.

Monti, E., Bassi, M. T., Papini, N., Riboni, M., Manzoni, M., Venerando, B., Croci, G., Preti, A., Ballabio, A., Tettamanti, G. and Borsani, G. (2000), Identification and expression of NEU3, a novel human sialidase associated to the plasma membrane, *Biochem J,* Vol. 349 No. Pt 1, pp. 343-351.

Monti, E., Preti, A., Venerando, B. and Borsani, G. (2002), Recent development in mammalian sialidase molecular biology, *Neurochem Res,* Vol. 27 No. 7-8, pp. 649-663.

Munoz, L. E., Lauber, K., Schiller, M., Manfredi, A. A. and Herrmann, M. (2010), The role of defective clearance of apoptotic cells in systemic autoimmunity, *Nat Rev Rheumatol,* Vol. 6 No. 5, pp. 280-289.

Cell Surface Glycans at SLE – Changes During Cells Death, Utilization for Disease Detection
and Molecular Mechanism Underlying Their Modification

89

Nakano, V., Fontes Piazza, R. M. and Avila-Campos, M. J. (2006), A rapid assay of the
sialidase activity in species of the Bacteroides fragilis group by using peanut lectin
hemagglutination, *Anaerobe,* Vol. 12 No. 5-6, pp. 238-241.

Nevinsky, G. A. and Buneva, V. N. (2003), Catalytic antibodies in healthy humans and
patients with autoimmune and viral diseases, *J Cell Mol Med,* Vol. 7 No. 3, pp. 265-
276.

Nevinsky, G. A. and Buneva, V. N. (2005), Natural Catalytic Antibodies - Abzymes, in Prof.
Dr. Ehud, K. (Ed.), *Catalytic Antibodies,* pp. 505-569.

Nimmerjahn, F., Anthony, R. M. and Ravetch, J. V. (2007), Agalactosylated IgG antibodies
depend on cellular Fc receptors for in vivo activity, *Proc Natl Acad Sci U S A,* Vol.
104 No. 20, pp. 8433-8437.

Orlinick, J. R. and Chao, M. V. (1998), TNF-Related Ligands and Their Receptors, *Cellular
Signalling,* Vol. 10 No. 8, pp. 543-551.

Parekh, R., Isenberg, D., Rook, G., Roitt, I., Dwek, R. and Rademacher, T. (1989), A
comparative analysis of disease-associated changes in the galactosylation of serum
IgG, *J Autoimmun,* Vol. 2 No. 2, pp. 101-114.

Parekh, R. B., Dwek, R. A., Sutton, B. J., Fernandes, D. L., Leung, A., Stanworth, D.,
Rademacher, T. W., Mizuochi, T., Taniguchi, T., Matsuta, K. and et al. (1985),
Association of rheumatoid arthritis and primary osteoarthritis with changes in the
glycosylation pattern of total serum IgG, *Nature,* Vol. 316 No. 6027, pp. 452-457.

Paul, S., Li, L., Kalaga, R., Wilkins-Stevens, P., Stevens, F. J. and Solomon, A. (1995), Natural
catalytic antibodies: peptide-hydrolyzing activities of Bence Jones proteins and VL
fragment, *J Biol Chem,* Vol. 270 No. 25, pp. 15257-15261.

Paul, S., Volle, D. J., Beach, C. M., Johnson, D. R., Powell, M. J. and Massey, R. J. (1989),
Catalytic hydrolysis of vasoactive intestinal peptide by human autoantibody,
Science, Vol. 244 No. 4909, pp. 1158-1162.

Planque, S., Nishiyama, Y., Taguchi, H., Salas, M., Hanson, C. and Paul, S. (2008), Catalytic
antibodies to HIV: physiological role and potential clinical utility, *Autoimmun Rev,*
Vol. 7 No. 6, pp. 473-479.

Ploegh, H. L. (1998), Viral Strategies of Immune Evasion, *Science,* Vol. 280 No. 5361, pp. 248-
253.

Pollack, S. J., Jacobs, J. W. and Schultz, P. G. (1986), Selective chemical catalysis by an
antibody, *Science,* Vol. 234 No. 4783, pp. 1570-1573.

Pradhan, D., Krahling, S., Williamson, P. and Schlegel, R. (1997), Multiple systems for
recognition of apoptotic lymphocytes by macrophages, *Mol. Biol. Cell,* Vol. 8 No. 5,
pp. 767-778.

Reutelingsperger, C. P. and Christiaan Peter, M. (1998), Method for detecting and/or
optionally quantifying and/or separating apoptotic cells in or from a sample, in,
United States, pp. 1-9.

Rook, G. A., Steele, J., Brealey, R., Whyte, A., Isenberg, D., Sumar, N., Nelson, J. L., Bodman,
K. B., Young, A., Roitt, I. M. and et al. (1991), Changes in IgG glycoform levels are
associated with remission of arthritis during pregnancy, *J Autoimmun,* Vol. 4 No. 5,
pp. 779-794.

Sashchenko, L. P., Khaidukov, S. V., Kozyr, A. V., Luk'yanova, T. I., Gabibov, A. G.,
Suchkov, S. V., Bobik, T. V., Alekberova, Z. S. and Gnuchev, N. V. (2001), Caspase-

dependent cytotoxicity of anti-DNA autoantibodies, *Dokl Biochem Biophys*, Vol. 380, pp. 313-315.

Savill, J., Fadok, V., Henson, P. and Haslett, C. (1993), Phagocyte recognition of cells undergoing apoptosis, *Immunol.Today*, Vol. 14 No. 3, pp. 131-136.

Scanlan, C. N., Burton, D. R. and Dwek, R. A. (2008), Making autoantibodies safe, *Proc Natl Acad Sci U S A*, Vol. 105 No. 11, pp. 4081-4082.

Seyrantepe, V., Landry, K., Trudel, S., Hassan, J. A., Morales, C. R. and Pshezhetsky, A. V. (2004), Neu4, a novel human lysosomal lumen sialidase, confers normal phenotype to sialidosis and galactosialidosis cells, *J Biol Chem*, Vol. 279 No. 35, pp. 37021-37029.

Sinohara, H. and Matsuura, K. (2000), Does catalytic activity of Bence-Jones proteins contribute to the pathogenesis of multiple myeloma?, *Appl Biochem Biotechnol*, Vol. 83 No. 1-3, pp. 85-92; discussion 93-84, 145-153.

Stoika, R. S., Bilyy, R. O. and Antoniuk, V. O. (2006), Agglutination-based method for fast detection, isolation and quantification of apoptotic cells, in *WO/2007/053654* USA, UA, pp. 1-85.

Sun, M., Gao, Q. S., Kirnarskiy, L., Rees, A. and Paul, S. (1997), Cleavage specificity of a proteolytic antibody light chain and effects of the heavy chain variable domain, *J Mol Biol*, Vol. 271 No. 3, pp. 374-385.

Taguchi, H., Planque, S., Nishiyama, Y., Szabo, P., Weksler, M. E., Friedland, R. P. and Paul, S. (2008), Catalytic antibodies to amyloid beta peptide in defense against Alzheimer disease, *Autoimmun Rev*, Vol. 7 No. 5, pp. 391-397.

Tartaglia, L. A. and Goeddel, D. V. (1992), Two TNF receptors, *Immunology Today*, Vol. 13 No. 5, pp. 151-153.

Tramontano, A., Janda, K. D. and Lerner, R. A. (1986), Catalytic antibodies, *Science*, Vol. 234 No. 4783, pp. 1566-1570.

van den Eijnde, S. M., Luijsterburg, A. J., Boshart, L., De Zeeuw, C. I., van Dierendonck, J. H., Reutelingsperger, C. P. and Vermeij-Keers, C. (1997), In situ detection of apoptosis during embryogenesis with annexin V: from whole mount to ultrastructure, *Cytometry*, Vol. 29 No. 4, pp. 313-320.

Vermijlen, D., Froelich, C. J., Luo, D., Suarez-Huerta, N., Robaye, B. and Wisse, E. (2001), Perforin and granzyme B induce apoptosis in FasL-resistant colon carcinoma cells, *Cancer Immunology, Immunotherapy*, Vol. 50 No. 4, pp. 212-217.

Yamaguchi, K., Hata, K., Koseki, K., Shiozaki, K., Akita, H., Wada, T., Moriya, S. and Miyagi, T. (2005), Evidence for mitochondrial localization of a novel human sialidase (NEU4), *Biochem J*, Vol. 390 No. Pt 1, pp. 85-93.

Regulatory T Cell Deficiency in Systemic Autoimmune Disorders – Causal Relationship and Underlying Immunological Mechanisms

Fang-Ping Huang and Susanne Sattler

Division of Immunology and Inflammation, Department of Medicine,
Imperial College London,
Great Britain

1. Introduction

Systemic lupus erythematosus (SLE), formerly named 'disseminated lupus erythematosus', is an organ-non-specific autoimmune disease that has a largely unknown aetiology. Multiple susceptibility genes as well as environmental factors are found to be involved in the lupus pathogenesis (multi-factorial) [1, 2]. Also known as the prototype of autoimmune diseases, lupus is very intriguing both clinically and immunologically for its systemic nature and complexity in pathogenesis. The disease is characterized by multi-organ involvement and presence of autoantibodies to a variety of self antigens, particularly of the nuclear components [3]. Deposition of the immune complexes may trigger complement activation causing tissue damages. The broad auto-reactivities and hyperactivity of B cells are known to be predominately T cell-dependent [4], but the cellular and molecular mechanisms underlying such a systemic loss of B and T cell tolerance are yet to be fully understood. In contrast to B cell hyperactivity [5], reduced Interleukin 2 (IL-2) production and aberrant responsiveness of T cells are characteristic of SLE [6, 7]. Moreover, impaired cellular immunity, complement deficiency, defects in the clearance of dying cells by macrophages [8-10], roles of DC and the disrupted mechanisms of tolerance induction [11-14] are among many immunological characteristics of, or potential mechanisms proposed for, the disease.

2. Regulatory T cells

Regulatory T cells (Treg) belong to a specialized group or subsets of CD4+ T cells with immunoregulatory capacity, which have been shown to play many important roles in maintaining peripheral tolerance [15, 16]. Treg can actively suppress self–reactive lymphocytes that escape central tolerance. The so-called naturally occurring Treg cells (nTreg), which constitutively express high levels of surface IL-2 receptor α chain (IL-2Rα, CD25) [17, 18], are originated from the thymus. Mice deficient in the CD4+CD25hi Treg cells developed a multi-systemic autoimmune disease, including gastritis, oophoritis, arthritis, and thyroiditis. Co-transfer of Treg cells with self-reactive cells could prevent the development of experimentally-induced autoimmune diseases [17, 19]. Another relatively more specific marker of Treg cells is the intracellular molecule Foxp3 (forkhead box P3). The Foxp3 gene is crucial in the development and function of Treg cells in both humans [20, 21] and mice [22-24], and defective Foxp3 expression generates strong activation of the immune system resulting in multi-organ autoimmune diseases [25, 26]. Foxp3 transduction has been shown to convert naive CD4+CD25- T cells into CD25+ regulatory cells with suppressive activity [22]. Expression of Foxp3 can also be induced in CD4+CD25- T cells upon activation [27] or in the presence of TGF-ß [28, 29]. These findings suggest that the microenvironment could influence the expression of Foxp3 during an immune response, inducing and promoting the expansion of peripheral Treg, also known as the inducible or adaptive Treg cells [27].

Treg may exert their immunosuppressive effects through cell-cell contacts and by the release of immunosuppressive cytokines such as IL-10 and TGF-β [30]. More recently, IL-35 has been identified to be the very cytokine not only directly associated with Treg functions but also their peripheral expansion [31, 32] [33, 34], including the induction of a unique human Treg subset (iT$_R$35) which could exert its immunosuppressive functions in an IL-35-dependent, but IL-10, TGF-β and Foxp3-independent, mechanism. Thus, although the induction and activation of Treg may be individually and cumulatively antigen-driven [35], these cells can suppress T effector cell (Teff) activation in an antigen non-specific manner [36, 37], e.g. by the release of immunosuppressive cytokines and via their inhibitory effects on antigen presenting cells (APC), DC in particular [38]. Indeed, the lack of Treg has been associated with many organ-specific autoimmune diseases [15, 17, 39] and, more recently, systemic autoimmune disorders including SLE [40-90].

3. Aberrant Treg frequencies and functions associated with lupus disorders

In recent years, Treg aberrations have been widely demonstrated in both SLE patients [40, 41, 43-48, 51-67, 71-80, 82-86, 88] and lupus mouse models [42, 49, 50, 68-70, 81, 87, 89-98]. These studies provided thus a plausible explanation for the systemic nature of the disease. A lack of Treg-mediated immune regulation in lupus is now a general consensus, although there have been differences in the findings as to whether a reduced Treg frequency [40-46, 49-53, 58-61, 68, 71-75, 82-84, 88, 90], defective Treg functions [44, 48, 53, 57, 59, 60, 66, 70, 76, 80, 89, 90] or both, or alternatively an insensitivity of the Treg target cells [66, 67, 70, 89, 99], are truly accountable.

By using CD25 as the marker, an early study by Crispin and colleagues first showed that, in lupus patients with active disease, the frequencies of Treg (CD4+CD25+/bright) were significantly decreased, while T cells with an activated T helper (Th) effector phenotype (CD4+CD69+) increased [40]. An imbalance of Treg versus Teff was therefore proposed as a potential mechanism of disease development, and similar findings from many subsequent clinical studies mentioned above also confirmed this notion. Since IL-2 receptor (IL-2R) can be up-regulated on activated effector T and B lymphocytes too, the use of CD25 (alpha chain of IL-2R) as a Treg marker has understandably its limitation. Nevertheless, the identification of Foxp3, a relatively more specific if not exclusive marker of Treg, later allowed further verifications for the proposed link between Treg aberrations and systemic autoimmunity [49-51, 53, 57, 61, 68, 71, 73, 74, 76, 83, 88, 100].

However, there have also been controversial findings from other studies showing that the frequency of Treg cells, either defined as CD4+CD25bright or CD4+Foxp3+, could be normal

[48, 66, 67, 70, 85, 86] or even increased [47, 54-56, 58, 62-65, 69, 74, 76-79, 81] in lupus disease. Instead, some of these studies suggested that Treg were functionally defective and less capable of suppressing those potentially auto-reactive lymphocytes in lupus patients [44, 48, 53, 57, 59, 60, 66, 76, 80], and the mouse models [70, 89, 90]. Again, alternative findings demonstrating lupus Treg being functionally normal [49, 50, 62, 67, 85], or at least normal in majority of patients tested [48, 64], or even enhanced in some way [68, 80, 87] added further confusion as well as interest to the matter.

Upon a closer examination, these seemingly discrepant findings can in fact be logically explained. Two most critical issues to be addressed are about the true causal relationship between the Treg changes and disease kinetics, and the complex underlying immunological mechanisms involved as discussed below.

4. Treg deficiency in systemic autoimmunity – the mutually causative relationship

In terms of disease kinetics, for example, low Treg frequencies are often found to be associated with SLE patients having active, but less so inactive, disease [40, 45, 83], or in patients on certain anti-inflammatory drugs undergoing clinical remission [47, 55, 56, 86]. Considering the multi-factorial nature, variability in disease onset and genetic heterogeneity of human lupus, however, it is also not surprising to note that such clinical association has not been always an obvious case [43, 48, 54, 62, 64].

Nevertheless, findings from studies using animal models especially inbred strains of mice which develop spontaneously a lupus like disease have offered some useful insights in this regard. The MRL/MpJ-*lpr/lpr* (MRL/*lpr*) mice develop spontaneously an age-dependent lupus-like disease and have been widely used as an animal model of human lupus. We have previously shown how the characteristic age-dependent biphasic changes of Treg frequency in the mice could reflect vividly a desperate, though eventually failed, attempt of the immune system trying to control auto-aggression [68]. After an early increase, Treg frequency (ratio) within the total CD4 T cell population in the peripheral lymphoid organs rapidly declined with age (**Fig. 1A-1B**), followed immediately by the onset and exacerbation of clinical disease [68], yet the total Treg number were in general higher compared to those in the control MRL/+ mouse strain (**Fig. 1C**).

Interestingly, in a similar study, it was demonstrated that peripheral Treg frequency in the NZB/W F1 strain of mice, another spontaneous lupus mouse model, was rather reduced at young age. In contrast, in the aged and diseased mice, a higher Treg frequency was detected in the renal draining lymph nodes, though also decreased in the spleen, as compared to normal BALB/c mice [50]. This may again reflect the differences in severity and kinetics of disease progression, in relation to the age-dependent Treg cell changes, between the MRL/*lpr* and NZB/W F1 strains. As shown in **Fig. 1C**, the total Treg numbers were constantly higher in the MRL/lpr strain too. This suggests that it is the Treg:Teff balance, rather than absolute Treg number, which is more relevant and critical to the disease kinetics. Such balance appears to have been maintained in the young MRL/*lpr* mice at least until 2-3 months of age, a stage prior to the development of overt clinical disease [2]. Compared to the MRL/*lpr* strain, NZB/W F1 mice develop a relatively milder clinical disease and at a much later stage [2]. The increased Treg frequency in the NZB/W F1 diseased mice could also reflect similarly the ongoing feedback regulatory mechanism yet relatively more sustainable in this mouse strain.

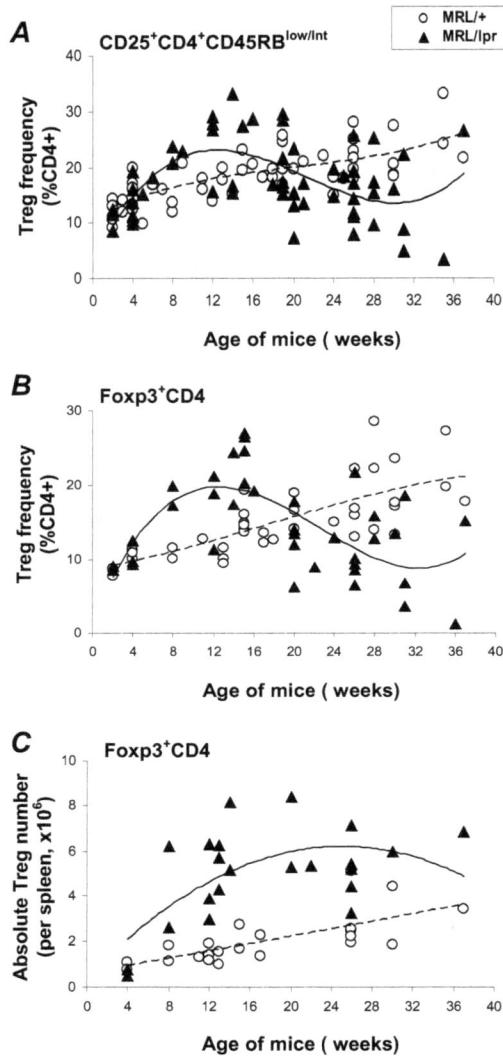

(Data from EJI 2008. **38**:1664-76 with permission)

Fig. 1. **Age-dependent bi-phasic changes of splenic Treg frequency in MRL/lpr mice.**
Freshly isolated splenocytes were stained for CD4, CD25, CD45RB and Foxp3 in different
combinations, and analyzed by multicolor flow cytometry. Treg cells were identified by
means of **(A)** CD4+CD25hiCD45RBlow/Int and **(B**, and **C)** CD4+Foxp3+, and shown as the
percentage of total CD4+ cell population (**A**, and **B**) and absolute Treg number per spleen
(**C**) for each mouse. Data shown are Treg frequencies calculated from individual mice of
different age (female), of the MRL/+ (open circles, n=58) and MRL/**lpr** (filled triangles,
n=60) strains respectively, where each symbol represents one individual animal.

In other words, although the original defect(s) leading to the initiation of lupus may differ in SLE patients and these different lupus mouse models, changes in Treg versus Teff can be a true reflection of the capacity, or limitation, of the immune system trying to control the pathogenic autoimmune responses.

5. Defective Treg-mediated suppression in systemic autoimmunity – the underlying immunological mechanisms

The next important question concerns the complex immunological mechanisms underlying Treg deficiency in lupus disorders. Defects in the Teff cells and DC in particular have been found to contribute either directly or indirectly to the aberrant Treg-mediated suppression. These include abnormal Teff and DC functional status, and their expression of, or responsiveness to, certain cytokines critically involved in Treg and/or Teff functions.

5.1 Teff resistance

It was demonstrated that Teff cells isolated from lupus patients were less susceptible to Treg-mediated suppression [66, 67], and the level of resistance inversely correlated with patients' clinical disease activities [67]. Similar findings have also been shown in several lupus-prone mouse strains [70, 89, 99]. Based on their findings, the authors concluded that it was the enhanced resistance of responder cells (i.e. Teff), rather than defects in Treg themselves, that was to be blamed for the defective Treg-mediated suppression. A lack of Fas-mediated Teff activation induced cell death (AICD) and low surface expression of T cell inhibitory molecules (e.g. CTLA-4), or their ligands (CD80, CD86) on APC, are among the possible mechanisms proposed.

Moreover, it was also shown that the aberrant resistance of Teff could be associated with the activation state or lineage-commitment of Teff cells. While Treg isolated from the autoimmune BALB/c-lpr/lpr and gld/gld Fas/FasL-deficient mice could block naïve T cell activation and differentiation into the Th1 phenotype, they were unable to suppress those pre-existing lineage-committed IFN-γ-producing effector Th1 cells [99].

5.2 Lack of Teff-derived soluble factors essential for Treg functions & expansion

However, soluble factors produced by Teff cells are also known to be crucial for normal Treg functions. IL-2 produced by activated Teff, for example, is an essential growth factor for Treg cell differentiation and proliferation, and a potent inducer of Treg IL-10 expression [101]. We have previously demonstrated that, in two unrelated lupus mouse models, IL-2 deficiency is responsible for an early and progressive defect in T cell proliferation, which could be restored by exogenous IL-2 [7]. The cytokine was indeed later found to be able to restore Treg expansion and functions, both in vitro and *in vivo*, in the lupus mice [68, 87]. In other words, under normal physiological conditions, the Treg-mediated suppressive action has to be 'endorsed' by their 'target cells' too. When such a 'mutual agreement' is no longer in order, i.e. the lack of 'informed consent' from their target cells, Treg cells are left functionally powerless allowing subsequently the rapid expansion of autoreactive T and B cells.

5.3 Imbalanced peripheral Treg versus Teff expansion

The imbalance between Treg and Teff, including Th1 [99], expansion has provided a good basis and some mechanistic explanations for the systemic nature of lupus disorders [14, 68].

Th17 is another subset of specialized T helper cells, which produce the signature cytokine IL-17, or IL-17A. IL-17 mediates various inflammatory responses such as recruitment of monocytes and neutrophils [102], T cell infiltration and activation [103], induction of further proinflammatory cytokine expression [104] and, Th17 as a new pathogenic cell type, has been implicated in many autoimmune inflammatory diseases (reviewed in [105]). IL-17 producing Th17 cells also contribute to the pathogenesis and development of SLE. Several groups have shown that the numbers of Th17 cells and notably the ratio between Th17 and Treg were altered in SLE patients [75, 82, 106-108]. The number of Th17 cells in the blood of SLE patients was elevated [82] and accordingly serum IL-17 levels were increased [82, 109, 110]. However, the changes in the number of Th17 cells itself did not seem to correlate with lupus disease development, whereas the ratio between Treg and Th17 cells had a very clear inverse correlation with disease activity, especially in those patients with acute nephritis [107]. Moreover, the low Treg:Th17 ratios were also found to be restorable following clinical treatment that controlled disease activity [108].

5.4 Cytokines differentially involved in driving Treg & Teff differentiation

Naive CD4+ T helper cells can be induced to differentiate into Th1, Th2, Th17 and Treg phenotypes depending to the local cytokine milieu. The presence of IL-12 signalling through STAT-4 (signal transduction and activator of transcription-4) drives towards Th1, whereas IL-4 (signalling through STAT-6) skews towards Th2 [111]. Interestingly, the differentiation of pro-inflammatory Th17 and anti-inflammatory Treg cells, two seemingly mutually exclusive cell types, follows a very similar pattern. Differentiation into both of these T cell subsets requires TGF-β, a cytokine capable of inducing expression of Foxp3 and RORγt, which are essential transcription factors for the development of Treg and Th17 cells, respectively [28, 112]. Under homeostatic non-inflammatory conditions, TGF-β induces only Treg, as Treg expressed Foxp3 itself is capable of suppressing Th17 development by binding to RORγt and thereby inhibiting its activity as a transcriptional activator [113]. Only in the presence of certain potent pro-inflammatory cytokines including IL-6, IL-21 and IL-23, the Foxp3 mediated inhibition of RORγt can be abrogated and differentiation into Th17 cells initiated [113, 114].

5.5 Roles of DC

Aberrant DC functions play evidently crucial roles in lupus disease induction, e.g. by driving the pathogenic Th1 type of responses [14] or skewing Teff versus Treg expansion [68]. **Fig. 2A** shows clearly that the DC generated from MRL/lpr mice are functionally defective in driving Treg, but not Teff, cell expansion. The importance of Treg:Th17 ratio for lupus disease activity has also been highlighted by work performed by Kang et al on the role of tolerogenic DC. The authors showed that injection of lupus-prone mice with a nucleosomal histone peptide epitope (H4$_{71-94}$) induced TGF-β producing Treg while suppressing inflammatory Th17 cells, with a general increase in survival. This was attributed to the induction of tolerogenic DC which produced enhanced levels of TGF-β, but decreased IL-6 expression [115]. Another study by Wan et al also pointed to the role of IL-6 produced by DC in blocking Treg function, and its genetic linkage (sle1) in mice originated from the NZM2410 lupus mouse strain [90]. In addition, aberrant expression of Type 1 interferon (IFN-α) by APC has also been shown to block Treg functions contributing to the Treg versus Teff imbalance in lupus disease [65, 81, 116].

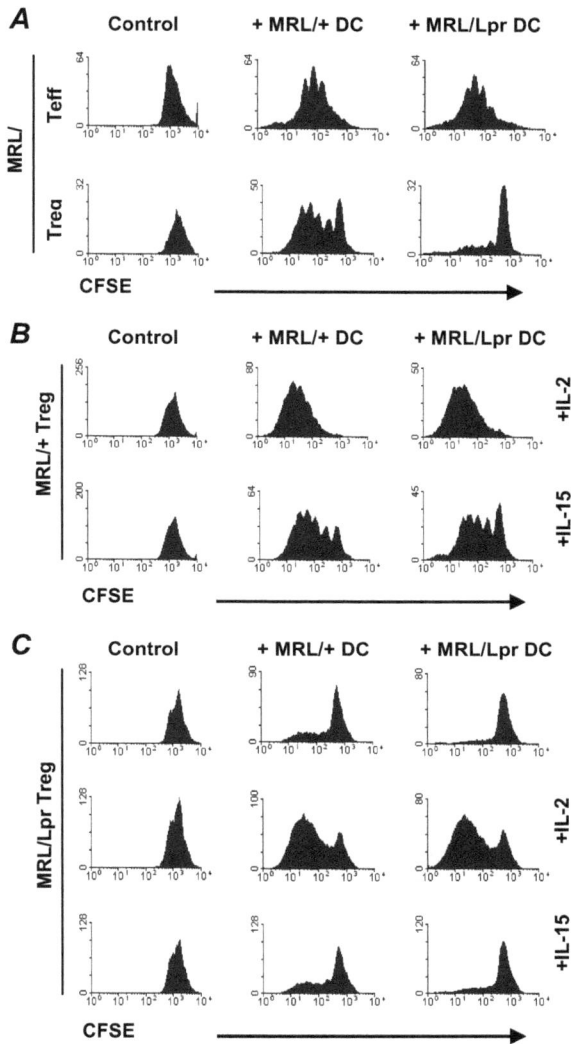

(Data from EJI 2008. 38:1664-76 with permission)

Fig. 2. **Defects in DCs and Treg cells of MRL/lpr mice.** *A. MRL/lpr DCs are defective in promoting Treg but not Teff cell proliferation.* Treg and Teff cells were purified from spleens of MRL/+ mice (3-month, female), and DCs were generated from bone marrow precursor cells of age-sex-matched MRL/+ or MRL/**lpr** mice (3-month, female). After labeling with CFSE, the Treg or Teff cells were stimulated with anti-CD3 mAb for 5 days, in the presence or absence of live MRL/**lpr** or MRL/+ DCs (as indicated in the graphs). *B. Restoration of Treg promoting capacity of MRL/lpr DCs by exogenous IL-2 and IL-15.* The CSFE-labeled splenic Treg cells purified from MRL/+ mice (as described in A) were stimulated with anti-CD3 mAb for

5 days, in the presence or absence of live MRL/**lpr** or MRL/+ DCs, and with or without addition of recombinant mouse IL-2 (10 ng/ml) or IL-15 (40 ng/ml), as indicated in the respective graphs. *C. Restoration of a defect in MRL/lpr Treg proliferation by IL-2, but not IL-15.* CSFE-labeled splenic Treg cells purified from MRL/**lpr** mice were stimulated with anti-CD3 mAb for 5 days, in the presence or absence of live MRL/**lpr** or MRL/+ DCs, and with or without addition of recombinant mouse IL-2 (10 ng/ml) or IL-15 (40 ng/ml). Cell division (CFSE dilution) was determined by flow cytometry. Controls were cells stimulated in the same way but in the absence of DCs. CM: culture medium control. Data shown were representative FACS profiles of more than 3 repeated experiments.

5.6 Possible Treg intrinsic defects

Furthermore, certain intrinsic defects associated with Treg themselves might also be involved [68]. IL-15 is a pleiotropic cytokine akin to IL-2 [117, 118], which is produced by monocytic cells including DC [119, 120] rather than T cells. IL-15 mediates its functions through the β- and γ-chains of the IL-2 receptor together with an unique IL-15 α-chain, and is known to be involved in the regulation of normal differentiation and expansion of T cells including Treg [121]. While the defect of MRL/lpr DC in driving expansion of the wild type (MRL/+) control Treg mentioned above (**Fig. 2A**) could be restored by adding exogenous IL-2 or IL-15 (**Fig. 2B**), the MRL/lpr Treg though also restorable by IL-2 failed completely to respond to IL-15 (**Fig. 2C**). These findings suggest that the MRL/lpr Treg possibly have an intrinsic defect as well in their responsiveness to the IL-2-like non-T cell-derived cytokine. It would also be very interesting to know how these cells may respond to other factors, such as IL-35 known to be closely associated with Treg functions [32].

6. Therapeutic implications of Treg in systemic autoimmune disorders

As discussed above, though also a result of overt autoimmune response itself, the lack of Treg mediated immune regulation contributes evidently to the early onset and kinetics of lupus disease development. Normalization of Treg frequencies and functions by restoring the Treg:Teff balance, may therefore prove to be clinically beneficial, hence a reasonable treatment strategy for the human disease. This concept has recently been tested in animal models by direct adoptive transfer of *ex vivo* derived, or *in vitro* expanded, Treg with encouraging results [68, 96, 122]. The treated mice had significantly delayed clinical disease as evident by delayed onset of glomerulonephritis, reduced proteinuria and skin lesions, and prolonged mouse survival [68, 96, 122].

Besides reconstitution of the Treg population by adoptive transfer, potential treatment methods to achieve an *in vivo* expansion of endogenous Treg and a normalization of the ratio between Treg and Teff, might be as diverse as the initial reasons for the deficiency in the Treg population. Accordingly, it has been shown that administration of rIL-2 promotes the proliferation of endogenous Treg and delays the progression of established disease, most likely by re-establishing the homeostatic balance of Treg and effector T cells [87]. Supporting evidence from earlier studies also indicates that tolerance induction by injecting various tolerogenic peptides [91, 115, 123], anti-thymocyte globulin agents [95], or oral administration of anti-CD3 antibodies [97], are all associated with *in vivo* Treg expansion.

It needs to be clearly pointed out that, while transfer of Treg may be beneficial against autoimmune syndromes [68], severe side effects such as infections following excessive (high dose) Treg treatment especially in non-adult mice can also occur (Yang et al, unpublished observations). Therefore, similar to the use of any immunosuppressive drug, caution should be taken about potential side effects of the treatment, for patients of young ages in particular.

7. Concluding remarks

In summary, immune regulation by Treg is an important mechanism against systemic autoimmunity, and a general lack of Treg-mediated suppression is evident in lupus disorder. Different findings from studies of lupus patients and various animal disease models about the aberrant changes in Treg frequency and functionality reflect vividly the disease kinetics, severity, and often the on-going desperate attempts of the immune system to control auto-aggression. Clarification of their true causal relationship is undoubtedly very important not only for our understanding of the complex disease mechanisms, but also for rational design of therapeutic strategies for our patients.

8. Acknowledgements

We wish to thank Dr Cui-Hong Yang and Dr Lina Tian for some of their important findings mentioned in this book chapter. We would also like to acknowledge the funding support which we have received for our research projects. SS is supported by the Arthritis Research UK (ARUK18523). FPH is currently supported by the Higher Education Funding Council UK (HEFC UK), and has received research funding support from the Arthritis Research UK (ARUK18523), the Hong Kong Research Grant Committee (RGC HKU 7246/01M, 7291/02M, 7410/03M, 7397/04M, 7580/06M), the MacFeat Bequest Fund (Glasgow) and the Li Ka Sheng Academic Foundation (Shantou). All correspondence should be addressed to FPH (fp.huang@imperial.ac.uk, or fphuang@hkucc.hku.hk)

9. References

[1] Vyse, T.J. and B.L. Kotzin, *GENETIC SUSCEPTIBILITY TO SYSTEMIC LUPUS ERYTHEMATOSUS*. Annu. Rev. Immunol., 1998. 16(1): p. 261-292.

[2] Theofilopoulos, A.N. and F.J. Dixon, *Murine models of systemic lupus erythematosus*. Adv Immunol, 1985. 37: p. 269-390.

[3] Mills, J.A., *Systemic lupus erythematosus*. N Engl J Med, 1994. 330(26): p. 1871-9.

[4] Rahman, A. and D.A. Isenberg, *Systemic lupus erythematosus*. N Engl J Med, 2008. 358(9): p. 929-39.

[5] Lipsky, P.E., *Systemic lupus erythematosus: an autoimmune disease of B cell hyperactivity*. Nat Immunol, 2001. 2(9): p. 764-6.

[6] Altman, A., et al., *Analysis of T cell function in autoimmune murine strains. Defects in production and responsiveness to interleukin 2*. J Exp Med, 1981. 154(3): p. 791-808.

[7] Huang, F.P. and D.I. Stott, *Restoration of an early, progressive defect in responsiveness to T-cell activation in lupus mice by exogenous IL-2*. Autoimmunity, 1993. 15(1): p. 19-29.

[8] Manderson, A.P., M. Botto, and M.J. Walport, *The role of complement in the development of systemic lupus erythematosus*. Annu Rev Immunol, 2004. 22: p. 431-56.

[9] Cook, H.T. and M. Botto, *Mechanisms of Disease: the complement system and the pathogenesis of systemic lupus erythematosus*. Nat Clin Pract Rheumatol, 2006. 2(6): p. 330-7.

[10] Pickering, M.C., et al., *Prevention of C5 activation ameliorates spontaneous and experimental glomerulonephritis in factor H-deficient mice.* Proc Natl Acad Sci U S A, 2006. 103(25): p. 9649-54.

[11] Matsumoto, K., et al., *Defect in negative selection in lpr donor-derived T cells differentiating in non-lpr host thymus.* J Exp Med, 1991. 173(1): p. 127-36.

[12] Mok, C.C. and C.S. Lau, *Pathogenesis of systemic lupus erythematosus.* J Clin Pathol, 2003. 56(7): p. 481-90.

[13] Watanabe-Fukunaga, R., et al., *Lymphoproliferation disorder in mice explained by defects in Fas antigen that mediates apoptosis.* Nature (London), 1992. 356(6367): p. 314-7.

[14] Ma, L., et al., *Systemic autoimmune disease induced by dendritic cells that have captured necrotic but not apoptotic cells in susceptible mouse strains.* Eur J Immunol, 2005. 35(11): p. 3364-75.

[15] Sakaguchi, S., *Naturally arising CD4+ regulatory t cells for immunologic self-tolerance and negative control of immune responses.* Annu Rev Immunol, 2004. 22: p. 531-62.

[16] Wing, K. and S. Sakaguchi, *Regulatory T cells exert checks and balances on self tolerance and autoimmunity.* Nat Immunol, 2010. 11(1): p. 7-13.

[17] Sakaguchi, S., et al., *Immunologic self-tolerance maintained by activated T cells expressing IL-2 receptor alpha-chains (CD25). Breakdown of a single mechanism of self-tolerance causes various autoimmune diseases.* J Immunol, 1995. 155(3): p. 1151-64.

[18] Saoudi, A., et al., *The thymus contains a high frequency of cells that prevent autoimmune diabetes on transfer into prediabetic recipients.* J Exp Med, 1996. 184(6): p. 2393-8.

[19] Asano, M., et al., *Autoimmune disease as a consequence of developmental abnormality of a T cell subpopulation.* J Exp Med, 1996. 184(2): p. 387-96.

[20] Yagi, H., et al., *Crucial role of FOXP3 in the development and function of human CD25+CD4+ regulatory T cells.* Int Immunol, 2004. 16(11): p. 1643-56.

[21] Bacchetta, R., et al., *Defective regulatory and effector T cell functions in patients with FOXP3 mutations.* J Clin Invest, 2006. 116(6): p. 1713-22.

[22] Hori, S., T. Nomura, and S. Sakaguchi, *Control of regulatory T cell development by the transcription factor Foxp3.* Science, 2003. 299(5609): p. 1057-61.

[23] Fontenot, J.D., M.A. Gavin, and A.Y. Rudensky, *Foxp3 programs the development and function of CD4+CD25+ regulatory T cells.* Nat Immunol, 2003. 4(4): p. 330-6.

[24] Khattri, R., et al., *An essential role for Scurfin in CD4+CD25+ T regulatory cells.* Nat Immunol, 2003. 4(4): p. 337-42.

[25] Brunkow, M.E., et al., *Disruption of a new forkhead/winged-helix protein, scurfin, results in the fatal lymphoproliferative disorder of the scurfy mouse.* Nat Genet, 2001. 27(1): p. 68-73.

[26] Gambineri, E., T.R. Torgerson, and H.D. Ochs, *Immune dysregulation, polyendocrinopathy, enteropathy, and X-linked inheritance (IPEX), a syndrome of systemic autoimmunity caused by mutations of FOXP3, a critical regulator of T-cell homeostasis.* Curr Opin Rheumatol, 2003. 15(4): p. 430-5.

[27] Curotto de Lafaille, M.A., et al., *CD25- T cells generate CD25+Foxp3+ regulatory T cells by peripheral expansion.* J Immunol, 2004. 173(12): p. 7259-68.

[28] Chen, W., et al., *Conversion of peripheral CD4+CD25- naive T cells to CD4+CD25+ regulatory T cells by TGF-beta induction of transcription factor Foxp3.* J Exp Med, 2003. 198(12): p. 1875-86.

[29] Fantini, M.C., et al., *Cutting edge: TGF-beta induces a regulatory phenotype in CD4+CD25- T cells through Foxp3 induction and down-regulation of Smad7.* J Immunol, 2004. 172(9): p. 5149-53.

[30] Kitani, A., et al., *Transforming growth factor (TGF)-beta1-producing regulatory T cells induce Smad-mediated interleukin 10 secretion that facilitates coordinated immunoregulatory activity and amelioration of TGF-beta1-mediated fibrosis.* J Exp Med, 2003. 198(8): p. 1179-88.

[31] Niedbala, W., et al., *IL-35 is a novel cytokine with therapeutic effects against collagen-induced arthritis through the expansion of regulatory T cells and suppression of Th17 cells.* Eur J Immunol, 2007. 37(11): p. 3021-9.

[32] Collison, L.W., et al., *The inhibitory cytokine IL-35 contributes to regulatory T-cell function.* Nature, 2007. 450(7169): p. 566-9.

[33] Seyerl, M., et al., *Human rhinoviruses induce IL-35-producing Treg via induction of B7-H1 (CD274) and sialoadhesin (CD169) on DC.* Eur J Immunol, 2009.

[34] Collison, L.W., et al., *IL-35-mediated induction of a potent regulatory T cell population.* Nat Immunol, 2010. 11(12): p. 1093-101.

[35] Tarbell, K.V., S. Yamazaki, and R.M. Steinman, *The interactions of dendritic cells with antigen-specific, regulatory T cells that suppress autoimmunity.* Semin Immunol, 2006. 18(2): p. 93-102.

[36] Thornton, A.M. and E.M. Shevach, *CD4+CD25+ immunoregulatory T cells suppress polyclonal T cell activation in vitro by inhibiting interleukin 2 production.* J Exp Med, 1998. 188(2): p. 287-96.

[37] Yu, P., et al., *Specific T regulatory cells display broad suppressive functions against experimental allergic encephalomyelitis upon activation with cognate antigen.* J Immunol, 2005. 174(11): p. 6772-80.

[38] Yamazaki, S., et al., *Dendritic cells expand antigen-specific Foxp3+ CD25+ CD4+ regulatory T cells including suppressors of alloreactivity.* Immunol Rev, 2006. 212: p. 314-29.

[39] Saoudi, A., et al., *The physiological role of regulatory T cells in the prevention of autoimmunity: the function of the thymus in the generation of the regulatory T cell subset.* Immunol Rev, 1996. 149: p. 195-216.

[40] Crispin, J.C., A. Martinez, and J. Alcocer-Varela, *Quantification of regulatory T cells in patients with systemic lupus erythematosus.* J Autoimmun, 2003. 21(3): p. 273-6.

[41] Liu, M.F., et al., *Decreased CD4+CD25+ T cells in peripheral blood of patients with systemic lupus erythematosus.* Scand J Immunol, 2004. 59(2): p. 198-202.

[42] Wu, H.Y. and N.A. Staines, *A deficiency of CD4+CD25+ T cells permits the development of spontaneous lupus-like disease in mice, and can be reversed by induction of mucosal tolerance to histone peptide autoantigen.* Lupus, 2004. 13(3): p. 192-200.

[43] Fathy, A., et al., *Diminished CD4+CD25+ T-lymphocytes in peripheral blood of patients with systemic lupus erythematosus.* Egypt J Immunol, 2005. 12(1): p. 25-31.

[44] Miyara, M., et al., *Global natural regulatory T cell depletion in active systemic lupus erythematosus.* J Immunol, 2005. 175(12): p. 8392-400.

[45] Lee, J.H., et al., *Inverse correlation between CD4+ regulatory T-cell population and autoantibody levels in paediatric patients with systemic lupus erythematosus.* Immunology, 2006. 117(2): p. 280-6.

[46] Mellor-Pita, S., et al., *Decrease of regulatory T cells in patients with systemic lupus erythematosus.* Ann Rheum Dis, 2006. 65(4): p. 553-4.

[47] Suarez, A., et al., *Enrichment of CD4+ CD25high T cell population in patients with systemic lupus erythematosus treated with glucocorticoids.* Ann Rheum Dis, 2006. 65(11): p. 1512-7.

[48] Alvarado-Sanchez, B., et al., *Regulatory T cells in patients with systemic lupus erythematosus.* J Autoimmun, 2006. 27(2): p. 110-8.

[49] Hsu, W.T., J.L. Suen, and B.L. Chiang, *The role of CD4CD25 T cells in autoantibody production in murine lupus.* Clin Exp Immunol, 2006. 145(3): p. 513-9.

[50] Scalapino, K.J., et al., *Suppression of disease in New Zealand Black/New Zealand White lupus-prone mice by adoptive transfer of ex vivo expanded regulatory T cells.* J Immunol, 2006. 177(3): p. 1451-9.

[51] Barath, S., et al., *The severity of systemic lupus erythematosus negatively correlates with the increasing number of CD4+CD25(high)FoxP3+ regulatory T cells during repeated plasmapheresis treatments of patients.* Autoimmunity, 2007. 40(7): p. 521-8.

[52] Barath, S., et al., *Measurement of natural (CD4+CD25high) and inducible (CD4+IL-10+) regulatory T cells in patients with systemic lupus erythematosus.* Lupus, 2007. 16(7): p. 489-96.

[53] Lyssuk, E.Y., et al., *Reduced number and function of CD4+CD25highFoxP3+ regulatory T cells in patients with systemic lupus erythematosus.* Adv Exp Med Biol, 2007. 601: p. 113-9.

[54] Lin, S.C., et al., *The quantitative analysis of peripheral blood FOXP3-expressing T cells in systemic lupus erythematosus and rheumatoid arthritis patients.* Eur J Clin Invest, 2007. 37(12): p. 987-96.

[55] Sfikakis, P.P., et al., *Increased expression of the FoxP3 functional marker of regulatory T cells following B cell depletion with rituximab in patients with lupus nephritis.* Clin Immunol, 2007. 123(1): p. 66-73.

[56] Vallerskog, T., et al., *Treatment with rituximab affects both the cellular and the humoral arm of the immune system in patients with SLE.* Clin Immunol, 2007. 122(1): p. 62-74.

[57] Valencia, X., et al., *Deficient CD4+CD25high T regulatory cell function in patients with active systemic lupus erythematosus.* J Immunol, 2007. 178(4): p. 2579-88.

[58] Bonelli, M., et al., *Foxp3 expression in CD4+ T cells of patients with systemic lupus erythematosus: a comparative phenotypic analysis.* Ann Rheum Dis, 2008. 67(5): p. 664-71.

[59] Bonelli, M., et al., *Quantitative and qualitative deficiencies of regulatory T cells in patients with systemic lupus erythematosus (SLE).* Int Immunol, 2008. 20(7): p. 861-8.

[60] Lee, H.Y., et al., *Altered frequency and migration capacity of CD4+CD25+ regulatory T cells in systemic lupus erythematosus.* Rheumatology (Oxford), 2008. 47(6): p. 789-94.

[61] Zhang, B., et al., *Reduction of forkhead box P3 levels in CD4+CD25high T cells in patients with new-onset systemic lupus erythematosus.* Clin Exp Immunol, 2008. 153(2): p. 182-7.

[62] Zhang, B., et al., *Clinical significance of increased CD4+CD25-Foxp3+ T cells in patients with new-onset systemic lupus erythematosus.* Ann Rheum Dis, 2008. 67(7): p. 1037-40.

[63] Azab, N.A., et al., *CD4+CD25+ regulatory T cells (TREG) in systemic lupus erythematosus (SLE) patients: the possible influence of treatment with corticosteroids.* Clin Immunol, 2008. 127(2): p. 151-7.

[64] Yates, J., et al., *Natural regulatory T cells: number and function are normal in the majority of patients with lupus nephritis.* Clin Exp Immunol, 2008. 153(1): p. 44-55.

[65] Yan, B., et al., *Dysfunctional CD4+,CD25+ regulatory T cells in untreated active systemic lupus erythematosus secondary to interferon-alpha-producing antigen-presenting cells.* Arthritis Rheum, 2008. 58(3): p. 801-12.

[66] Vargas-Rojas, M.I., et al., *Quantitative and qualitative normal regulatory T cells are not capable of inducing suppression in SLE patients due to T-cell resistance.* Lupus, 2008. 17(4): p. 289-94.

[67] Venigalla, R.K., et al., *Reduced CD4+,CD25- T cell sensitivity to the suppressive function of CD4+,CD25high,CD127 -/low regulatory T cells in patients with active systemic lupus erythematosus.* Arthritis Rheum, 2008. 58(7): p. 2120-30.

[68] Yang, C.H., et al., *Immunological mechanisms and clinical implications of regulatory T cell deficiency in a systemic autoimmune disorder: Roles of IL-2 versus IL-15.* Eur J Immunol, 2008. 38: p. 1664-1676.

[69] Abe, J., et al., *Increased Foxp3(+) CD4(+) regulatory T cells with intact suppressive activity but altered cellular localization in murine lupus.* Am J Pathol, 2008. 173(6): p. 1682-92.

[70] Parietti, V., et al., *Function of CD4+,CD25+ Treg cells in MRL/lpr mice is compromised by intrinsic defects in antigen-presenting cells and effector T cells.* Arthritis Rheum, 2008. 58(6): p. 1751-61.

[71] Atfy, M., et al., *Impact of CD4+CD25high regulatory T-cells and FoxP3 expression in the peripheral blood of patients with systemic lupus erythematosus.* Egypt J Immunol, 2009. 16(1): p. 117-26.

[72] Banica, L., et al., *Quantification and molecular characterization of regulatory T cells in connective tissue diseases.* Autoimmunity, 2009. 42(1): p. 41-9.

[73] Barreto, M., et al., *Low frequency of CD4+CD25+ Treg in SLE patients: a heritable trait associated with CTLA4 and TGFbeta gene variants.* BMC Immunol, 2009. 10: p. 5.

[74] Suen, J.L., et al., *Altered homeostasis of CD4(+) FoxP3(+) regulatory T-cell subpopulations in systemic lupus erythematosus.* Immunology, 2009. 127(2): p. 196-205.

[75] Yang, J., et al., *Th17 and natural Treg cell population dynamics in systemic lupus erythematosus.* Arthritis Rheum, 2009. 60(5): p. 1472-83.

[76] Bonelli, M., et al., *Phenotypic and functional analysis of CD4+ CD25- Foxp3+ T cells in patients with systemic lupus erythematosus.* J Immunol, 2009. 182(3): p. 1689-95.

[77] Dai, Z., et al., *Normally occurring NKG2D+CD4+ T cells are immunosuppressive and inversely correlated with disease activity in juvenile-onset lupus.* J Exp Med, 2009. 206(4): p. 793-805.

[78] Yang, H.X., et al., *Are CD4+CD25-Foxp3+ cells in untreated new-onset lupus patients regulatory T cells?* Arthritis Res Ther, 2009. 11(5): p. R153.

[79] Yan, B. and Y. Liu, *The Nature of Increased Circulating CD4CD25Foxp3 T Cells in Patients with Systemic Lupus Erythematosus: A Novel Hypothesis.* Open Rheumatol J, 2009. 3: p. 22-4.

[80] Gomez, J., et al., *Conserved anti-proliferative effect and poor inhibition of TNFalpha secretion by regulatory CD4+CD25+ T cells in patients with systemic lupus erythematosus.* Clin Immunol, 2009. 132(3): p. 385-92.

[81] Scaglione, B.J., et al., *Regulatory T cells as central regulators of both autoimmunity and B cell malignancy in New Zealand Black mice.* J Autoimmun, 2009. 32(1): p. 14-23.

[82] Henriques, A., et al., *Frequency and functional activity of Th17, Tc17 and other T-cell subsets in Systemic Lupus Erythematosus.* Cell Immunol, 2010. 264(1): p. 97-103.

[83] Habibagahi, M., et al., *Quantification of regulatory T cells in peripheral blood of patients with systemic lupus erythematosus.* Rheumatol Int, 2010.

[84] Chen, D.Y., et al., *The associations of circulating CD4(+)CD25(high) regulatory T cells and TGF-beta with disease activity and clinical course in patients with adult-onset Still's disease.* Connect Tissue Res, 2010. 51(5): p. 370-7.

[85] Mesquita, D., et al., *Systemic lupus erythematosus exhibits a dynamic and continuum spectrum of effector/regulatory T cells.* Scand J Rheumatol, 2011. 40(1): p. 41-50.

[86] Ma, J., et al., *The imbalance between regulatory and IL-17-secreting CD4+ T cells in lupus patients.* Clin Rheumatol, 2010. 29(11): p. 1251-8.

[87] Humrich, J.Y., et al., *Homeostatic imbalance of regulatory and effector T cells due to IL-2 deprivation amplifies murine lupus.* Proc Natl Acad Sci U S A, 2010. 107(1): p. 204-9.

[88] Xing, Q., et al., *Elevated Th17 cells are accompanied by FoxP3+ Treg cells decrease in patients with lupus nephritis.* Rheumatol Int, 2011.

[89] Monk, C.R., et al., *MRL/Mp CD4+,CD25- T cells show reduced sensitivity to suppression by CD4+,CD25+ regulatory T cells in vitro: a novel defect of T cell regulation in systemic lupus erythematosus.* Arthritis Rheum, 2005. 52(4): p. 1180-4.

[90] Wan, S., C. Xia, and L. Morel, *IL-6 produced by dendritic cells from lupus-prone mice inhibits CD4+CD25+ T cell regulatory functions.* J Immunol, 2007. 178(1): p. 271-9.

[91] Kang, H.K., et al., *Very low-dose tolerance with nucleosomal peptides controls lupus and induces potent regulatory T cell subsets.* J Immunol, 2005. 174(6): p. 3247-55.

[92] Reilly, C.M., et al., *The histone deacetylase inhibitor trichostatin A upregulates regulatory T cells and modulates autoimmunity in NZB/W F1 mice.* J Autoimmun, 2008. 31(2): p. 123-30.

[93] Tago, F., et al., *Repeated 0.5-Gy gamma irradiation attenuates autoimmune disease in MRL-lpr/lpr mice with suppression of CD3+CD4-CD8-B220+ T-cell proliferation and with up-regulation of CD4+CD25+Foxp3+ regulatory T cells.* Radiat Res, 2008. 169(1): p. 59-66.

[94] Sharabi, A. and E. Mozes, *The suppression of murine lupus by a tolerogenic peptide involves foxp3-expressing CD8 cells that are required for the optimal induction and function of foxp3-expressing CD4 cells.* J Immunol, 2008. 181(5): p. 3243-51.

[95] Kaplan, J., et al., *Therapeutic benefit of treatment with anti-thymocyte globulin and latent TGF-beta1 in the MRL/lpr lupus mouse model.* Lupus, 2008. 17(9): p. 822-31.

[96] Scalapino, K.J. and D.I. Daikh, *Suppression of glomerulonephritis in NZB/NZW lupus prone mice by adoptive transfer of ex vivo expanded regulatory T cells.* PLoS One, 2009. 4(6): p. e6031.

[97] Wu, H.Y., et al., *Suppression of murine SLE by oral anti-CD3: inducible CD4+CD25-LAP+ regulatory T cells control the expansion of IL-17+ follicular helper T cells.* Lupus, 2009. 18(7): p. 586-96.

[98] Zhang, J.L., et al., *CD3 mAb treatment ameliorated the severity of the cGVHD-induced lupus nephritis in mice by up-regulation of Foxp3+ regulatory T cells in the target tissue: kidney.* Transpl Immunol, 2010. 24(1): p. 17-25.

[99] Hondowicz, B.D., et al., *Autoantibody production in lpr/lpr gld/gld mice reflects accumulation of CD4+ effector cells that are resistant to regulatory T cell activity.* J Autoimmun, 2008. 31(2): p. 98-109.

[100] Cuda, C.M., et al., *Murine lupus susceptibility locus Sle1a controls regulatory T cell number and function through multiple mechanisms.* J Immunol, 2007. 179(11): p. 7439-47.

[101] Scheffold, A., J. Huhn, and T. Hofer, *Regulation of CD4+CD25+ regulatory T cell activity: it takes (IL-)two to tango.* Eur J Immunol, 2005. 35(5): p. 1336-41.

[102] Witowski, J., et al., *IL-17 stimulates intraperitoneal neutrophil infiltration through the release of GRO alpha chemokine from mesothelial cells.* J Immunol, 2000. 165(10): p. 5814-21.

[103] Albanesi, C., A. Cavani, and G. Girolomoni, *IL-17 is produced by nickel-specific T lymphocytes and regulates ICAM-1 expression and chemokine production in human keratinocytes: synergistic or antagonist effects with IFN-gamma and TNF-alpha.* J Immunol, 1999. 162(1): p. 494-502.

[104] Schwarzenberger, P., et al., *Requirement of endogenous stem cell factor and granulocyte-colony-stimulating factor for IL-17-mediated granulopoiesis.* J Immunol, 2000. 164(9): p. 4783-9.

[105] Xu, S. and X. Cao, *Interleukin-17 and its expanding biological functions.* Cell Mol Immunol. 2010 May, 7(3): p. 164-74.

[106] Wong, C.K., et al., *Hyperproduction of IL-23 and IL-17 in patients with systemic lupus erythematosus: implications for Th17-mediated inflammation in auto-immunity.* Clin Immunol, 2008. 127(3): p. 385-93.

[107] Xing, Q., et al., *Elevated Th17 cells are accompanied by FoxP3+ Treg cells decrease in patients with lupus nephritis.* Rheumatol Int. 2011 Jan 18. [Epub ahead of print]

[108] Ma, J., et al., *The imbalance between regulatory and IL-17-secreting CD4+ T cells in lupus patients.* Clin Rheumatol. 2010 Nov; 29(11): p. 1251-8.

[109] Mok, M.Y., et al., *The relation of interleukin 17 (IL-17) and IL-23 to Th1/Th2 cytokines and disease activity in systemic lupus erythematosus.* J Rheumatol. 2010 Oct; 37(10): p. 2046-52.

[110] Chen, X.Q., et al., *Plasma IL-17A is increased in new-onset SLE patients and associated with disease activity.* J Clin Immunol. 2010 Mar; 30(2): p. 221-5.

[111] Nelms, K., et al., *The IL-4 receptor: signaling mechanisms and biologic functions.* Annu Rev Immunol, 1999. 17: p. 701-38.

[112] Mangan, P.R., et al., *Transforming growth factor-beta induces development of the T(H)17 lineage.* Nature, 2006. 441(7090): p. 231-4.

[113] Zhou, L., et al., *TGF-beta-induced Foxp3 inhibits T(H)17 cell differentiation by antagonizing RORgammat function.* Nature, 2008. 453(7192): p. 236-40.

[114] Bettelli, E., et al., *IL-10 is critical in the regulation of autoimmune encephalomyelitis as demonstrated by studies of IL-10- and IL-4-deficient and transgenic mice.* J Immunol, 1998. 161(7): p. 3299-306.

[115] Kang, H.K., M. Liu, and S.K. Datta, *Low-dose peptide tolerance therapy of lupus generates plasmacytoid dendritic cells that cause expansion of autoantigen-specific regulatory T cells and contraction of inflammatory Th17 cells.* J Immunol, 2007. 178(12): p. 7849-58.

[116] Golding, A., et al., *Interferon-alpha regulates the dynamic balance between human activated regulatory and effector T cells: implications for antiviral and autoimmune responses.* Immunology, 2010. 131(1): p. 107-17.

[117] Grabstein, K.H., et al., *Cloning of a T cell growth factor that interacts with the beta chain of the interleukin-2 receptor.* Science, 1994. 264(5161): p. 965-8.

[118] McInnes, I.B., et al., *The role of interleukin-15 in T-cell migration and activation in rheumatoid arthritis [see comments].* Nat Med, 1996. 2(2): p. 175-82.

[119] Ruckert, R., et al., *Dendritic cell-derived IL-15 controls the induction of CD8 T cell immune responses.* Eur J Immunol, 2003. 33(12): p. 3493-503.

[120] Ohteki, T., et al., *Essential roles of DC-derived IL-15 as a mediator of inflammatory responses in vivo.* J Exp Med, 2006. 203(10): p. 2329-38.

[121] Koenen, H.J., E. Fasse, and I. Joosten, *IL-15 and cognate antigen successfully expand de novo-induced human antigen-specific regulatory CD4+ T cells that require antigen-specific activation for suppression.* J Immunol, 2003. 171(12): p. 6431-41.

[122] Su, H., et al., *Transforming growth factor-beta1-induced CD4+CD25+ regulatory T cells in vitro reverse and prevent a murine lupus-like syndrome of chronic graft-versus-host disease.* Br J Dermatol, 2008. 158(6): p. 1197-209.

[123] Sharabi, A., et al., *A peptide based on the complementarity-determining region 1 of an autoantibody ameliorates lupus by up-regulating CD4+CD25+ cells and TGF-beta.* Proc Natl Acad Sci U S A, 2006. 103(23): p. 8810-5.

Postinfectious Autoimmune Syndrome as a Key Factor in Chronization of the Infectious Disease

Natalia Cherepahina, Murat Agirov, Jamilyia Tabaksoeva,
Kusum Ahmedilova and Sergey Suchkov
First Moscow State Medical University
Russian State Medical University
Russia

1. Introduction

Disturbances in immune tolerance provoke autoimmune aggression, i.e., a specific immune response to auto-Ags with subsequent development of an autoimmune syndrome or an autoimmune disease (Suchkov et al., 2007).

A crucial role in formation of autoimmune syndromes and progression of autoimmune diseases is played by inborn (in the first place, HLA-associated) predisposition coupled with impaired immune responsiveness of the invaded organism. Noteworthy, initiation and progression of autoaggressive reactions cannot be triggered without preliminary activation of signaling reaction cascades, which include:

i. polyclonal activation of autoreactive cytotoxic T lymphocytes (CTL) by super-Ag (multimolecular protein complexes composed of microbial Ags, Ags and/or haptens of the carrier or intermediary drug-related metabolites) demonstrating broad spectrum of epitopes;

ii. release of sequestered or intramolecular (cryptic) autoepitopes after the tissue damage or organ injures during the inflammatory process;

iii. anti-idiotypic Ab formation that can damage own tissue and promote autoaggression;

iv. effect of mimicking epitopes (microbial Ags cross-reacting with autoepitopes of human tissues and organs).

Of particular interest in this respect is so-called *molecular mimicry*. Its biological mechanism is based on cross-reactivity, i.e., ability of the infected organism to cross-react, by virtue of structural homology between its auto-Ags and microbial Ags, with the microbial antigen thereby triggering miscellaneous immune reactions. Under these conditions, the role of autoaggressors is played simultaneously by two different groups of Ags, namely, mimicking Ags of the microbial pathogen and patient's own autoAgs. Their interactions form the clinical picture of the postinfectious autoimmune syndrome (PIFA), one of main clinical variants of syndromeal immune pathology (Paltsev et al., 2009a).

Today, the key role of the immune system in the pathogenesis of chronically relapsing infectious diseases (CRID) leaves no doubt. Their clinical course is controlled by an immense variety of factors and their combinations among which the immunologic syndrome (IS) reflecting the origin and severity of disturbances in immune homeostasis occupies a special niche. The concept of IS is not new in principle and is widely met in the current literature.

However, the term "*clinico-immunological syndrome*" (CIS) is far less explicit and needs to be supplemented with a pathogenetically rationalized, clinically significant formulaic definition encompassing the tremendous body of evidence accumulated thus far in the modern literature (Paltsev et al., 2009b) (Fig. 1).

CLINICAL CRITERIA
- Causal factor
- Lingering or chronic course of inflammatory processes (irrespective of localization) associated with frequent relapses
- Activation of conditionally pathogenic microflora, mixed infections; changes in the infectious pathogen during progression of the disease; involvement of other internal organs in autoimmune process
- Resistance to antibacterial therapy

CRITERIA OF STRUCTURAL IMMUNODEFICIENCY
- Clinical picture
- Deterioration of parameters reflecting populational magnitude and functional activity of lymphocytes, their subpopulations and non-specific protective factors to levels below the physiological level
- Diagnostically significant deterioration of 2–3 parameters in one component of the immune system or associated disturbances

CRITERIA OF FUNCTIONAL IMMUNODEFICIENCY
- Clinical picture
- Laboratory findings (content and functional activity of T and B lymphocytes, monocytes/macrophages and their subpopulations and other significant nonspecific protective factors)

Fig. 1. Clinical and immunological criteria of PIFSI

PIFSI – postinfectious secondary immunodeficiency syndrome.
In this section, we shall consider one of the most important clinical aspects of CIS, viz., *postinfectious CIS (PICIS)* whose role for practitioners in clinical medicine can hardly be overestimated. PICIS being a form of secondary (*syndromal*) immune pathology associated with the underlying (infectious) disease is provoked by a variety of factors including infectious pathogens of various etiology, clinical progression and complication of the disease proper, or inadequately applied antimicrobial therapy. The most common forms of this syndrome are as follows:
i.   postinfectious secondary immunodeficiency syndrome (PIFSI);
ii.   (ii) postinfectious autoimmune syndrome (PIFA);
iii. autoimmune syndrome coupled with postinfectious secondary immunodeficiency (PIFASID) (Suchkov et al., 2004).
Predisposition to one or another form of syndromeal immune pathology depends on a great number of genetically determined factors, which play a key role in the formation of patient's own immune resources. Its functional activity is controlled by coordinated functioning of *innate* and *adaptive* immune mechanisms; however, their role in the development and chronization of infectious processes is still open to question, which strongly impedes the construction of state-of-art immunopathogenetic models (Fig. 2).

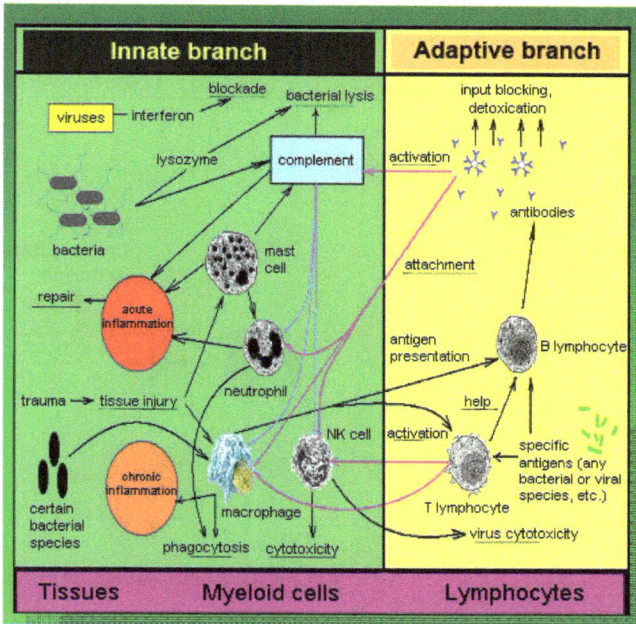

Fig. 2. The innate and adaptive branches of immunity.

In this context, analysis of major immunopathologic manifestations in patients with PICIS-related chronically relapsing infectious diseases and construction of basic algorithms for state-of-art immunogenetic diagnostic protocols becomes a prime target for clinical medicine.

Human immune system is a complex physiological mechanism whereby the human organism protects itself from exogenous etiopathogenic attacks. Its functional activity is provided by two types of protective immune mechanisms, one of which is *specific* and the other one is *nonspecific*. The main outcome of the immune response to etiopathogenic attacks is formation of two populations of regulatory T helper cells (Th cells). The Th population is further subdivided into Th1 cells responsible for activation of effector links of cell-mediated immunity (macrophages and cytotoxic T lymphocytes/CTL) and Th2 cells exerting control over antibody (AB) production (McGuirk & Mills, 2002) (Fig. 3).

However, the key factor in determining a particular type of the immune response and, correspondingly, a particular form of CIS, is localization (*extracellular* or *intracellular*) of the etiopathogen (Fig. 4).

The latter circumstance is of particular importance from both pathogenetic and clinical points of view, since the majority of currently known pathogenic microorganisms can escape from immune control and, in doing so, change the scenario of genetically programmed immune responsiveness thereby provoking unpredictable complications for the patient and hindering physician's attempts to implement adequate treatment strategies (Azikury, 1985; Aitpaev & Seisembekov, 1987).

Two major disturbances in immune responsiveness are presently recognized as causal factors in chronization of infectious diseases and formation of PICIS:

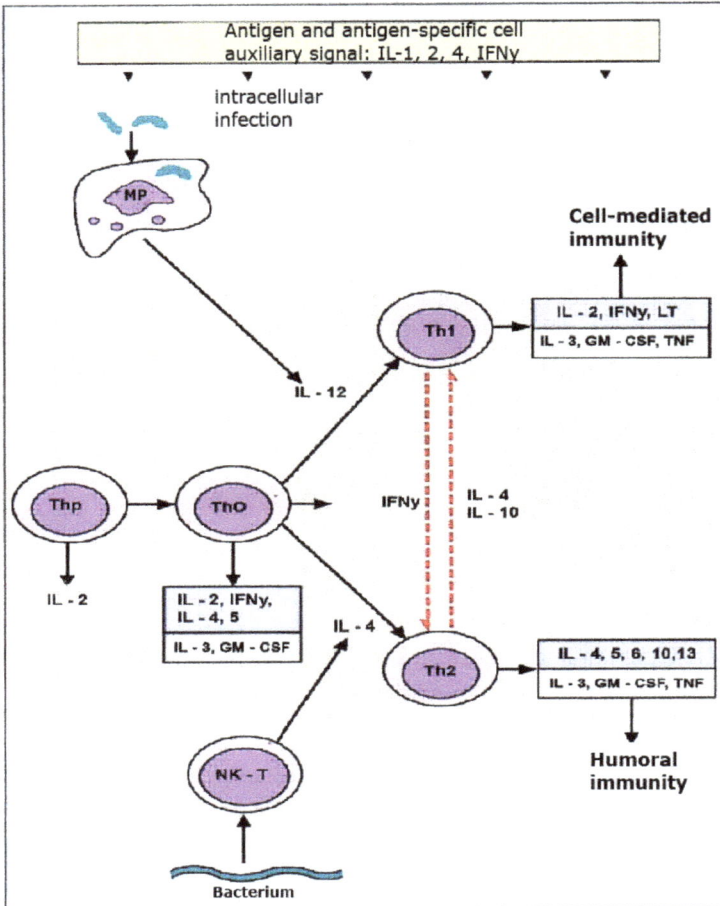

Note: In the presence of IL-4, precursor Th0 cells are transformed into Th2 cells whose main function consists in activation of humoral immunity and production of definite classes of cytokins, viz., IL-3, IL-4, IL-5, IL-6, IL-10, IL-13, TNF, etc. Under the action of IL-12, Th0 precursors are transformed into Th2 cells stimulating the production of other cytokin populations, e.g., IL-2, IL-3, IFN –γ, TNF-α, TNF-β, etc., able to activate cell-mediated immune responses. Other Th1/Th2 classes are represented by natural killer cells (NK cells), helper T cells (Th cells), granulocytic macrophageal colony-stimulating factors (GM-CSF), interferon (IFN), interleukin (IL), macrophages (MØ) and tumor necrosis factor (TNF).

Fig. 3. The pathways of formation of Th1/Th2 lymphocytes.

i.   deficiency of effector links of immunity with predominant involvement of the T link (as in the case of isolated forms of PIFSI);
ii. disbalance of intercellular immunoregulatory mechanisms responsible for the formation of associated forms of syndromeal immune pathologies, e.g., PIFA and PIFASID).

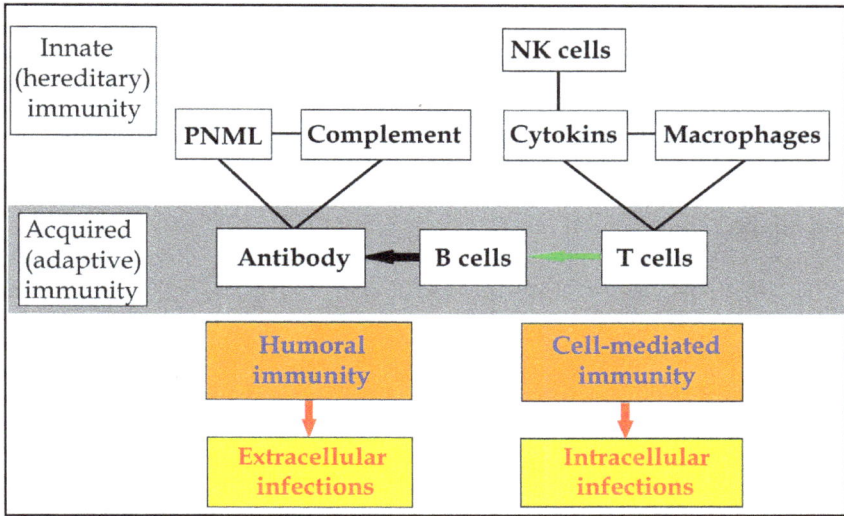

Note: PMNL and NK are polymorphonuclear leukocytes and natural killer cells, respectively.

Fig. 4. The contribution of the innate and adaptive branches of immunity to control over intra- and extracellular infections.

2. Clinical manifestations of PICIS in the framework of clinical models of CRID

As targets for our investigation, we chose three classical models of CRID, namely, intracranial infectious inflammatory pathologies (ICIIP), chronic pyelonephrites (CPN) and myocardites (M). All these pathologies have one common feature (i.e., association with a concrete organ or a tissue), but differ from one another both topically and pathogenetically. Although the panel of immunologic disturbances varies substantially depending on the clinical form of PICIS, immune statuses of patients and clinical manifestations of the diseases are very similar (Antonov & Tsinzerling, 2001; Borisov, 2000; Kukhtevich et al., 1997; Morozov, 2001; Paukov, 1996).

2.1 Immunopathological factors as biomarkers and biopredictors of chronization of infectious diseases
2.1.1 Inflammation mediators as PICIS-related factors
Emergence and accumulation, in patient's blood, of inflammation markers whose concentration reaches the highest level in patients with PIFA and degresses in the direction from PIFASID to PIFSI are the most common markers of chronization of infectious diseases and formation of syndromeal immune pathologies (Mazo et al., 2007; Litvinov et al., 2008; Zhmurov et al., 2000; Rumyantsev & Goncharova, 2000).

2.1.2 Abnormalities in the innate branch of immunity as a PICIS-related factor
Miscellaneous shifts in the innate branch of immunity play a no less important role in chronization of infectious diseases. Thus, pronounced suppression of innate immune

mechanisms is a salient feature of PIFSI, while PIFA and PIFASID are distinguished for disproportions in individual links of innate immunity and/or disbalance in the functional activity of its specific mechanisms (Bauer et al., 2001; Bingen-Bidois et al., 2002; Blackwell et al., 1987; Carballido et al., 2003; Dantzer & Wollman, 2003).

Complement deficiency. In patients with PIFA and PIFASID, outbursts of activity in the C5 and C5a components of the complement are usually observed against the background of stable operation of the majority of other links of the immune system (PIFA) or pronounced disproportions between them (PIFASID).

Deficiency of phagocytosis and cytotoxicity mechanisms. To factors responsible for chronization of infectious diseases, one may relate oppositely directed changes in phagocytosis and cytotoxicity parameters. In PIFSI, both mechanisms are strongly suppressed, while in PIFA and PIFASID relative stability of certain components of both systems is concomitant with disproportions in other components.

Deficiency of dendritic cells. Dendritic cells (DCs) are among the most essential regulatory factors in the innate branch of immunity. In patients with PIFSI, the specific contribution of these cells is rather small, while in case of PIFASID and PIFA DCs play a prominent role and show a tendency for activation (Sanaev et al., 2008; Cherepakhina et al., 2009).

2.1.3 Abnormalities in the adaptive branch of immunity as a PICIS-related factor

Deficiency of T cell-mediated immunity. Among other disturbances in the adaptive branch of immunity, special attention should be given to differently directed changes in T cell-mediated immunity. PIFSI, for example, is characterized by enhanced suppression of T cell functions resulting from disproportions in immunoregulatory components and massive apoptosis of T cells. In contrast, activation of T cell-mediated immunity is critical for PIFA and PIFASID, being more pronounced for the former and less pronounced for the latter.

Deficiency of humoral immunity. Suppression of humoral immunity is a characteristic feature of PIFSI, while PIFA and PIFASID are associated with its activation. The activating effect of quantitative and qualitative (functional) mechanisms of humoral immunity is especially apparent in PIFA, while in patients with PIFASID this effect is far less expressed.

Disproportions in the cytokin spectrum of the blood. PIFSI is associated with significant reduction of the population of antiinflammatory cytokins, while in PIFA this population is predominant. PIFASID is characterized by general disproportions in the cytokin spectrum at large (Cherepakhina et al., 2010a).

3. PICIS and its main clinical forms

3.1 PIFSI

The main clinical manifestations of PIFSI are related to disturbances in antimicrobial protective mechanisms due to deficiency of the innate branch of immunity and development of secondary immune pathologies in the adaptive branch of immunity. The latter manifest themselves as chronically relapsing infectious diseases of bacterial or mixed origin (Shogenov et al., 2006).

3.2 PIFA

During induction and progression of CRID, some autoreactive CTL cross-reacting with microbial antigens (Ags) in the paradigm of the infectious process undergo activation by hazardous factors including *molecular mimicry* (Khitrov et al., 2007a; Fujinami et al., 2006; Rose & Mackay, 2000; Benoist & Mathis, 2001). Its consequences are especially apparent during recognition of determinant autoAgs by T cells and subsequent formation of the PIFA syndrome (Fig. 5). The latter attack any target organ or tissue of the infected organism by a rocket mechanism. The risk of PIFA development increases dramatically with increasing incidence of infectious diseases and the panel of infecting pathogens (*mixed* infections).

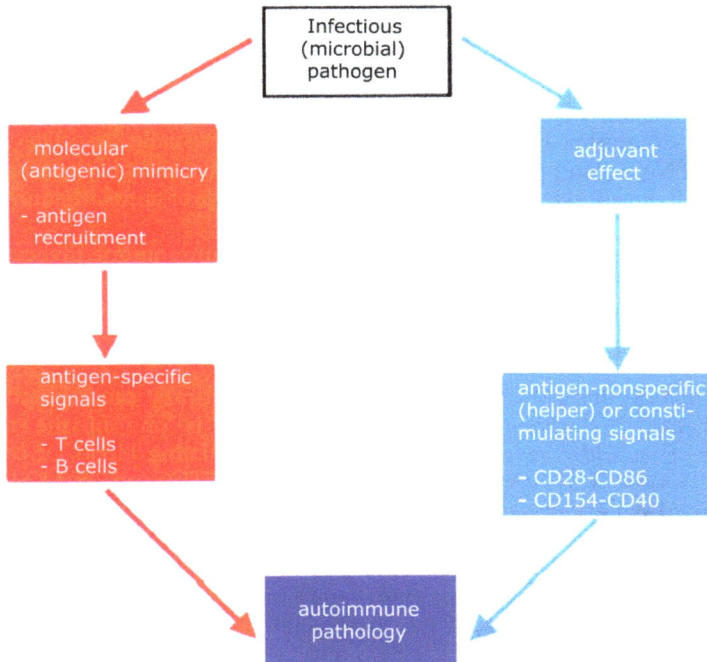

Note: The primary infectious (microbial) pathogen triggers a postinfectious autoimmune syndrome (PIFA) through activation of two different mechanisms: (i) depletion of intrinsic (antigenic) molecular mimicry pools of cross-reacting (mimicking) antigenic determinants of the infecting pathogen (red arrows); (b) generation, by the infectious pathogen, of antigen-nonspecific signals (blue arrows) able to induce inflammation and thus enhance immune responsiveness (so-called adjuvant effect).

Fig. 5. A schematic representation of the postinfectious autoimmune syndrome (PIFA).

There exist at least three different interpretations for the relatedness of the infectious process to the risk of PIFA in response to activation of autoreactive clones of T and B lymphocytes, namely: (i) stimulation by microbial *superAgs*; (ii) secretion of *cryptic* (intramolecular) autoAg determinants in response to cell damage induced by persisting infections and (iii) molecular mimicry. These pathogenetic mechanisms are not mutually exclusive and play a crucial role in definite (as a rule, early) steps of PIFA-related CRID. The main triggering factors in the PIFA initiation step are: (i) antigenic activity of the microbial pathogen and (ii) tropism of the microbial pathogen towards definite cell populations, organs and tissues as targets for its cytopathic effect (Vturin et al., 1994; Manges et al., 2004).

Contrary to PIFSI, all classes of antimicrobial ABs (antibacterial, antiviral, antiparasitic, etc.) are morbid in PIFA. Although in the majority of patients the incidence and titers of antibacterial and antiviral ABs are more or less identical, in certain forms of CRID (e.g., CPN or M) antiparasitic ABs are detected in highest titers, while in patients with other pathologies (e.g., ICIIP) they are absent. These findings can be attributed to clinical manifestations of the underlying diseases rather than to inadequate functioning of triggering mechanisms of PIFA) (Cherepakhina et al., 2010b).

Indeed, autoaggression provoked by insufficient coordination between two branches of immunity and hyperfunction of its adaptive branch is a dominant feature of PIFA. Its unique feature is a vast repertoire of antiorganic and antitissue autoABs responsible for *multiseropositivity* and specific autoimmune inflammation markers, e.g., anti-B7-HI autoABs) (Khitrov et al., 2007).

By illustration, antimyelin and antineuronal autoABs are usually associated with ICIIP. Patients with CPN contain predominantly anti-THG autoABs as highly specific markers of autoimmune inflammation in renal tissue, while the presence of anti-KM autoABs indicates AIM (Miller et al., 1970).

To the most informative models of PIFA one may relate autoimmune myocarditis (AIM), autoimmune encephalomyelitis (AEM), ICIIP, rheumatoid arthritis (PA), autoimmune hepatitis (AIHe), autoimmune colienteritis (AICE), autoimmune pancreatitis (AIPCT), autoimmune gastritis (AIGa), autoimmune (streptococcal) glomerulonephritis (AGN), CPN, etc.

Autoimmune myocarditis (AIM) usually develops in genetically predisposed individuals infected with the Coxsackievirus-3 virus (CVB3) and is one of the most typical manifestations of *molecular mimicry*. The presence, in circulating blood, of cardiomyosin-autoreactive cytotoxic T lymphocytes (KM-autoreactive CTL) and anti-KM autoABs is prerequisite to AIM development. Their interactions in patients with *PIFA* or *PIFASID* initiate myocardial lesions in response to enhanced secretion of sequestered autoAgs (Shogenov et al., 2010) (Fig. 6).

In type I diabetes mellitus (DM I), *insulitis* develops in genetically predisposed individuals at the earliest (preclinical) stages of the disease (as a rule, against the background of infection with the Coxsackie-4 virus (CVB4)), and is further transformed into PIFA. This pathological process is mediated by autoreactive CTL and autoABs against islet autoAgs. Their coordinated functioning initiates the destruction (direct or indirect) of beta cells, e.g., through secretion of cytokins, generation of free radicals or apoptosis of beta cells, eventually resulting in *PIFA* or *PIFASID*.

The main causal factors in initiation of chronically relapsing autoimmune colienteritis (AICE) are mimicking AGs of microbial or dietary origin. These AGs are localized in the intestinal lumen where they activate immune cells of intestinal mucosa. Having penetrated into these cells, AGs begin to interact with tissue immunocytes (most frequently, with lymphocytes and DCs) thereby triggering adaptive immune responses. Innate immune resources also become activated under the stimulating effect of microbial products due to activation of specific surface receptors of intestinal epithelium. This reaction cascade stimulates the secretion of numerous cytokins and chemokins able to activate immunocytes of intestinal mucosa. Activation of antigen-presenting cells (APC) (e.g., DCs) initiate enhanced production of Th1 cells (Crohn's disease) or atypical Th2 cells (ulcerative colitis). In addition to major cytokins stimulating the activity of Th1 cells (IL-12, IL-18, etc.), activated macrophages give rise to a great diversity of antiinflammatory cytokins (IL-1, IL-6,

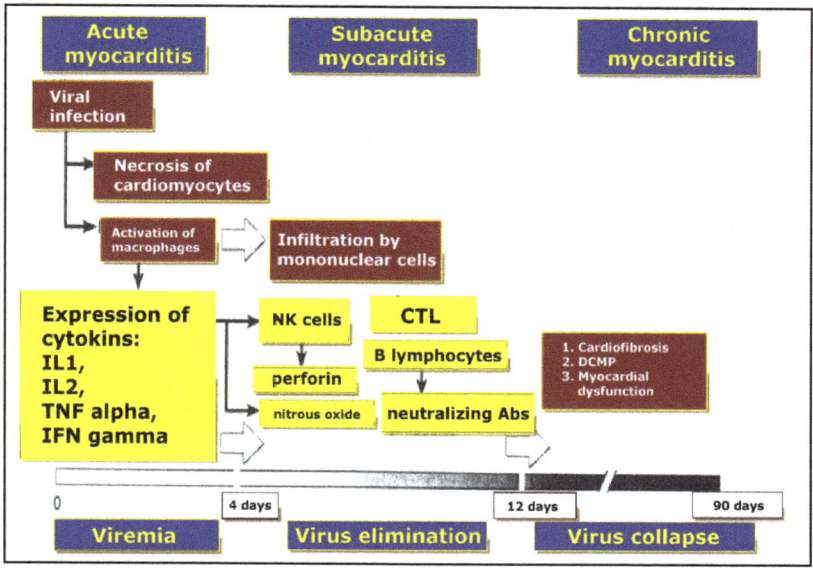

Note: AB – antibody; CTL – cytotoxic T lymphocyte; IFN - interferon; IL – interleukin; NK – natural killer cell; DCMП – dilated cardiomyopathy.

Fig. 6. Initiation and progression of myocarditis

TNF alpha, etc.) endowed with an ability to stimulate the activity of different cell populations (including endothelial cells) in inflammation foci by promoting enhanced migration of lymphocytes, fibroblasts and epithelial cells from the vascular network to inflammation niduses, which significantly deteriorates the clinical picture of autoimmune nidal inflammation (Khaitov & Pinegin, 2000; Bach, 2005).

3.3 PIFASID
A salient feature of this syndrome is equal contribution of associated abnormalities to both branches of immunity. Its clinical picture is distinguished for mixed-type immunopathology, viz., autoimmune syndrome coupled with immunodeficiency and concurrent deterioration of antiinfectious protection.

4. Associative correlation between clinical manifestations of PICIS and CRID

The associativity between microbial infection and various immunopathological states with PICIS can be correlative or causal. In patients with CRID, syndromal forms of immune pathologies depend critically on the stage of the inflammatory process occurring in target organs or tissues and general chronization of the disease (Sanaev et al., 2007).

For example, early stages of CRID are concomitant with PIFSI (› 50%), whereas the contribution of PIFA and PIFASID does not exceed 20%. At the subsequent stages, the clinical picture is different, viz., the contribution of the autoimmune syndrome increases dramatically (to 50% at the intermediate stages (PIFA) and to 60% at the final stage (PIFASID).

The correlation between the stage of CRID and the form of PICIS is also characterized by the involvement of an additional (third) component, viz., clinical form or variant of CRID. Here are several analytical examples related to:

1. *clinical form of CRID.* In patients with primary pyelonephritis (PPNP) and infectious myocarditis (IM), PIFSI is detected in 75% of cases, whereas in patients with secondary pyelonephrites (SPNP) and AIM the contribution of PIFSI is notably decreased (to 25%) giving way to autoaggression (the contribution of PIFA and PIFASID increases to 60% and 85%, respectively);

2. *stage of CRID.* At early stages (< 3 months for CPN and < 1 month for myocarditis (M)), PIFSI is detected in 40% of cases; however, at later stages of CRID its share decreases appreciably, while that of autoimmune syndromes increases in contrast;

3. *rate of progression and chronization of CRID.* In patients with relapsing or rapidly progressing CRID (e.g., ICIIP or AIM), the contribution of PIFSI does not exceed 32-36%, while the share of autoimmune syndromes reaches 80-100%. In such patients, persistent forms of meningoencephalitis (e.g., ICIIP) or AIM associated with myocardial dystrophies are predominant.

These findings suggest that PIFSI is not only the outcome of the infectious process, but also represents a factor responsible for its lingering and chronically relapsing course. Further progression and *chronization* of CRID are controlled by postinfectious autoaggression factors, such as PIFA and PIFASID.

5. Clinico-immunological criteria of PICIS and state-of-art immunogenetic diagnostic algorithms

So far, there is no unique set of criteria for adequate assessment of immune statuses of patients with different forms of PICIS, most probably, due to immense diversity of clinical manifestations of syndromal immunopathologies and factors responsible for their emergence. Moreover, existing laboratory protocols for assessing immune statuses are nonspecific and do not include specific analyses of microbial pathogens (Vinnitskij, 2002; Kolesnikov et al., 2001; Cherepakhina et al., 2010c).

With this in mind and in order to procure adequate evaluation of many syndromal immune pathologies, we developed a series of clinical and immunologic tests and criteria for more precise diagnosis of PICIS. The criteria for constructing immunogram charts include:

i.   *screening of abnormalities in the innate branch of immunity* (selective markers of phagocytosis, natural cytotoxicity (NCT), basic functional parameters of DC- and Ag-presenting cells (APC) and complement components (if necessary);

ii. *screening of abnormalities in the adaptive branch of immunity* (selective markers of effector or regulatory links of the immune system, serotyping of blood elements for anti-organic and anti-tissue autoABs concurrently with identification of Abs against mimicking Ag determinants of infecting pathogens).

The main criteria in the etiotropic diagnosis step (design of microbial landscape maps) include:

i.   identification and localization of microbial gene pools;

ii. serological profiles of antimicrobial ABs.

The novel diagnostic ideology is based on a combination of two categories of investigations:

i.   pathogenetically oriented diagnosis of PICIS and (ii) etiotropic diagnosis of microbial pathogens as the main causal factors of PICIS.

The most efficient technological strategies will be based on:

i.   at the *immunodiagnostics* stage (cytofluorimetric analysis of processing and presentation of AGs on the surface of APC, monitoring of antiorganic and antitissue autoAB pools, analysis of metabolic profiles of individual cells, etc.);

ii. *etiotropic diagnostics* (combination of conventional techniques for culturing microbial cells with advanced molecular diagnostics strategies based on sequencing of microbial genomes, screening of biological fluids and tissues for antimicrobial ABs, etc.).

6. Conclusion

Morbidity from infectious pathologies (e.g., CRID), in the first place, those provoked by viruses, conditionally pathogenic ("opportunistic") microflora and/or pathogens endowed with atypical properties including muiltiple resistance to antibacterial drugs, is steadily increasing. Among other things, CRID-affected individuals are characterized by lowering general immune responsiveness concurrent with unusual forms of immune responses to the clinical course of the infectious pathology. Studies in this field including our own investigations established that PICIS is one of the most important clinical manifestations of CRID, since it determines, in many features, the progression and chronization of underlying pathologies and their possible complications. The *monosyndromal* dominant form of PICIS in patients with CRID is PIFSI. However, more than 30% of CRID patients suffer from more specific forms of PICIS concomitant with autoimmune aggression (PIFA) or from combined immunopathological forms (e.g., PIFASID).

Clinical forms of PICIS and, correspondingly, immunologic disturbances in patients with CRID correlate associatively with the clinical picture of the disease. It is not excluded that chronization of infectious inflammatory processes involves a general sequence of pathogenetically important factors, which differ in inner architechtonics of each of PICIS variants and thus demonstrate their high criterial significance.

Future progress in clinical immunology and immune biotechnology may open up fresh opportunities for introduction into routine clinical practice of advanced protocols for immunogenetic diagnostics of PICIS-related infectious diseases and design of state-of-art treatment-and-rehabilitation protocols based on the use of the most advanced immunogenetic tools and strategies.

7. References

Suchkov S.V.; Shogenov Z.S. & Khitrov A.N. (2007). Postinfectious autoimmune syndrome: features of pathogenesis and modern protocols of clinical immunogenodiagnostics. *Therapeutic Archives*. Vol.79, No.4, (April 2007), pp. 71-76, ISSN 0040-3660

Paltsev M.A.; Cherepakhina N.E. & Suchkov S.V. (2009). Postinfectious clinical immunologic syndrome: foundations of etiopathogenesis and strategy of immunogenodiagnostics. *Bulletin of the Russian Academy of Medical Sciences*. Vol.10, (October, 2009), pp. 25-31, ISSN 0869-6047

Paltsev M.A. Clinical and immune-mediated syndrome (CAIMS) in clinical practice: features and strategies in immune and molecular diagnostics. (2009). *New Horizons in Allergy, Asthma & Immunology*, pp. 177-181, ISBN 978-88-7587-505-3, Dubai, UAE, April 24-27, 2009

Suchkov S.V.; Blagoveschenskij S.V. & Vinnitskij L.I. (2004). Modern aspects of immunopathogenesis and immunocorrection in patients with intracranial infectious inflammatory diseases. *Allergology and Immunology*. Vol.5, No.2, (2004), pp. 323-330, ISSN 1562-3637

McGuirk P. & Mills K.H. Pathogen-specific regulatory T cells provoke a shift in the Th1/Th2 paradigm in immunity to infectious diseases. (2002). *Trends in Immunology*. Vol.23, No.9, (September 2002), pp. 450-455, ISSN 1471-4906

Azikury O.I. Cellular and humoral immunity at pyelonephritis. (1985). *Urology and Nephrology*. Vol.2, (March 1985), pp. 10-11, ISSN 0042-1154

Aitpaev B. K. & Seisembekov T.Z. (1987). Cellular and humoral factors of nonspecific resistance and immunologic reactivity at chronic pyelonephritis. *Therapeutic Archives*. Vol.8, (August 1987), pp. 59-63, ISSN 0040-3660

Antonov V.P. & Tsinzerling V.A. Contemporary status of the problem of chronic and slow neuroinfections. (2001). *Archieves of Pathology*. Vol.63(1), (January 2001), pp. 47-51, ISSN 0004-1955

Borisov I.A. Pyelonephritis. (2000). In: *Nephrology*, Tareeva I.E. (Ed.), pp. 383-399, Medicine, ISBN 5-225-04195-7, Moscow, Russia

Kukhtevich A.V.; Gordovskaya N.B. & Kozlovskaya N.L. Pyelonephritis. *Russian Medical Journal*. Vol.5, No.23, (December 1997), pp. 54-62, ISSN 0869-7760

Morozov A.V. Chronic infection of urinary tract (pathogenesis, diagnostic and treatment principles). *Russian Medical Journal*. Vol.9, No.23, (December 2001), pp. 1074-1077, ISSN 0869-7760

Paukov V.S. Immunology and morphology of chronic inflammation. *Achieves of Pathology*. Vol.58(1), (January 1996), pp. 28-33, ISSN 0869-7760

Mazo E.B.; Vinnitskij L.I. & Litvinov V.A. (2007). Chronic pyelonephritis: features of immunopathogenesis and its' clinical and diagnostical values. *Therapeutic Archives*. Vol.79(1), (January 2007), pp. 85-89, ISSN 0040-3660

Litvinov V.A.; Cherepakhina N.E. & Suchkov S.V. (2008). Chronic pyelonephritis: features of immunopathogenesis and principles of clinical immunogenetic diagnostics. *Physician*. Vol.1, (January 2008), pp. 12-17, ISSN 0236-3054

Zhmurov V.A.; Oskolkov V.A. & Malishevskij M.V. (2000). Correlation between immunogenetic markers and metabolic processes at chronic pyelonephritis. *Urology*. Vol.3, (2000), pp. 9-13, ISSN 0042-1154

Rumyantsev A.S. & Goncharova I.S. Etiology and pathogenesis of pyelonephritis. *Nephrology*. Vol.4, No.3, (2000), pp. 40-52, ISSN 1561-6274

Bauer J.; Rauschka H. & Lassmann H. Inflammation in the nervous system: the human perspective. *Glia*, Vol.36, No.2, (November 2001), pp. 235-243, ISSN 1098-1136

Bingen-Bidois M.; Clermont O. & Bonacorsi S. Phylogenetic analysis and prevalence of urosepsis strains of Escherichia coli bearing pathogenicity island-like domains. *Infect Immun*. Vol. 70, No.6, (June 2002), pp. 3216-3226, ISSN 1098-5522

Blackwell C.C.; May S.J. & Brettle R.P. Secretor state and immunoglobulin levels among women with recurrent urinary tract infections. *J Clin Lab Immunol*. Vol.22, No.3, (1987), pp. 133-137, ISSN 0141-2760

Carballido J.A.; Alvarez-Mon M. & Olivier C. Inflammatory pathology in urology. Standardization. *Actas Urol Esp*. Vol.27, No.3, (March 2003), pp. 173-179, ISSN 0210-4806

Dantzer R. & Wollman E.E.   Relationships between the brain and the immune system. *J Soc Biol.* Vol.197, No.2, (2003), pp. 81-88, ISSN 0037-766X

Sanaev A.O.; Kachkov I.A. & Vinnitskij L.I. (2008). Immunomonitoring and immunorehabilitation in case of intracranial infectious inflammatory diseases. *Russian Journal of Immunology.* Vol.2(11), No.1, (2008), pp. 78-82, ISSN 1028-7221

Cherepakhina N.E.; Shogenov Z.S. & Elbeik T. (2009). Postinfectious clinical-and-immunologic syndrome and its place in clinical practice. *Therapeutic Archives.* Vol.81(1), No.12, (December 2009), pp. 71-78, ISSN 0040-3660

Cherepakhina N.E.; Tabaksoeva D.A. & Suchkov S.V. (2010). Associative relation of microbial factor and postinfectious clinical-and-immunologic syndrome in case of chronic relapsing diseases. *Clinical Microbiology and Antimicrobial Chemotherapy.* Vol.12, No.2, suppl.1, (2010), p. 54, ISSN 1684-4386

Shogenov Z.S.; Cherepakhina N.E. & Suchkov S.V. (2006). Immunogenetic diagnostics and postinfectious immunodeficiency syndrome in physicians' practice. *Clinical Laboratory Diagnostics.* Vol.11, (November 2006), pp. 36-43, ISSN 0869-2084

Khitrov A.N.; Shogenov Z.S. & Suchkov S.V. (2007). Molecular mimicry phenomenon and its place in postinfectious autoimmune syndrome (PIFA) pathogenesis. *Molecular Medicine.* Vol.4, (2007), pp. 24-32, ISSN 1728-2918

Fujinami R.S.; von Herrath M.G. & Christen U. Molecular mimicry, bystander activation, or viral persistence: infections and autoimmune disease. *Clin. Microbiol. Rev.* Vol.19, No.1, (January 2006), pp. 80-94, ISSN 0893-8512

Rose N.R. & Mackay I.R.   Molecular mimicry: a critical look at exemplary instances in human diseases . *Cell Mol. Life Sci.* Vol.57, No.4 (April 2000), pp. 542-551, ISSN 1420-682X

Benoist C. & Mathis D.   Autoimmunity provoked by infection: how good is the case for T cell epitope mimicry?   *Nat. Immunol.* Vol.2, No.9, (September 2001), pp. 797-801, ISSN 1529-2908

Vturin B.V.; Delektorskij V.V. & Kovalchuk V.K. Pathogenic mechanisms of bacteria at different infections. (1994). *Archives of pathology.* Vol.56, No.5, (September 1994), pp. 10-15, ISSN 0004-1955

Manges A.R.; Dietrich P.S. & Riley L.W. Multidrug-resistant Escherichia coli clonal groups causing community-acquired pyelonephritis. *Clin Infect Dis.* Vol.38, No.3, (February 2004), pp. 329-334, ISSN 0934-9723

Cherepakhina N.E.; Maksimenko D.M. & Suchkov S.V. (2010). Microbial landscape and its value for the modern model of immunopathogenesis of chronic relapsing infectious diseases. *Proceedings of the III World asthma & COPD forum and World forum of pediatrics*, pp. 99-102, ISBN 978-88-7587-558-9, Dubai, UAE, April 24-27, 2010

Khitrov A.N.; Shogenov Z.S. & Tretyak E.B. (2007). Postinfectious immunodeficiency and autoimmunity: pathogenic and clinical values and implications. *Expert Review of Clinical Immunology.* Vol.3, No.3, (May 2007), pp. 323-331, ISSN 1744-666X

Miller T.E.; Smith J.W. & Lehmann J.W. Autoimmunity in chronic experimental pyelonephritis. *J Infect Dis.* Vol.122, No.3, (September 1970), pp. 191-195, ISSN 1344-6304

Shogenov Z.S.; Akhmedilova K.A. & Tabaksoeva D.A. Features of immunopathogenesis and chronization of myocarditis as the basis of immunogenetic diagnostic and immunogenetic monitoring protocols development. *Russian cardiology journal.* Vol.6(86), (November 2010), pp. 76-87, ISSN 1560-4071

Khaitov R.M. & Pinegin B.V. Contemporary conceptions of safeguard of host organism against infection. *Immunology.* Vol.1, (January 2000), pp. 61-64, ISSN 0206-4952

Bach J.F. Infections and autoimmunity. *Rev. Med. Interne.* Vol.1, (October 2005), pp. 32-34, ISSN 0248-8663

Sanaev A.O.; Kachkov I.A. & Vinnitskij L.I. (2007). Modern aspects of immunotherapy at intracranial infectious inflammatory diseases therapy by example of brain abscesses. *Allergology and Immunology.* Vol.8, No.4, (2007), pp. 384-387, ISSN 1562-3637

Vinnitskij L.I. Diagnostic facilities of contemporary immune technologies in surgical clinic. (2002) *Allergology and Immunology.* Vol.3, No.1, (2002), pp. 198-203, ISSN 1562-3637

Kolesnikov A.P.; Khabarov A.S. & Kozlov V.A. (2001). Diagnostics and differentiated treatment of secondary immunodeficiencies. *Therapeutic Archives.* Vol.73(4), (April 2001), pp. 55-59, ISSN 0040-3660

Cherepakhina N.E.; Maksimenko D.M. & Suchkov S.V. (2010). Strategy of immunotherapy and immunorehabilitation of chronic relapsing infectious. *International Journal on Immunorehabilitation.* Vol.12, No.2, (May 2010), p. 139, ISSN 1562-3629

7

Contribution of Peroxynitrite, a Reactive Nitrogen Species, in the Pathogenesis of Autoimmunity

Rizwan Ahmad[1] and Haseeb Ahsan[2]
[1]Department of Biochemistry, Oman Medical College, Sohar,
[2]Department of Biochemistry, Faculty of Dentistry, Jamia Millia Islamia, New Delhi,
[1]Sultanate of Oman
[2]India

1. Introduction

Peroxynitrite is a member of reactive nitrogen species that also includes nitric oxide ($\cdot$NO) and nitrogen dioxide radical ($NO_2\cdot$). Peroxynitrite is a reactive nitrogen species and an anion with the formula ($ONOO^-$). It is an unstable 'valence isomer' of nitrate (NO_3^-), making it an oxidant and nitrating agent. Because of its oxidizing properties, peroxynitrite can damage a wide range of molecules in cells, including DNA and proteins (1). It is produced by the body in response to a variety of environmental toxins, stress, ultraviolet light and many other stimuli. It is also produced in the body due to ischemia/ reperfusion injury and inflammation (2, 3). *In vivo,* peroxynitrite is formed in the macrophages, endothelial cells, platelets, leukocytes, neurons, etc by the reaction between $O_2\cdot^-$ and $\cdot$NO (4, 5). Tissue inflammation and chronic infection lead to the overproduction of $\cdot$NO and $O_2\cdot^-$, which rapidly combine to yield peroxynitrite: $O_2\cdot^- + \cdot NO \rightarrow ONO_2^-$. Endothelial $\cdot$NO synthase (eNOS) is responsible for most of the vascular $\cdot$NO produced. The eNOS oxidizes its substrate L-arginine to L-citrulline and $\cdot$NO. A functional eNOS requires dimerization of the enzyme, the substrate L-arginine, and an essential cofactor, BH4 (5,6,7,8-tetrahydro-L-biopterin). The $O_2\cdot^-$ produced can react with vascular $\cdot$NO to form peroxynitrite. Diminished levels of BH4 promote $O_2\cdot^-$ production by eNOS. The transformation of eNOS from a vasoprotective enzyme to a contributor to oxidative stress has been observed in several *in vitro* systems, animal models of cardiovascular diseases and in patients with cardiovascular risk factors (6). In inflammation or septic shock, $\cdot$NO is also synthesized by the inducible $\cdot$NO synthase (iNOS), an isoform that is expressed in many cell types including vascular endothelial cells, vascular smooth muscle and inflammatory cells in response to pro-inflammatory cytokines. Peroxynitrite, can be formed intravascularly in various disease conditions when there is overproduction of either $\cdot$NO or $O_2\cdot^-$ (7). The intravascular formation of peroxynitrite can result in oxidative modifications of plasma and vessel wall proteins including the formation of protein-3-nitrotyrosine. Protein tyrosine nitration in plasma or vessel wall proteins may be indicative of peroxynitrite formation, and constitutes a good biomarker of $\cdot$NO-derived oxidant production in the vascular space. Detection of 3-nitrotyrosine *in vivo* has attracted considerable interest not only as a biomarker of peroxynitrite formation but also as a predictor of vascular risk (8).

Peroxynitrite is a potent oxidant and nitrating species formed by rapid reaction of two free radicals – nitric oxide and superoxide anion (9). It can modify variety of biomolecules but possesses high affinity for tyrosine residues in proteins, and 3-nitrotyrosine is a relatively specific marker of peroxynitrite mediated damage to proteins (10). Other markers of peroxynitrite-induced protein modifications are; cysteine oxidation, oxidation/nitration of tryptophan and tyrosine, protein carbonyls, dityrosine and fragmentation. In view of numerous reports on detection of significant amount of 3-nitrotyrosine in various pathological conditions, the significance of non-enzymatic tyrosine nitration in health and disease has become a subject of great interest. Protein nitration has been observed in atherosclerosis, hypertension, Parkinson's, Huntington's and Alzheimer's disease (11-13), multiple sclerosis (14), autoimmune myocarditis (15), systemic lupus erythematosus (SLE) (16) and rheumatoid arthritis (17). Furthermore, self proteins become immunologically active if their structure is altered. Accumulations of a variety of chemically modified proteins have been reported in inflamed tissues or apoptotic cells (18).

Histones are highly conserved proteins but poorly immunogenic. These positively charged proteins were found to be immunogenic after acetylation or complexation with RNA. Autoantibodies against histones are present as often as anti-DNA antibodies in SLE. It has been demonstrated that anti-native DNA autoantibodies are commonly co-present with anti-histone autoantibodies and may react with each of the five chromatin-associated histones and also with H3–H4 and H2A–H2B complex (19). However, importance of anti-histone antibodies in SLE is confounded by discrepancies in their reported prevalence, isotype, specificity and correlation with symptoms. Over expression of inducible nitric oxide synthase enzyme has been seen in numerous tissues of active SLE patients, *vis-à-vis* higher level of serum nitrotyrosine. Nitrotyrosine serves as a long-term indicator of peroxynitrite-mediated protein modification and it is not affected by endogenous source of NOx or serum thiol (20). The *in vivo* nitration of histones (as shown in cultured cells exposed to nitric oxide donors and mutatect tumour tissues) appears to be a potentially useful marker for demonstrating extended exposure of cells/tissues to NO derived reactive nitrogen species. The generation of peroxynitrite by activated macrophages, neutrophils and endothelial cells and presence of nitrotyrosine in human tissues, fluids and in animal models of various diseases needs further investigation on protein-peroxynitrite interactions (21).

2. Cellular biochemistry and pathology

Peroxynitrite is a relatively long-lived oxidant that may serve as an important cytotoxic agent. Its biological effects are due to its reactivity toward a large number of molecules including lipids, amino acids, and nucleic acids. It is involved in tissue damage in a number of pathophysiological conditions such as neurodegenerative diseases, cardiovascular disorders, etc. (1-3). Evidence suggests that most of the cytotoxicity attributed to nitric oxide is due to peroxynitrite, produced from the reaction between the free radical species, $\cdot NO$ and $O_2^{\cdot -}$. Peroxynitrite interacts with lipids, DNA and proteins causing oxidative damage and other free radical induced chain reactions. These reactions trigger cellular responses such as cell signaling, oxidative injury, committing cells to necrosis or apoptosis. *In vivo*, peroxynitrite generation represents a crucial pathological mechanism in conditions such as stroke, myocardial infarction, chronic heart failure, diabetes, inflammation, neurodegenerative disorders and cancer. Even though nucleic acid antigens are by themselves poorly immunogenic, their antigenicity can be enhanced by modification through different free radicals (8).

Peroxynitrite exhibits unique chemical reactivities such as protein nitration, DNA strand breakage, base modification, etc., which may have cytotoxic effects and also lead to mutagenesis. It is thought to be involved in both cell death and an increased cancer risk (8-22,23). The reaction of peroxynitrite with lipids leads to peroxidation (malondialdehyde and conjugated diene formation) and formation of nitrito-, nitro-, nitrosoperoxo-, and nitrated lipid oxidation derivatives (24-26). Peroxynitrite is a particularly effective oxidant of aromatic molecules, thioethers and organosulfur compounds that include free amino acids and polypeptide residues.

The reaction of various amino acids with peroxynitrite leads to the following products: 1) cysteine and glutathione are converted to disulfides; 2) methionine is converted to sulfoxide or is fragmented to ethylene and dimethyl disulfides. Dimethyl sulfoxide is oxidized to formaldehyde; and 3) tyrosine and tryptophan undergo one electron oxidation to radical cations, which are hydroxylated, nitrated and dimerized (27-29). Exposure of amino acids, peptides and proteins to ionizing radiation such as gamma radiation and peroxynitrite in the presence of O_2, give rise to hydroperoxides. These hydroperoxides decompose to oxygen and carbon centered radicals on exposure to copper (Cu+) and other transition metal ions. Hydroperoxide formation on nuclear proteins results in oxidative damage to associated DNA. These hydroperoxide-derived radicals react readily with pyrimidine DNA bases and nucleosides to form adduct species, for example 8-oxo-dG. This adduct is highly mutagenic and induces G:C to T:A transversions in human DNA after replication (30).

A change in the structure of DNA could either be due to radiation or due to interaction with different free radicals (31). Since there are many polybasic compounds in the vicinity of DNA, there exists a possibility of their interaction with DNA on exposure to radiation or free radicals. Lysine and arginine-rich histones in nucleosomes on modification by environmental agents form histone-DNA adducts, making it immunogenic. It appears that the pathogenic anti-DNA autoantibodies are generated through some modified epitopes on nucleic acids (32-34). Prominent DNA modifications induced by exposure to peroxynitrite include the formation of 8-nitro-guanine and 8-oxyguanine, as well as the induction of single-strand breaks (35). Peroxynitrite reacts significantly only with guanine, which upon oxidation and nitration leads to mutagenicity and strand breaks, respectively. Peroxynitrite also damages DNA by covalent bond formation and removal of DNA bases (36).

Purine nucleotides are vulnerable to oxidation and to adduct formation (37,38). Peroxynitrite is a mutagenic agent with a potential to produce nitration, nitrosation and deamination of DNA bases. Methylation of cytosine in DNA is important for the regulation of gene expression and normal methylation patterns are altered by the carcinogenic effect of peroxynitrite (39). Prominent DNA modifications induced by peroxynitrite include the formation of 8-nitro-guanine and 8-oxyguanine, as well as the induction of single strand breaks (40). DNA single strand breaks generated by peroxynitrite leads to activation of the nuclear enzyme, poly (ADP-ribose) synthetase (PARS), which can trigger cellular suicidal pathway. Single strand breaks generated by peroxynitrite can arise from two processes: 1) sugar damage, which involves abstraction of hydrogen leading to the formation of sugar radical or 2) base damage, which rapidly depurinates to generate abasic sites, finally resulting in single strand breaks (41). Peroxynitrite is mutagenic in the *supF* gene inducing G to T transversions and deletions clustered at the 5′ end of the gene. The mutagenicity of peroxynitrite is believed to result from chemical modifications at guanine leading to miscoding (42). Carcinogenesis is induced by altered DNA or tissue damage, mutations and chromosomal aberrations (43,44). Peroxynitrite is a mutagenic agent with the potential to produce nitration, nitrosation and deamination reactions on DNA bases. It reacts significantly only with guanine, which upon oxidation and nitration leads to mutagenicity and strand breaks, respectively (45,46). Peroxynitrite levels are elevated in inflammation and infection and play an important role in autoimmunity and carcinogenesis (Figure 1). It damages tumor suppressor genes and leads to the expression of proto-oncogenes. Peroxynitrite induced DNA damage leading to mutations has been strongly implicated in carcinogenesis (47) (Figure 1).

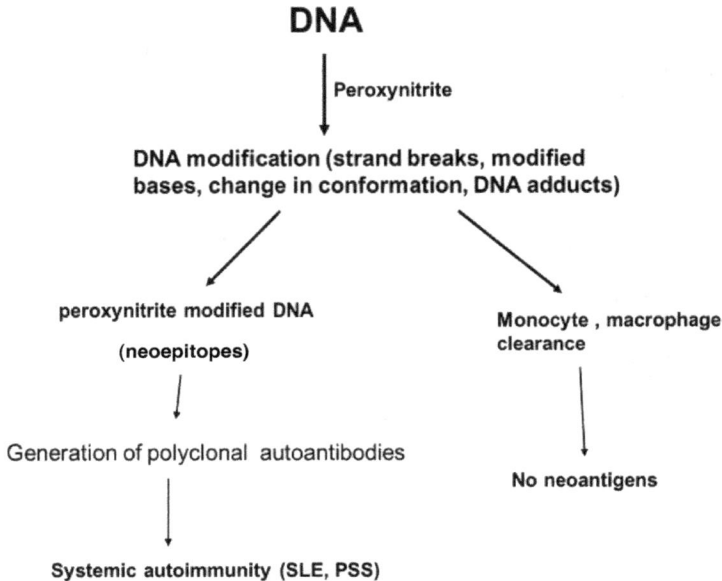

DNA

Peroxynitrite

DNA modification (strand breaks, modified bases, change in conformation, DNA adducts)

peroxynitrite modified DNA

(neoepitopes)

Monocyte , macrophage clearance

Generation of polyclonal autoantibodies

No neoantigens

Systemic autoimmunity (SLE, PSS)

Fig. 1. The role of peroxynitrite, a reactive nitrogen species, in the etiopathogenesis of autoimmune disorders, such as systemic lupus erythematosus (SLE) and progressive systemic sclerosis (PSS).

Proteins are targets of reactive nitrogen species such as peroxynitrite and NO_2. Among the various amino acids in proteins, tryptophan residues are especially susceptible to attack by reactive nitrogen species (48). Peroxynitrite is capable of oxidizing protein and non-protein sulfhydryl (-SH) groups including lipid peroxidation and reactivity with aromatic amino acid side chain in proteins to form nitroadducts (49). Peroxynitrite induced tyrosine nitration may lead to dysfunction of nitrated proteins, SOD, cytoskeletal proteins, neuronal tyrosine hydroxylase, cytochrome P450 and prostacyclin synthase (50-53). Oxidation of critical -SH groups is responsible for the inhibition of mitochondrial and cytosolic aconitase and other critical enzymes in the mitochondrial respiratory chain (54). Peroxynitrite mediated nitration of myofibrillar creatine kinase activity may lead to contractile dysfunction of the heart (55). Peroxynitrite-modified cellular proteins are subject to accelerated degradation via the proteosome (56).

Adducts arise from the chemical modification of bases in DNA or amino acids in proteins by toxic chemicals and high energy UV radiation. Many chemicals known to be carcinogenic in humans have been shown to form adducts. Ultraviolet radiation is regarded as one of the major environmental factors responsible for the photoconjugation of DNA with amino acid residues. Lysine is an amino acid of particular interest as a potential participant in DNA-protein photo-cross-linking. Nearly 60% of thymine and cytosine bases in DNA are modified due to lysine photoaddition and approximately every helical turn of DNA contains one lysine molecule in the photobound state (57). It appears to enhance the antigenicity of the DNA-lysine adduct, suggesting possible roles of peroxynitrite-induced neoepitopes in damaged DNA in the production of autoantibodies in cancer patients (58).

Ahmad et al have characterised the peroxynitrite treated human-DNA lysine photoadduct (59). We have investigated the photochemical addition of lysine to native DNA in view of its potential importance in the photo-cross-linking of histones to DNA in chromatin. The C-2 carbon atom of thymine in DNA undergoes a covalent photoaddition reaction with the ε-amino group of lysine on UV irradiation to form a DNA-lysine photoconjugate or photoadduct (57). The UV spectroscopic analysis of the DNA-lysine photoadduct showed hyperchromism, indicating either the formation of single-stranded breaks in DNA or "breathing" of a double-stranded polymer at the site of lysine conjugation. Peroxynitrite caused substantial damage to the DNA-lysine adduct as evident from the hyperchromicity of the spectral curve, which could be attributed to the generation of strand breaks (Figure 2A). On peroxynitrite modification, the hypochromicity increased, which may be due to the shielding effect of lysine, limiting the sites for peroxynitrite action. Hypochromicity may also be attributed to the extensive cross-linking between peroxynitrite and the DNA-lysine adduct (31).

As shown in Figure 2B, the fluorescence emission intensity (FI) was highest for native DNA (curve 1) and least for the DNA-lysine photoadduct (curve 3). However, on peroxynitrite modification there was a change in the emission intensity, as seen in the figure (curve 2). A decrease in FI of 45.2% for the DNA-lysine photoadduct in comparison to the peroxynitrite-modified DNA-lysine adduct was observed from fluorescence spectroscopy measurements. Loss of FI of 21.3% in the peroxynitrite-modified adduct with respect to native DNA is indicative of the loss of structural integrity in DNA and generation of single-strand regions (59). The UV absorption and fluorescence characteristics of native and modified lysine photoadduct have been summarized in Table 1.

Properties	Native DNA	Native adduct	Modified adduct
A260/280 ratio	1.74	1.20	1.01
Melting temperature (°C)	75	70	85
Hyperchromicity (%)	–	52	84
Loss of FI (%)	–	76.1	21.3

Table 1. Absorption and fluorescence characteristics of native DNA, DNA-lysine photoadduct (native adduct) and peroxynitrite-modified photoadduct (modified adduct)

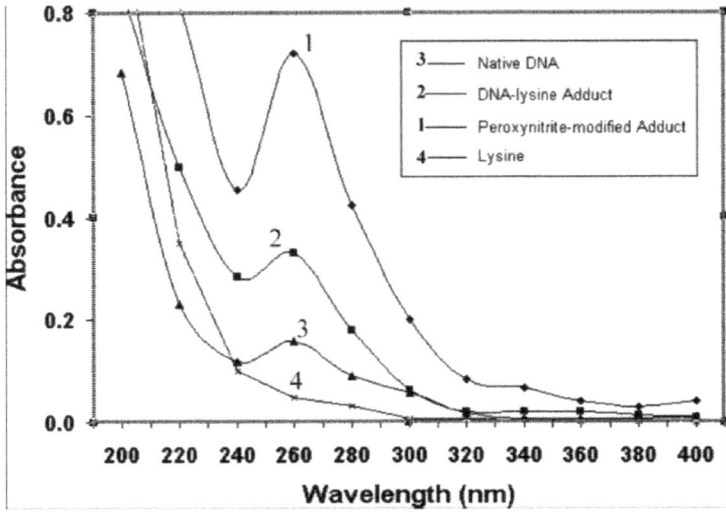

(a)

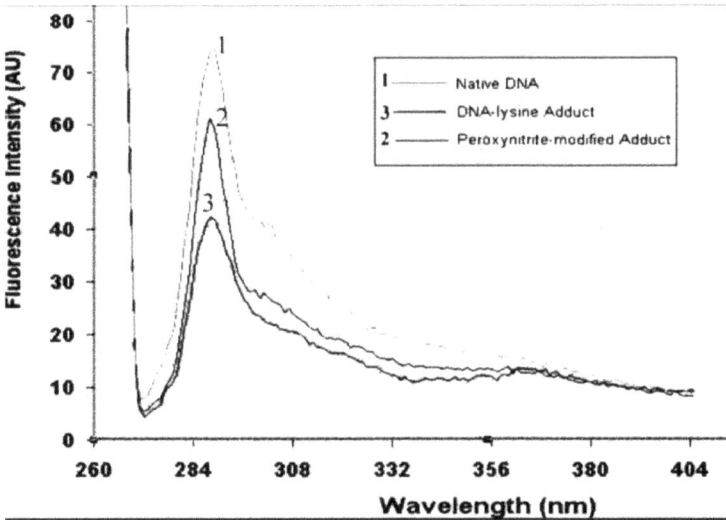

(b)

Fig. 2. UV absorption spectra of native DNA (curve 3), DNA-lysine photoadduct (curve 2) and peroxynitrite-modified adduct (curve 1). **2B:** Fluorescence spectra of native DNA (curve 1), DNA-lysine photoadduct (curve 3), and peroxynitrite-modified adduct (curve 2).

The melting profile of the DNA-lysine photoadduct reveals that the ultraviolet radiation induced covalent incorporation of lysine into the native DNA. The photoaddition of lysine to DNA might have obliterated the favorable A = T and G = C pairing interaction of double helical native DNA (57), thus decreasing the duplex melting temperature (Tm) by 5°C relative to the fully paired parent native DNA. In the study, on peroxynitrite treatment, the Tm of the DNA-lysine adduct increased by 15°C with respect to the native DNA-lysine photoadduct (Figure 3). This may be due to shielding of the available sites for peroxynitrite action by lysine. Hence, more energy would be needed to break the covalent bonding between lysine and the DNA bases in order to denature the double helix (59).

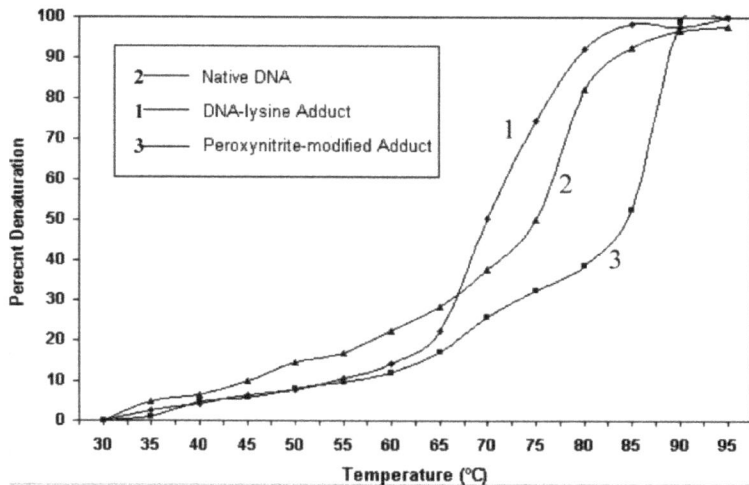

Fig. 3. Thermal melting profile of native DNA (curve 2), DNA-lysine photoadduct (curve 1), and peroxynitrite-modified photoadduct (curve 3).

Biological significance of tyrosine nitration has generated much interest among biomedical scientists because abnormal generation of 3-nitrotyrosine *in vivo* in diverse pathological conditions have been proved without doubt. Peroxynitrite is a strong oxidant that can oxidize a variety of biomolecules including proteins and non-protein thiol, protein sulphides, lipids and deoxyribose. The markers of oxidative damage to proteins include mainly carbonyls of lysine, arginine, threonine and proline, oxidized tryptophan, tyrosine and cysteine residues and fragmented protein. One persistent footprint left by peroxynitrite is nitration of phenolic ring of tyrosine residues in protein. The resultant 3-nitrotyrosine is a relatively specific marker of nitrosative stress. A recent study on repair of protein nitration in rat tissues by 3-nitrotyrosine denitrase activity suggests that a tyrosine nitration–denitration pathway participates in nitric oxide/peroxynitrite dependent signal transduction, a phenomenon similar to phosphorylation–dephosphorylation system. The reports suggest that 3-nitrotyrosine has importance not only as biomarker of nitrogen mediated tissue injury but also as a means to gain insight into molecular mechanisms of nitric oxide related physiological and pathophysiological phenomena. Furthermore, hypernitrotyrosinemia has also been reported in various inflammatory diseases including SLE, Sjogren's syndrome, vasculitis and rheumatoid arthritis (60).

Alteration of DNA or proteins resulting from photomodification or peroxynitrite could lead to the development of antibodies or mutations to modified DNA. Therefore, the DNA-lysine photoadduct and modified photoadduct could have important implications in various pathophysiological conditions such as toxicology, carcinogenesis, and autoimmune phenomena (57).

3. Autoimmune phenomenon

Manifestations of autoimmunity are often complex and heterogenous. It has been postulated that the immune response against host antigens could be due to genetic predisposition, exaggerated B cell activity, cross-reactivity between foreign and host antigens, etc. The foreign antigens arise as a consequence of infection, inflammation, drug administration, environmental factors, free radicals, etc (57,61). It has been established that not only oxygen but nitrogen free radicals play an important role in the pathogenesis of several human diseases. Reactive nitrogen species is produced by the reaction of nitric oxide with superoxide. Nitric oxide radical participate in some pathological conditions such as arthritis, vasculitis, asthma, hypertension, etc. It is also an unstable molecule like oxygen free radical but less reactive and can react with proteins (31).

Two diseases that are considered as a prototype for systemic autoimmunity are systemic lupus erythematosus (SLE) and rheumatoid arthritis (RA). SLE is a multi-systemic disorder characterized by a variety of autoantibodies and abnormal lymphocyte function that are responsible for many of the clinical manifestations important in diagnosis. A hallmark of SLE is the presence of antinuclear antibodies (ANA). ANA are prototype autoantibodies that mark the course of rheumatic diseases (62). Because of the close association between ANA and clinical diagnosis, these antibodies have become a key component in the evaluation of patients. These antibodies target a diverse range of macromolecules including DNA, RNA, proteins and protein-nucleic acid (PNA) complexes. Antibodies to DNA have been particularly associated with SLE which is considered to be a prototype autoimmune disease. Native DNA is no longer regarded as the antigen initiating the disease mainly immunization with nDNA does not produce SLE like symptoms. A few of the possible candidates could be polynucleotides, denatured DNA, RNA or modified DNA. While antibodies to single stranded DNA are formed in several inflammatory complexes including RA; antibodies to double stranded DNA serve as an immunochemical marker in the diagnosis of SLE (63). Serum obtained form SLE individuals have been shown to possess anti-DNA antibodies of diverse antigenic specificity. These anti-DNA autoantibodies have been used to evaluate therapeutic effect and clinical features of SLE patients (64,65).

The origin of autoantibody remains an enigma and the production of anti-DNA antibodies is even more complicated. Even though nucleic acid antigens are themselves poorly immunogenic, their antigenicity can be enhanced by modification with agents such as free radicals. Autoantibodies produced against such modified macromolecule are the hallmark of systemic human disease, SLE. B cell hyperactivity and the production of pathogenic autoantibodies is the main immunonological event in the pathogenesis of this disease. One approach to study the pathogenesis of SLE and determine how the autoantibody response is initiated and sustained is to analyse variable genes expressed by antibodies. Quantification of this repertoire has revealed the presence of a specific expansion of IgG clonotypes that impart reactivity with disease related autoantigens. The amino acid and nucleotide sequence of autoantibodies derived from human lupus present in immune complexes and renal eluates of subjects with active disease show features of diversification with a high rate of replacement or silent mutations and the clustering of mutations in the hypervariable region. This distinctive feature implies that a pure polyclonal activation cannot be the only mechanism responsible for autoantibody production. An antigen-driven process is more likely to play a role in their generation. It has been suggested that the antibodies may be stimulated by nucleic acid antigens or pathogens. B cells whose paratopes have complementary determining regions (CDR) which are formed by amino acids that can promote DNA binding may be selectively stimulated by nucleic acid related structures (31). A number of studies support the role of free radicals in the initiation and progression of autoimmune response. Therefore, in chronic inflammatory diseases, peroxynitrite generated by phagocytic cells may cause damage to DNA and proteins, generating neoepitopes that lead to the production of antibodies cross-reacting with nDNA or histone proteins. Modification of native DNA or proteins by peroxynitrite might also lead to the generation of neoepitopes on the molecule, and may be one of the factors for the induction of the immune responses as seen in an autoimmune disease like systemic lupus erythematosus (SLE) (58). The peroxynitrite modified human DNA was found to be highly immunogenic in rabbits inducing high titre immunogen specific antibodies (Figure 4). The data demonstrate that the antibodies, though cross-reactive with various nucleic acids and polynucleotides, preferentially bind peroxynitrite-modified epitopes on DNA (58).

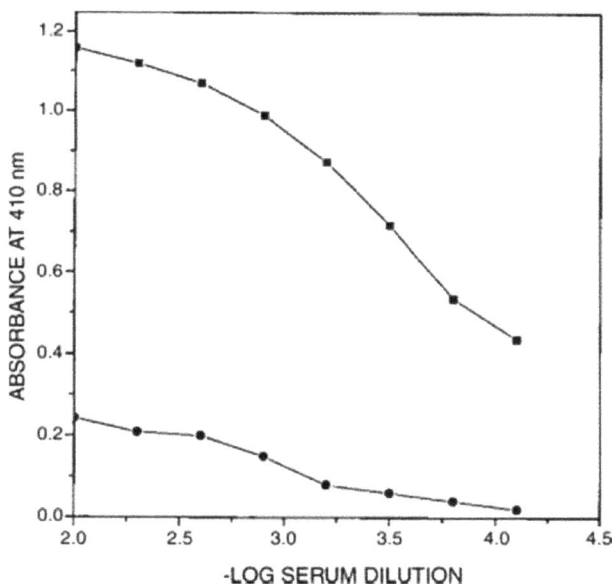

Fig. 4. Antigenicity of peroxynitrite modified human DNA. Direct binding ELISA of anti-peroxynitrite-human DNA antisera (○) and pre-immune sera (●). The microtitre plates were coated with peroxynitrite modified-human DNA (2.5 μg/ml).

DNA is a non-immunogenic entity, but any significant unrepaired alteration in its basic structure could render it "foreign," leading to the activation of immune pathways. A change in the structure of DNA could either be due to radiation or interaction with different free radicals. NO and its derivatives are among the radicals known to interact with DNA and are primarily involved in deamination of DNA bases. Peroxynitrite, on the other hand, leads to more extensive damage than that caused by an equivalent dose of ·NO. Formation occurs both intracellularly inside macrophages and extracellularly, and causes DNA strand breaks and modification of guanine (66). The two main products identified from the reaction of deoxyguanosine with peroxynitrite are 8-oxodeoxyguanine and 8-nitroguanine. The former has long been regarded as a reliable biomarker for monitoring DNA damage in studies with various oxidizing agents. The peroxynitrite-modified DNA has been shown to acquire immunogenicity and was suspected to be one of the causes for generation of autoantibodies in cancer and autoimmune disorders (12,67). The peroxynitrite modified DNA is a potent immunizing stimulus, inducing high-titer immunogen-specific antibodies in rabbits. Peroxynitrite modification might have generated potential neoepitopes against which antibodies are raised. The analysis of cross-reactivity indicates that anti-peroxynitrite-DNA IgG is immunogen-specific, showing various extents of cross-reactivity attributable to sharing of common antigenic determinants. The common antigenic determinants between peroxynitrite-DNA and nDNA could possibly be the sugar-phosphate backbone, since peroxynitrite attacks DNA and causes single strand breaks through sugar fragmentation. Induced antibodies also recognized synthetic polynucleotides, representing A/B conformations, with a preference for the B-form (12). Elevated levels of ·NO in systemic lupus erythematosus (SLE) patients suggest a role for ·NO in the pathogenesis of the disease. Murine models of SLE demonstrate abnormally high levels of ·NO compared with normal mice, whereas systemic blockade of ·NO production reduces disease activity. Elevated serum nitrate levels correlate with indices of disease activity and, along with serum titers of anti-(ds DNA) antibodies, serve as indicators of SLE (68-69). Auto-antibody production in SLE has been attributed to either selective stimulation of autoreactive B-cells by self-antigens or antigens crossreactive with self. The persistence of anti-DNA antibodies in SLE patients, despite systems to suppress self-recognition, suggests that the response is driven by an antigen resembling nDNA. The DNA damage by peroxynitrite is far more lethal than that caused by ·NO alone, leading to the perturbations in nDNA that render it immunogenic. This modified DNA might therefore play a role in the induction of circulating anti-DNA autoantibodies in various autoimmune disorders including SLE (12,59)

Histones are small, highly conserved cationic proteins which bind DNA. They are weak immunogen because of their conserved nature. Histones are major constituent of cells' chromatin and remain confined to nucleus. However, after apoptosis they may appear in circulation as nucleosomes. Incidence of autoantibodies against histone H1, H2A, H2B, H3 and H4 are 60%, 53%, 48%, 36% and 29.5% respectively in the sera of SLE patients (70). Histones also act as autoantigens in humorally-mediated paraneoplastic diseases (71). Furthermore, anti-histone antibodies have also been reported in polymyositis / dermatomyositis (72).

As peroxynitrite reaction involves free radical intermediates, it may favor cross-linking and aggregation during nitration. The extent of cross-linking depends on type of reagent used, protein concentration, type of protein and solvent conditions including pH. The exact chemical nature of the cross-linking is disputed but linkage of side chains of tyrosine residue is the common answer. Formation of tyrosyl radical by peroxynitrite and its reaction with another tyrosyl radical (on same or different histone molecule) may generate O,O'-dityrosine covalent cross-links. Peroxynitrite induces an array of modifications in H2A structure namely-tyrosine nitration, formation of protein carbonyl, dityrosine and cross-linking. Such gross structural changes might favor polymerization of native epitopes of H2A histone into potent immunogenic neo-epitopes. The histone proteins are conserved proteins and act as weak immunogens. However, they show strong immunogenicity after acetylation and alterations in amino acid structure or sequence can generate neo-epitopes on self proteins causing and immune attack. The oxidative and nitrative action of peroxynitrite confers additional immunogenicity on H2A histone and probably there is a direct correlation between nitration and immunogenicity. In another words, peroxynityrite-modified H2A still has some old epitopes which are scattered among neo-epitopes. Hence, immunization with peroxynityrite-modified H2A may produce polyspecific antibodies which can recognize both old and neo-epitopes or altogether there are two types of antibodies, one recognizing nitrated neo-epitopes and other binding exclusively with old epitopes (73).

The mechanism of autoantibody production in diseases such as SLE has not yet been clearly identified. If antigen selection is an important aspect of differentiation, the nature of the stimulating antigen also remains to be determined. The origin of antibodies remains obscure, although modified DNA appears to be a causative factor in RA and SLE. It is possible that the production of autoantibodies may be the result of free radical attack on DNA or histone proteins causing changes at the macromolecule level. It is therefore postulated that in chronic inflammatory diseases, free radicals generated by phagocytic cells may cause damage to DNA and proteins and antibodies to self-antigen are produced. Also, a defect in the control of apoptosis and delayed clearance of apoptotic debris provide sustained interaction between free radicals and macromolecules, generating neoepitopes which subsequently result in autoimmunity and generating polyspecific autoantibodies (73). Sera of animals immunized with native and peroxynitrite-modified histones were tested on polysorp wells coated with respective immunogens (Figure 5). Modification by 100 µm peroxynitrite conferred more high immunogenicity on H2A histone (73).

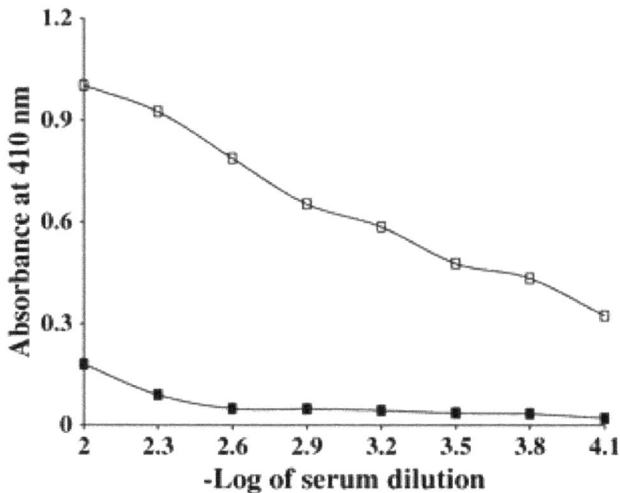

Fig. 5. Antigenicity of peroxynitrite modified proteins. Direct binding ELISA of experimentally induced antibodies against peroxynitrite-modified H2A (□) and native histone H2A (■).

Accumulation of a variety of post-translationally modified self-proteins during inflammation may lead to generation or unmasking of new antigenic epitopes that in turn activate B-and/or T-cells, thereby impairing or bypassing immunological tolerance. Peroxynitrite-modified H2A histone could act as an autoantigen leading to generation of anti-H2A histone antibodies. It is envisaged that anti-histone antibodies seen in a sub-group of SLE patients might originate from immunological activity of peroxynitrite-modified histones due to their protection from digestion by normal proteolytic machinery (61). In the context of anti-histone antibodies in drug induced lupus erythematosus, it is quite possible that the drug itself might mimic reaction(s) pathway(s) leading to abnormal synthesis of peroxynitrite. The peroxynitrite may then modify the structure of histone making it immunogenic (76).

Hence, alteration of DNA or proteins resulting from photomodification or peroxynitrite could lead to the development of antibodies or mutations to modified DNA. Therefore, the DNA-lysine photoadduct and modified photoadducts could have important implications in toxicology, carcinogenesis, and autoimmune phenomena. Hence, understanding the pathophysiology of peroxynitrite could lead to important therapeutic interventions against this increasingly important and physiologically relevant reactive nitrogen species.

4. References

[1] Szabo C. Multiple pathways of peroxynitrite cytotoxicity. Toxicol Lett. (2003) 140–141: 105–112.

[2] Pacher P, Beckman JS, Liaudet L. Nitric oxide and peroxynitrite in health and disease. Physiol Rev. (2007) 87(1): 315–424.

[3] Szabo C, Ischiropoulos H, Radi R. Peroxynitrite: biochemistry, pathophysiology and development of therapeutics. Nat Rev Drug Discov. (2007) 6(8): 662–80.

[4] Squadrito GL, Pryor WA . Oxidative chemistry of nitric oxide: the roles of superoxide, peroxynitrite, and carbon dioxide. Free Rad Biol Med (1998), 25(4-5):392-403.

[5] Radi R, Peluffo G, Alvarez MN, Naviliat M, Cayota A. Unraveling peroxynitrite formation in biological systems. Free Radic Biol Med. (2001) 30(5): 463–88.

[6] Forstermann U, Munzel T. Endothelial nitric oxide synthase in vascular disease: from marvel to menace. Circulation. (2006) 113(13): 1708–14.

[7] Romero N, Denicola A, Radi R. Red blood cells in the metabolism of nitric oxide-derived peroxynitrite. IUBMB Life. (2006) 58(10): 572–80.

[8] Ahmad R, Rasheed Z Ahsan H. Biochemical and cellular toxicology of peroxynitrite: implications in cell death and autoimmune phenomenon. Immunopharmacology and Immunotoxicology (2009) 18(7): 388–396.

[9] Pryor W A, Squandrito G I. Chemistry of peroxynitrite: aproduct from the reaction of nitrite oxide with superoxide. Am J Physiol. (1995),268, L699-22.

[10] Oshima H,Frisen M, Bruer I, Bartsch H. Nitrotyrosine as a marker for endogenous nitrosation and nitration of proteins. Food Chem Toxicol (1990), 28: 647-52.

[11] Good P F, Hsu A, Werner P, Perl DP, Olanow C W. Protein nitration in Parkinson's disease. J Neuropathol Exp Neurol (1998), 57:338-42.

[12] Browne S E, Ferrante R J , Beal M F. Oxidative stress in Huntington's disease, Brain Pathol. (1999): 147-63

[13] Smith M A, Richey harris P L, Sayre L M, Beckman J S, Perry G. Widespread peroxynitrite-mediated damage in Alzheimer's disease. J Neurosci (1997), 17:2653-7

[14] Bagasra O, Michaelis FH, Zheng YM et al. Activation of the inducible form of nitric oxide synthase in the brains of patients with multiple sclerosis. Proc Natl Acad Sci (USA) (1995), 92: 12041-5

[15] Bachmaier K, Nikolaus N, Pommerer C et al. iNOS expression and nitrotyrosine formation in the myocardium in response to inflammation is controlled by the interferon transcription factor 1. Circulation (1997), 96:585-91

[16] Oates J C, Christensen E F, Reilly C M, Self S E, Gilkeson G S. Prospective measure of serum 3-nitrotyrosine levels in systemic lupus erythmatosus:correlation with disease activity. Proc Assoc Am Physicians (1995), 111:611-21

[17] Kaur H,Halliwell B. Evidence for nitric oxide mediated oxidative damage in chronic inflammation. Nitrotyrosine in serum and synovial fluid from rheumatoid patients. FEBS Lett (1994),350:9-12

[18] Anderson S M. Post translational modification of self antigens: implications for autoimmunity.Curr Opin Immunol (2004), 16:753-8

[19] Olins A L, Olins D E. Stereo electron microscopy of the 25-nm chromatin fibres in isolated nuclei.J Cell Biol (1979), 81:260-5

[20] Monesteir M, Kortzin B L. Antibodies to histones in systemic lupus erythmatosus and drug-induced lupus syndromes. Rheum Dis Clin North Am (1992), 18: 415-536

[21] Haqqani A S, Kelly J F, Birnboin H C. Selective nitration of histone tyrosine residues *in vivo* mutatect tumors. J Biol Chem (2002), 277:3614-21

[22] Maeda H, Akaike T. Nitric oxide and oxygen radicals in infection, inflammation, and cancer. Biochemistry (Mosc). (1998) 63(7): 854–865.

[23] Ohshima H, Bartsch H. Chronic infections and inflammatory processes as cancer risk factors: possible role of nitric oxide in carcinogenesis. Mutat Res. (1994) 305(2): 253–264.

[24] Rubbo H. Nitric oxide and peroxynitrite in lipid peroxidation. Medicina (B Aires). (1998) 58(4), 361–366.

[25] Rubbo H, Freeman BA. Nitric oxide regulation of lipid oxidation reactions: formation and analysis of nitrogen-containing oxidized lipid derivatives. Methods Enzymol. (1996) 269: 385–394.

[26] Rubbo H, Radi R, Trujillo M, Telleri R, Kalyanaraman B, Barnes S, Kirk M, Freeman B A. Nitric oxide regulation of superoxide and peroxynitrite-dependent lipid peroxidation. Formation of novel nitrogen-containing oxidized lipid derivatives. J Biol Chem (1994) 269(42): 26066–26075.

[27] Ramezanian MS, Padmaja S, Koppenol WH. Nitration and hydroxylation of phenolic compounds by Peroxynitrite. Chem Res Toxicol. (1996) 9(1): 232–240.

[28] Ramezanian MS, Padmaja S, Koppenol WH Nitration and hydroxylation of phenolic compounds by Peroxynitrite. Methods Enzymol. (1996) 269: 195–201.

[29] Alvarez B, Radi R. Peroxynitrite reactivity with amino acids and proteins. Amino Acids. (2003) 25(3–4): 295–311.

[30] Luxford C, Morin B, Dean RT, Davies MJ Histone H1 and other protein- and amino acid-hydroperoxides can give rise to free radicals which oxidize DNA. Biochem J. (1999); 344(1), 125–134.

[31] Ahsan H, Ali A, Ali R (2003). Oxygen free radicals and systemic autoimmunity. Clin. Exp. Immunol. 131(3):398–404.

[32] Ahsan H, Abdi S, Ali A (2002) Recognition of DNA-arginine photoadduct by anti-DNA auto-antibodies in systemic lupus erythematosus. Ind. J. Med. Res. 115:201–211.

[33] Dixit K, Ahsan H, Ali A (2003) Polydeoxyribonucleotide C photoconjugated with lysine or arginine present unique epitopes for human anti-DNA autoantibodies. Hum. Immunol. 64(9): 880–886.

[34] Habib S, Moinuddin, Ali R (2006) Peroxynitrite modified DNA: a better antigen for systemic lupus erythematosus anti-DNA autoantibodies. Biotechnol. Appl. Biochem. 43(2): 65–70.

[35] Szabo C, Ohshima H (1997) DNA damage induced by peroxynitrite: subsequent biological effects. Nitric Oxide 1(7):373–385.

[36] Yermilov V, Rubio J, Becchi M, Friesen MD, Pignatelli B, Ohshima H (1995) Formation of 8-nitroguanine by the reaction of guanine with peroxynitrite *in vitro*. Carcinogenesis 16(9): 2045–2050.

[37] Douki T, Cadet J. Peroxynitrite mediated oxidation of purine bases of nucleosides and isolated DNA. Free Rad Res. (1996) 24(5): 369–380.

[38] Douki T, Cadet J, Ames BN. An adduct between peroxynitrite and 2'-deoxyguanosine: 4,5-dihydro-5-hydroxy-4-(nitrosooxy)-2'-deoxyguanosine. Chem Res Toxicol. (1996) 9(1): 3–7.

[39] Wiseman H, Halliwell B. Damage to DNA by reactive oxygen and nitrogen species: role in inflammatory disease and progression to cancer. Biochem J. (1996) 313(1): 17–29.

[40] Ohshima H, Virág L, Souza J, Yermilov V, Pignatelli B, Masuda M, Szabo C. Detection of certain peroxynitrite-induced DNA modifications. Methods Mol Biol. (2002) 186: 77–88.

[41] Ohshima H, Virág L, Souza J, Yermilov V, Pignatelli B, Masuda M, Szabo C. Detection of certain peroxynitrite-induced DNA modifications. Methods Mol Biol. (2002) 186: 77–88.

[42] Tretyakova NY, Burney S, Pamir B, Wishnok JS, Dedon PC, Wogan GN, Tannenbaum, SR. Peroxynitrite-induced DNA damage in the sup F gene: correlation with the mutational spectrum. Mutat Res (2000) 447(2): 287–303.

[43] Ames BN, Shigenaga MK, Gold LS. DNA lesions, inducible DNA repair, and cell division: three key factors in mutagenesis and carcinogenesis. Environ Health Perspect. (1993) 101(suppl 5): 35–44.

[44] Ames BN, Shigenaga MK, Hagen TM Oxidants, antioxidants, and the degenerative diseases of aging. Proc Natl Acad Sci (USA) (1993) 90(17): 7915–7922.

[45] Sawa T, Ohshima H. Nitrative DNA damage in inflammation and its possible role in carcinogenesis. Nitric Oxide. (2006) 14(2): 91–100.

[46] Yermilov V, Rubio J, Becchi M, Friesen MD, Pignatelli B, Ohshima H. Formation of 8-nitroguanine by the reaction of guanine with peroxynitrite *in vitro*. Carcinogenesis. (1995) 16(9): 2045–2050.

[47] Ohshima H. Genetic and epigenetic damage induced by reactive nitrogen species: implications in carcinogenesis. Toxicol Lett (2003) 140–141: 99–104.

[48] Suzuki T, Mower HF, Friesen MD, Gilibert I, Sawa T, Ohshima, H. Nitration and nitrosation of N-acetyl-L-tryptophan and tryptophan residues in proteins by various reactive nitrogen species. Free Rad Biol Med. (2004) 37(5): 671–681.

[49] Beckman JS, Koppenol WH. Nitric oxide, superoxide, and peroxynitrite: the good, the bad, and ugly. Am J Physiol. (1996) 271(5 Pt 1): C1424–1437.

[50] Beckman JS. Oxidative damage and tyrosine nitration from Peroxynitrite. Chem Res Toxicol. (1996) 9(5): 836–844.

[51] Beckman JS. Protein tyrosine nitration and peroxynitrite. FASEB J. (2002) 16(9): 1144.

[52] Greenacre SA, Ischiropoulos H. Tyrosine nitration: localisation, quantification, consequences for protein function and signal transduction. Free Rad Res. (2001) 34(6): 541–581.

[53] Ischiropoulos H, Zhu L, Chen J, Tsai M, Martin JC, Smith CD, Beckman JS. Peroxynitrite-mediated tyrosine nitration catalyzed by superoxide dismutase. Arch Biochem Biophy. (1992) 298(2): 431–437.

[54] Hausladen A, Fridovich I. Superoxide and peroxynitrite inactivate aconitases, but nitric oxide does not. J Biol Chem. (1994) 269(47): 29405–29408.

[55] Mihm MJ, Yu F, Carnes CA, Reiser PJ, McCarthy PM, Van Wagoner DR, Bauer JA Impaired myofibrillar energetics and oxidative injury during human atrial fibrillation. Circulation. (2001) 104(2): 174–180.

[56] Grune T, Blasig IE, Sitte N, Roloff B, Haseloff R, Davies KJ. Peroxynitrite increases the degradation of aconitase and other cellular proteins by proteasome. J Biol Chem. (1998) 273(18): 10857–10862.

[57] Islam N, Ali R. (1998) Immunological studies on DNA-lysine photoadduct. Biochem. Mol. Biol. Int. 45(3):453–464.

[58] Dixit K, Moinuddin, Ali A (2005) Immunological studies on peroxynitrite modified DNA. Life Sci. 77(21):2626–2642.

[59] Ahmad R, Rasheed Z, Kaushal E, Singh D, Ahsan H. Biochemical evaluation of human DNA-lysine photoadduct treated with peroxynitrite. Toxicol Mech Meth. (2008) 18(7): 589–595.

[60] Gong C X, Liu F, Grundke-Iqbal I, Iqbal K.Dysregulation of protein phosphorylation/dephosphorylation in Alzheimer's disease: atherapeutic target.J Biomed Biotechnol (2006), 2006:31825.

[61] Ahmad R, Alam K, Ali R. Antigen binding characteristics of antibodies against hydroxyl radical modified thymidine monophosphate. Immunol Lett (2000),71:111-115

[62] Pisetsky DS. Antinuclear antibodies. Diagn Lab Immunol (1994),14:371-85

[63] Isenberg D, Shenfeld Y.The origin and significance of anti-DNA antibodies.Immunol Today (1997),8:279-81

[64] Tan EM. Autoantibody to nuclear antigens (ANA):their immunobiology and medicine. Adv Immunol (1982),33:167-208

[65] Pollard KM, Jones JE, TanEM, Theofilopoulos AN, Dixon FJ, Rubin RL. Polynucleotide specificity of murine monoclonal anti-DNA antibodies. Clin Immunol Immunopathol (1986), 40:197-208.

[66] Burney S, Caulfield JL, Niles JC, Wishnok JS, Tannenbaum SR. The chemistry of DNA damage from nitric oxide and peroxynitrite. Mutat Res (1999),424 (1-2):37-49.

[67] Habib S, Moinuddin, Ali R. Acquired antigenicity of DNA after modification with peroxynitrite. Int J Biol macromol (2005),35(3-4):221-225.

[68] Wanchu A, Khullar M, Deodhar SD bambery P, Sud A. Nitric oxide synthesis is increased in patients with systemic lupus erythmatosus. Rheumatol Int. (1998),18(2):41-43.

[69] Oates JC, Ruiz P, Alexander A, Pippen AM, Gilkeson GS. Effect of late modulation of nitric oxide production on murine lupus. Clin Immunol Immunopathol. (1997), 83(1):86-92.

[70] Gheidira I, Andolsi H, Mankai A, Fabien N, Jeddi M. Anti-histone antibodies in systemic lupus erythmatosus, comparison of three assays:ELISA, dot blot and immunoblot. Pathol Biol (2006), 54: 148-54

[71] Marc M, Thomas M, Lothar B, Frank SL. Anti-histone antibodies in subacute sensory neuropathy. J Neurooncol (1991),11:71-75.

[72] Masahidi K, Hironobu I, Norhito Y, Shinichi S, Kanako K, Kunihiko T. Prevelance and antigen specificity of anti-histone antibodies in patients with polymyositis/ dermatomyositis. J Invest Dermatol (1999), 112:1523-747.

[73] Khan MA, Dixit K, Jabeen S, Moinuddin, Alam K. Impact of peroxynitrite modification on structure and immunogenicity of H2A histone. Scan J Immunol (2008), 69:99-109.

8

Gut Microbiota - "Lost in Immune Tolerance"

Serena Schippa and Valerio Iebba
Public Health and Infectious Diseases dept., 'Sapienza' University of Rome,
Italy

1. Introduction

"There are a number of immune-mediated diseases known to be increased in Inflammatory Bowel Diseases (IBD)", says Charles N. Bernstein, MD, from University of Manitoba, Canada. "The finding of an increased association of chronic inflammatory diseases with either form of IBD could suggest a common genetic predisposition, common causative triggers, or possibly the triggering of one inflammatory condition secondary to the treatment of a primary inflammatory condition" (Snook et al., 1989). IBD could be classified as auto-inflammatory disorders characterized by recurrent episodes of systemic inflammation, often manifested by fever, as well as inflammation of specific tissues, such as joints, skin, gut, and eyes. These disorders are caused by primary dysfunction of the innate immune system, without evidence of adaptive immune dysregulation. (Galeazzi et al., 2006). In order to find out common causative triggers, in autoimmune disorder and/or auto-inflammatory disorders we would think about the important role of the gut microbiota in human health. IBD spectrum, including Crohn's disease (CD) and Ulcerative colitis (UC) as the main phenotypes, is a multi-factorial pathology where auto-inflammatory background, genetic susceptibility, environmental factors and intestinal bacteria are the main proposed etiological triggers, and the intestinal tissue injury is principally caused by the immune tolerance loss against the intestinal microbiota.

The most numerous bacterial populations are in the gastrointestinal tract with a surprisingly total bacterial weight of 1.5 Kg. Although these populations are highly stable, they are still prone to perturbations by environmental insults (Sullivan et al., 2001), with important consequences for our physiology and, consequently, our health. In the evolution of human diseases some, that were once rare, have become common, while others have disappeared and new varieties have emerged. The hypothesis proposed by Martin J. Blaser to explain it postulates how changes in human ecology result in changes in the microbes that populate our bodies (Blaser & Falkow, 2009). In the past century, the human condition, especially in developed countries, has undergone dramatic changes that affect the transmission and maintenance of the indigenous microbiota. Partly responsible for an increased prevalence of allergic and autoimmune disorders in later years (Strachan, 1989; Cookson & Moffatt, 1997) could be the hygiene hypothesis, that is a diminished exposure of humans to parasites and pathogens. The lack of such exposition may cause the immune system to shift its immunological response away from a balance between type 1 and type 2 T-helper cells (Prescott et al., 1999). Studies on intestinal bacteria composition in IBD patients have reported an altered balance of beneficial versus aggressive microbial species (dysbiosis): this could lead to a pro-inflammatory luminal milieu driving chronic intestinal inflammation in a susceptible host. Many other autoimmune pathologies are being associated to an altered intestinal microflora. To date, several evidences on the role of the gut microbiota in shaping intestinal immune responses during health and disease have been collected. Immunological de-regulation is the cause of many non-infectious human diseases such as autoimmunity, allergy and cancer. The gastrointestinal tract is the primary site of interaction between the host immune system and microorganisms, both symbiotic and pathogenic. It has recently been proposed that the total information encoded by the mammalian genome is not sufficient to carry out all functions that are required to maintain health and that products of our microbiome are a crucial protection from various diseases. It is possible that alterations in the development or composition of the microbiota (dysbiosis) disturb the partnership between the microbiota and the human immune system, ultimately leading to altered immune responses that may underlie various human inflammatory and immune disorders. According to numerous recent studies there is a vast, intricate and unexpected level of interdependence between beneficial bacteria and the immune system. Recent studies have shown that, at least for experimental IBD, the disease spontaneously occurs when immune suppression is defective; thus, inflammation seems to be a default immunological state in the absence of regulation. In this chapter, after a description of the structure and function of the gut microbiota organ and his cross-talk with the human host, we shall give a description of the forces that contribute to the intestinal ecosystem stability. We shall report findings indicating how the host immune system responds to bacterial colonization of the gastrointestinal tract, indicating that disturbances in the bacterial microbiota will result in the deregulation of adaptive immune cells, which may underlie autoimmune disorders. "This raises the possibility that the mammalian immune system, which seems to be designed to control microorganisms is, in fact, itself controlled by microorganisms" (Round & Mazmanian, 2009). In conclusion, it seems conceivable that alterations in both structure and function of intestinal microbiota could be one of the "common causative triggers" of autoimmune and/or auto-inflammatory disorders.

2. Structure of the gut microbiota organ

The human body is colonized by a vast number of bacteria, archaea, viruses, and unicellular eukaryotes. This enormous number of microorganisms form complex communities, or microbiota, at various sites within the human body. In fact, humans have been proposed to be "meta-organisms" consisting of 10-fold greater numbers of bacterial than animal cells that are metabolically and immunologically integrated.

Human gut 'microbiota'

The gastrointestinal tract harbors the largest and most complex bacterial ecosystem in the human body (Hattori & Taylor, 2009; Neish, 2009). The majority of the gut microbiota is composed of strict anaerobes, which dominate the facultative anaerobes and aerobes by two to three orders of magnitude (Gordon & Dubos, 1970; Harris et al., 1976). An increasing gradient in bacterial concentration characterizes the human gastrointestinal tract, from stomach, to jejunum, ileum and colon, where the concentration peaks to 10^{11}-10^{12} bacterial cells per gram of stool (Ley et al., 2006; Leser & Molbak, 2009). The human intestinal microbial community is complex and is composed of at least 1,000 distinct bacterial species. For long times, our understanding of the composition of intestinal microbial communities was based on the enumeration and characterization of cultivable organisms. However, this approach left substantial gaps in the catalogue of intestinal bacterial species, as most gut organisms are resistant to culture by available methods. The recent development of molecular profiling methods allowed unprecedented knowledge into the intestinal microbial communities, leading to the identification of new bacterial species (Eckburg et al., 2005). Molecular profiling of the human intestinal microbiota has revealed a high level of variability between individuals at the bacterial species level. Although there have been over 50 bacterial phyla described to date (Schloss & Handelsman, 2004), the human gut microbiota is dominated only by Bacteroidetes and Firmicutes, whereas Proteobacteria, Verrucomicrobia, Actinobacteria, Fusobacteria, and Cyanobacteria are present in minor proportions (Eckburg et al., 2005). The intestinal Firmicutes are Gram-positive bacteria, dominated by species belonging to the Clostridia class, but also include Enterococcaceae and Lactobacillaceae families and *Lactococcus spp.* Intestinal Bacteroidetes are Gram-negative bacteria comprised of several Bacteroides species, including *Bacteroides thetaiotaomicron*, *Bacteroides fragilis* and *Bacteroides ovatus*. The remaining intestinal bacteria, accounting for less than 10% of the total population, belong to the Proteobacteria, Fusobacteria, Actinobacteria, Verrucomicrobia and Spirochaetes phyla and a bacterial group that is closely related to Cyanobacteria (Eckburg et al., 2005). The mucosal immune system must be able to flexibly and rapidly adapt to microbiota, the composition of which may change in unpredictable ways as a function of host diet or other interactions with the external environment. The adult-like structure of the gut microbiota is established after the two years of life, during which the gut ecosystem progresses from sterility to extremely dense colonization (Palmer et al., 2007). Through healthy adulthood, the bacterial density and diversity in the gut remains relatively stable over time, in spite of the continuous flow of intestinal content, reflecting the ability to maintain a high degree of homeostasis (Vanhoutte et al., 2004; Leser & Molbak, 2009). The adult microbiota shows an astonishing individual variability, and it is considered as unique as a fingerprint in terms of species and strains composition (Zoetendal et al., 1998; Eckburg et al., 2005; Ley et al., 2006). Age, sex, diet, lifestyle, and geographic origins influence the composition of the gut microbiota, but studies involving human adults with different relatedness, from genetically unrelated people to monozygotic twins, demonstrated that the impact of genotype may also be significant in shaping the gut bacterial ecosystem (Vaughan et al., 2000; Ley et al., 2005; Mueller et al., 2006; Khachatryan et al., 2008; Li et al., 2008). For example, European children with a fat-rich western-life diet, and Burkina Faso ones, with a fiber-rich dietary content, showed marked differences in fecal microbiota composition (De Filippo et al., 2010).

Shaped by millennia of co-evolution, host and bacteria have developed beneficial relationships, creating a suitable environment for mutualism.

Human gut 'microbiome'

Despite the remarkable host specificity in the gut community membership, a high degree of conservation in its expressed functions and metabolites has been reported (Mahowald et al., 2009). This suggests that the gut microbiota may be characterized by a marked "functional redundancy" to ensure that the key functions of the microbial community remain unaffected by the individual variability in terms of species composition (Gill et al., 2006). The existence of a "human core gut microbiome", defined as those genes which are common to the gut microbiomes of all or the majority of humans, has been hypothesized to be responsible for the functional stability of the gut microbiota (Turnbaugh & Gordon, 2009). On the contrary, a "human core gut microbiota", defined as a number of species which are common to all humans, could hardly be defined, since different combinations of species could fulfill the same functional roles (Tschop et al., 2009; Turnbaugh et al., 2009). A recent study from the MetaHIT consortium (Arumugam et al., 2011) identified three fecal enterotypes geographic- and ethnicity-independent, showing a limited number of equilibrated host-microbial relationships, that could respond differently to environmental endeavors. Aside to the core, the set of genes, present in smaller subsets of human, represents the "human variable microbiome". This wide variation from the core is the result of a combination of host-specific factors, such as genotype, physiological status, host pathologies, lifestyle, diet, environment, and the presence of transient populations of microorganisms that cannot persistently colonize the human gut. In return, core and variable components of the human microbiome influence different aspects of the human health, including nutrient responsiveness and immunity (Turnbaugh et al., 2007).

3. Function of the gut microbiota organ

It was given emphasis to the importance of an ecologic view of our relationships with microbes, where the mutual survival of harbored microbiota and human host is interdependent (Ley et al., 2006; Chow et al., 2010). The cross talk between environmental microbiologists and human microbiota researchers should be improved in order to better understand the relationships between human and his microbiota. Not much is known yet about the possible roles of microbes in human-associated communities outside the intestinal tract, but it becomes increasingly clear that the gut microbiota exerts many beneficial effects on the human body system. Our intestinal symbionts play many important roles in: nutrient digestion and synthesis; energy metabolism; vitamin synthesis; epithelial development, immune responses (Tappenden & Deutsch, 2007; Flint et al., 2007). In addition, host-microbe interactions are essential for the host's defense against pathogenic infections.

Trophic functions

Collectively, the flora has a metabolic activity equal to a virtual organ within an organ (Scheline, 1973; Sousa et al., 2008). In return, the intestinal microorganisms are provided with steady growth conditions and a constant stream of nutrients (Savage, 1977). The presence of an intestinal microbiota is not essential for survival of the host, but germ-free (GF) mice require 30% more energy in their diet (Wostmann, 1981), showing the rule of the indigenous microbiota in energy scavenging from food. This energy utilization by the gut microbiota works on different levels. Specialized intestinal bacteria synthesize enzymes that human cells lack for the digestion of plant polysaccharides. The intestinal microbial community is well equipped to degrade these biomolecules (Hooper et al., 2002; Robert & Bernalier-Donadille, 2003). Microbial fermentation generates butyrate and other short-chain fatty acids that the host can use as energy sources and that help maintain the integrity of the intestinal epithelium (Tappenden & Deutsch, 2007; Flint et al., 2007; Pryde et al., 2002). In addition to its direct role in increasing caloric uptake from diet, the presence of a gut microbiota regulates fat storage in the host (Greiner & Bäckhed, 2011), promoting the absorption of monosaccharides from the gut lumen (Bäckhed et al., 2004).

Host's defense development

The intestinal symbionts provide an important barrier to colonization by potential pathogens, called "colonization resistance," by competing for the same nutrients and attachment sites as intruding microorganisms. (Dethlefsen et al., 2007; Tappenden & Deutsch, 2007; van der Waaij et al., 1971; Stecher & Hardt, 2008). Furthermore, the presence of a microbiota stimulates the development of the mucosal immune system. Without the interaction host-microbiota, the intestinal surface is more sensitive to injury, and less capable of inducing repair of the damaged surface. The host epithelium and its immune cells do not simply tolerate commensal bacteria, but depend on them to maintain the architectural integrity (Rakoff-Nahoum et al., 2004).

4. Host immune system and gut microbiota organ

Macpherson & Harris report the intrinsic potential of the microbiota to stimulate both pro- and anti-inflammatory responses. The composition of the bacterial communities in the gut may linked to the correct functioning of the immune system (Macpherson & Harris, 2004). Recently it has been proposed that the mammalian genome information is not sufficient to achieve all functions required to maintain health, and that products of our microbiome are essential in protecting from different diseases (Zaneveld et al., 2008). It is possible that alterations in the development or composition of the microbiota could affect the cross-talk between microbiota and human immune system, in the end leading to altered immune responses that may trigger various human inflammatory disorders.

Germ-free animals show a defective development of gut-associated lymphoid tissues (Macpherson & Harris, 2004; Falk et al., 1998), of antibody production, and have fewer and smaller Peyer's patches and mesenteric lymph nodes (Bouskra et al., 2008; Abrams et al., 1963). These structures could be collectedly called "inducible structures", due to their ex-novo formation following the introduction of gut bacteria. This observable fact suggests a dynamic relationship between the immune system and the microbiota. Furthermore, gut bacteria have been shown to direct the glycosylation of surface proteins exposed in the lumen (Bry et al., 1996). The observations of developmental defects in germ-free mice at the tissue, cellular and molecular levels suggest that normal immune function may be impaired in the absence of the gut microbiota. An evolutionary alliance has been forged between mammals and beneficial bacteria that is crucial for maintaining the long-term survival of both. In other words our well-being seems to be dependent to the microorganisms we harbor. The evidence described above implicates microbiota ability in shaping immune responses during health and disease.

Physiological inflammation

The concept of 'physiological inflammation' was introduced as a normal response to colonizing flora. When the capacity to develop or maintain physiological intestinal inflammation is lost, pathological inflammation takes over, resulting in disease (Fiocchi, 2008). Recently it has been reported (Rescigno et al., 2008) the interplay between dendritic cells (DCs), intestinal epithelial cells (IECs) and luminal bacteria. It was demonstrated how a specific protein produced by IECs give instructions to DCs in order to give a mitigated response (physiological inflammation). Moreover, the NALP3 (NACHT domain-, leucine-rich repeat-, and PYD-containing protein 3) large cytoplasmic complex, called inflammasome, links the sensing of microbial products and metabolic stress to the activation of the proinflammatory cytokynes IL-1β (Interleukyne-1β) and IL-18 (Interleukyne-18). Inflammasome has been associated with several auto-inflammatory conditions (Martinon et al., 2009). An altered microbiota could exert its function on underlying mucosal immune system both directly, trough bacterial PAMPs (Pathogen-Associated Molecular Patterns), and indirectly, through bacterial products.

Bacterial role in maintaining bowel health

Several bacterial species have ability in control the inflammatory response. On this base, in the early 1900s, Ilya Mechnikov was the first to propose the use of live microorganisms to maintain bowel health and prolong life. Now, the term probiotic is used to describe dietary microorganisms that are beneficial to the health of the host (Sartor, 2004). Bacterial species can act on several cell types (epithelial cells, DCs and T cells), but recent evidence suggests that the induction of regulatory T cells (TReg) by these microorganisms is crucial to their ability to limit inflammation and/or auto-inflammatory disease. Moreover, it has been recently evaluated the potential role of *Faecalibacterium prausnitzii* on intestinal inflammation using cellular and animal models (Sokol et al., 2008). The authors found that stimulation by *F.prausnitzii* led to significantly lower IL-12 (Interleukyne-12) and IFN-γ (Interferon-γ) production levels and higher secretion of IL-10 (Interleukyne-10). Another gram negative bacterium linked to human innate immunity is *Bacteroides thetaiotaomicron*, able to elicit the over production of the small proline-rich protein-2 (sprr2a), an epithelial barrier fortifier, and the decay-accelerating factor (DAF), an apical epithelial inhibitor of complement-mediated cytolysis (Hooper et al., 2001). Moreover current evidence supports the idea that certain beneficial bacteria have evolved molecules (known as symbiosis factors) that induce protective intestinal immune responses. One of these is the polysaccharide A (PSA) produced by *Bacteroides fragilis,* which induces an immunoregulatory response that provides protection from inflammation induced by *Helicobacter hepaticus*. In particular, PSA suppresses pro-inflammatory interleukin-17 production by intestinal immune cells and protects from inflammatory disease through a functional requirement for interleukin-10-producing CD41 T cells (Mazmanian et al., 2008). Gut bacteria could also interact with the underlying immune system in an indirect fashion, through their metabolic products. It was reported (Segain et al., 2000) how short-chain fatty acids (SCAFs), and particularly *n*-butyric acid, could promote epigenetic changes in pro-inflammatory genes. A better knowledge of the complex microbial networks existing in the intestinal human ecosystem will be an important step to assess their interplay with sub-mucosal immune system (Gill et al., 2006).

Development of the intestinal microbiota

Recent papers (Palmer et al., 2007; Cucchiara et al., 2009) on development of the intestinal microbiota in infants revealed that in the first few days/weeks of life, the microbiota of newborns is highly variable and subject to waves of temporal fluctuations to coordinately assemble a stable microbiota. The first years of life are also a time of great post-natal development of the immune system. As the microbiota has marked influences on the immune system, deviations from the normal development of the microbiota (through modern strategies such as caesarean section, formula-based diet, hygiene, vaccination and use of antimicrobials in infants) may alter the outcome of immune development and potentially predispose individuals to various inflammatory diseases later in life. On the basis of clinical, epidemiological and immunological evidence, it seems possible that changes in the intestinal microbiota may be an essential factor in the incidence of numerous inflammatory disorders.

Equilibrium imbalance in gut microbiota

It is conceivable that the absence of beneficial microorganisms (owing to dysbiosis) that promote the appropriate development of the immune system leads to the induction of inflammatory responses and immune-mediated disease. We could asses that both autoimmune diseases and auto-inflammatory diseases, dysfunction of the innate immune system, without evidence of adaptive immune dysregulation, may be influenced by deviances from well-established microbial equilibria. Literature data established   that specific aspects of the adaptive immune system are influenced by intestinal commensal bacteria (Lee & Mazmanian, 2010). Elevated systemic antibodies towards commensal gut microbiota were found in auto-inflammatory condition as reported by a study conducted on Familiar Mediterranean Fever (FMF), an auto-inflammatory diseases. It has been shown that FMF is characterized by increased systemic reactivity against commensal gut microbiota. This is probably the consequence of hypersensitivity of the inflammasome in FMF that triggers the inflammation and contributes to the excessive translocation of bacteria and bacterial antigens through the gut barrier (Manukyan GP et al., 2008).Understanding the molecular mechanisms mediating host-microbiota symbiosis could redefine our vision of the evolution of adaptive immunity and, consequently, our approach in the treatment of numerous immunologic disorders.

5. The potential impacts of a disturbance on microbial gut composition and/or ecosystem processes

It is predictable that social and medical progress that affects the composition of the microbiota will also have consequences for our physiology and health. The microbial composition is generally sensitive to disturbance. Perturbations on microbial composition might have different results, depending on the resistance or resilience phenotype of the gut microbiota. Finally, a community whose composition is sensitive and not resilient might produce process rates similar to the original community if the members of the community are functionally redundant. Generally adult are more resistant, whilst children are more resilient, due to their developing microbiota till age of 7, when a 'climax' is reached (Cucchiara et al., 2009).

It has been proposed that improved hygiene, is at the origin of increased incidence of allergic and autoimmune diseases (Strachan, 1989; Bach, 2002). Some bacterial agents – notably those that co-evolved with us – are able to protect against a large spectrum of immune-related disorders. In 1998, about one in five children in industrialized countries suffered from allergic diseases such as asthma, allergic rhinitis or atopic dermatitis (International Study of Asthma and Allergies in Childhood, ISAAC committee, 1998). This proportion has tended to increase over the last 10 years, asthma becoming an 'epidemic' phenomenon (Masoli et al., 2004). As human health and longevity have improved in developed countries, new diseases have arisen without obvious explanation. Beginning in the nineteenth century and accelerating in the twentieth century, there have been dramatic changes in human ecology, including cleaner water, smaller families, an increase in the number of Caesarian sections, increased use of pre-term antibiotics, lower rates of breastfeeding and more than 60 years of widespread antibiotic use, particularly in young children, representing a deep microbiota perturbation (Dethlefsen & Relman, 2011). The 'hygiene hypothesis' has postulated that our decreased sampling of the microorganisms in food, air, water or soil is an important factor in modern allergic and metabolic diseases (Blaser, 2006). Our decreased sampling of the microorganisms could reflect the loss of our ancestral microorganisms. As the representation of particular species diminishes in one generation, the vertical transmission to the next generation (Nahar et al., 2009) will decrease. Several specific examples illustrate the concept that the loss of an indigenous microorganism will have consequences for the host. For example, as H. pylori is disappearing from human populations, reflecting both diminishing transmission and increasing antibiotic treatment , both 'idiopathic' peptic ulcer disease and gastric cancer rates are diminishing, which is clearly salutary. However, oesophageal reflux, barrett's oesophagus and adenocarcinoma are increasing, which is clearly deleterious (Pohl & Welch, 2005; el-Serag & Sonnenberg, 1998). We believe that the "hygiene" and the "disappearing" hypotheses , reported as alternatives, could instead coexist. In fact the changing in the in human macro ecology, improved by our decreased sampling of the microorganisms, could progressively affect the composition of our indigenous microbiota, which in turn influence human physiology and, ultimately, disease risk.

6. Intestinal microbiota and autoimmune disorders

The recent identification of symbiotic bacteria with potent anti-inflammatory properties, and their correlative absence during disease, suggests that certain aspects of human health may depend on the status of the microbiota. The medical and social reconsideration of the microbial world may have profound consequences for the health of our future generations. If improvements in hygiene and health care have altered the process by which a healthy microbiota is assembled and maintained, then patients with autoimmune and/or auto-inflammatory disorder should display signs of dysbiosis. This indeed seems to be the case, at least according to a growing number of studies that are now linking these diseases to alterations in the microbiota. The bacterial composition of the intestines of adult patients with IBD is known to differ from that of healthy controls (Frank et al., 2007). This is reported in IBD pediatric patients too (Conte et al., 2006). No infectious organisms have been conclusively shown to be the causative agents of IBD. This raises the possibility that the targets of inflammation in IBD are not pathogens and instead are pathobionts that are overrepresented during dysbiosis. In IBD a breakdown in immune tolerance to gut bacteria also exists (De Winter et al., 1999; Elson et al., 2007; Elson et al., 2000). The cause of this increase in immune stimulation is of great interest, and several lines of evidence indicate a fundamental role for commensal bacteria in the progression of disease (Sartor, 1997). Patients with IBD respond favorably to antibiotic treatment and fecal diversion, and have higher antibody titers against indigenous bacteria than unaffected individuals (Elson, 2000; Tannock, 2002). In addition, inflammatory lesions are more pronounced in areas of the intestine that contain the highest number of bacteria. It has been shown an increased expression of antimicrobial peptides (Cash et al., 2006), higher levels of antibodies towards mucosal bacteria (Furrie et al., 2004) and an exaggerated mucosal immune response particularly in active CD but also in UC directed against bacterial cytoplasmic proteins (Macpherson et al., 1996). Similar results were found in Celiac Disease, a multi-factorial disease where genetic factor together with environmental factors (gluten) participate to the pathology. Our group carried out a study on the characterization of the intestinal microbiota in pediatric Celiac patients before and after gluten-free diet (GFD). Our results showed a peculiar dominant microbiota associable to CD, significantly different before and after the GFD diet and to the control group (Schippa et al., 2010). Furthermore, the gastric ulcer due to *Helicobacter pilory* seems to be related to an enhanced level of auto-antibodies against gastric epithelial proteins (Ayada et al., 2009; Bergman et al., 2005; Sorrentino et al., 1998). In active Systemic Lupus Erythematosus (SLE) patients the quality of the colonization resistance (CR) of the intestinal micro flora is lower than in healthy individuals. A lower CR results in translocation of more species of foreign bacteria. Some of these bacteria may serve as antigen for the production of anti-bacterial antibodies cross reacting with DNA (Apperloo-Renkema et al., 1995). Among patients with Ankylosing Spondylitis (AS) it has been shown an over-expression of Toll-Like Receptor 4 (TLR4) and TLR5 genes in peripheral blood cells (PBC), providing further support for the importance of TLR subtypes responsive to Gram-negative bacteria in the pathogenesis of AS (Assassi et al., 2010). In the autoimmune arthritis disorder the causative etiologies of inflammation are: a genetic predisposition, life style, feeding, and allergy against foods and microorganisms. It has been reported (Mielants et al., 1996; Rodríguez-Reyna et al., 2009) an abnormal intestinal trans-epithelial permeability in these patients that allows a direct passage of undigested food particles and bacterial components in the blood stream, leading to an immune reaction around joints. This altered permeability could be due to the direct interaction existing between adherent intestinal bacteria and the tight junctions of intestinal epithelial cells, as reported in other pathologies (Weflen et al., 2009; Fasano & Nataro, 2004). Epidemiological studies have provided evidence for a link between altered intestinal microbiota to other allergic disorders, such as atopic eczema and rheumatoid arthritis (Penders et al, 2007; Kalliomaki & Isolauri, 2003). In 1999 an investigation of the role of intestinal bacteria in the development of asthma concluded that allergic children from Sweden and Estonia had lower levels of colonization by *Bacteroides spp.* and higher levels of colonization by aerobic microorganisms than non-allergic children from either region (Bjorksten, 1999). Although it is not clear whether dysbiosis is a cause or an effect of disease, it seems that deviations in the composition of the gut microbiota may be one factor underlying the development of disease in genetically predisposed individuals. The effects of the microbiota on the immune system are thus becoming increasingly evident.

7. Conclusion

Accumulating evidence from various sources suggests that the increase in autoimmune and/or auto-inflammatory diseases observed is partly caused by a decline in infectious diseases and progress in hygiene. In a healthy microbiota we will find a balanced composition of many classes of bacteria: a) symbionts, organisms with known health-promoting effects; b) commensals, permanent residents of this complex ecosystem, providing no benefits; c) pathobionts, also permanent residents of the microbiota with the potential to induce pathology. In conditions of dysbiosis there is an unnatural shift in the composition of the microbiota, which results in either a reduction in the numbers of symbionts and/or an increase in the numbers of pathobionts. Overall bacterial richness is reduced, but some microbial taxa may benefit from the inflammatory conditions and increase in abundance. The causes for this are not entirely clear, but are likely to include recent societal advances in developed countries. In addition to the classic pathogenic species, we propose that another kind of pathogenicity exists in the gut: one in which the whole community is "pathogenic" when its emergent properties contribute to disease. In a "pathogenic community" no single microbe is pathogenic alone. Instead, the community assemblage is an environmental risk factor that contributes to a disease state. A microbial community will be pathogenic within the context of other risk factors, such as host genotype, diet, and behavior. A "pathogenic community" could be formed as results of improvements in hygiene and health care, all factors that have altered the process by which a healthy microbiota is assembled and maintained. Thus, patients with autoimmune and/or auto-inflammatory disorder should display signs of dysbiosis in their intestinal microbiota. Genetic and habitual factors shape the composition of the microbiota, which in turn shapes the immune system of individuals that are predisposed to inflammatory disease. The recent identification of symbiotic bacteria with potent anti-inflammatory properties, and their correlative absence during disease, suggests that certain aspects of human health may depend on the status of the microbiota. We can asses that the disruption of the cross-talk between humans and microbes, the "lost in immune tolerance", could be one of the factors leading to the development of a diseases status. The millenary human-microbes co-evolution led to a complete interdependence between harbored microbiota and human host. Understanding the intricate network existing in this complex ecosystem will be a necessary step, in order to give insights on autoimmune and/or auto-inflammatory diseases.

8. References

Abrams, GD, Bauer H & Sprinz H. Influence of the normal flora on mucosal morphology and cellular renewal in the ileum. A comparison of germ-free and conventional mice. *Lab. Invest.* 1963 Mar;12:355-64.

Apperloo-Renkema HZ, Bootsma H, Mulder BI, Kallenberg CG & van der Waaij D. Host-microflora interaction in systemic lupus erythematosus (SLE): circulating antibodies to the indigenous bacteria of the intestinal tract. *Epidemiol Infect.* 1995 Feb;114(1):133-41.

Arumugam M, Raes J, Pelletier E, Le Paslier D, Yamada T, Mende DR, Fernandes GR, Tap J, Bruls T, Batto JM, Bertalan M, Borruel N, Casellas F, Fernandez L, Gautier L, Hansen T, Hattori M, Hayashi T, Kleerebezem M, Kurokawa K, Leclerc M, Levenez F, Manichanh C, Nielsen HB, Nielsen T, Pons N, Poulain J, Qin J, Sicheritz-Ponten T, Tims S, Torrents D, Ugarte E, Zoetendal EG, Wang J, Guarner F, Pedersen O, de Vos WM, Brunak S, Doré J, Consortium M, Weissenbach J, Ehrlich SD, Bork P; MetaHIT Consortium (additional members), Antolín M, Artiguenave F, Blottiere HM, Almeida M, Brechot C, Cara C, Chervaux C, Cultrone A, Delorme C, Denariaz G, Dervyn R, Foerstner KU, Friss C, van de Guchte M, Guedon E, Haimet F, Huber W, van Hylckama-Vlieg J, Jamet A, Juste C, Kaci G, Knol J, Lakhdari O, Layec S, Le Roux K, Maguin E, Mérieux A, Melo Minardi R, M'rini C, Muller J, Oozeer R, Parkhill J, Renault P, Rescigno M, Sanchez N, Sunagawa S, Torrejon A, Turner K, Vandemeulebrouck G, Varela E, Winogradsky Y & Zeller G. Enterotypes of the human gut microbiome. *Nature.* 2011 Apr 20. [Epub ahead of print]

Assassi S, Reveille JD, Arnett FC, Weisman MH, Ward MM, Agarwal SK, Gourh P, Bhula J, Sharif R, Sampat K, Mayes MD & Tan FK. Whole-blood Gene Expression Profiling in Ankylosing Spondylitis Shows Upregulation of Toll-like Receptor 4 and 5. *J Rheumatol.* 2010 Oct 15. [Epub ahead of print]

Ayada K, Yokota K, Kawahara Y, Yamamoto Y, Hirai K, Inaba T, Kita M, Okada H, Yamamoto K & Oguma K. Immune reactions against elongation factor 2 kinase: specific pathogenesis of gastric ulcer from *Helicobacter pylori* infection. *Clin Dev Immunol.* 2009;2009:850623. Epub 2009 Jul 14.

Bach JF, The effect of infections on susceptibility to autoimmune and allergic diseases, *N. Engl. J. Med.* 347 (2002) 911–920.

Bäckhed F, Ding H, Wang T, Hooper LV, Koh GY, Nagy A, Semenkovich CF & Gordon JI. The gut microbiota as an environmental factor that regulates fat storage. *Proc Natl Acad Sci U S A.* 2004 Nov 2;101(44):15718-23. Epub 2004 Oct 25.

Bergman MP, Vandenbroucke-Grauls CM, Appelmelk BJ, D'Elios MM, Amedei A, Azzurri A, Benagiano M & Del Prete G. The story so far: *Helicobacter pylori* and gastric autoimmunity. *Int Rev Immunol.* 2005 Jan-Apr;24(1-2):63-91.

Bjorksten B. The environmental influence on childhood asthma. *Allergy.* 1999;54 Suppl 49:17-23.

Blaser MJ & Falkow S. What are the consequences of the disappearing human microbiota? *Nat Rev Microbiol.* 2009 Dec;7(12):887-94. Epub 2009 Nov 9.

Blaser, MJ. Who are we? Indigenous microbes and the ecology of human diseases. *EMBO Rep.* 2006;7,956–960.

Bouskra D, Brézillon C, Bérard M, Werts C, Varona R, Boneca IG & Eberl G. Lymphoid tissue genesis induced by commensals through NOD1 regulates intestinal homeostasis. *Nature.* 2008 Nov 27;456(7221):507-10. Epub 2008 Nov 5.

Bry L, Falk PG, Midtvedt T & Gordon JI. A model of host–microbial interactions in an open mammalian ecosystem. *Science.* 1996 Sep 6;273(5280):1380-3.

Cash HL, Whitham CV, Behrendt CL & Hooper LV. Symbiotic bacteria direct expression of an intestinal bactericidal lectin. *Science.* 2006 Aug 25;313(5790):1126-30.

Chow J, Lee SM, Shen Y, Khosravi A & Mazmanian SK. Host-bacterial symbiosis in health and disease. *Adv Immunol.* 2010;107:243-74.

Conte MP, Schippa S, Zamboni I, Penta M, Chiarini F, Seganti L, Osborn J, Falconieri P, Borrelli O & Cucchiara S. Gut-associated bacterial microbiota in paediatric patients with inflammatory bowel disease. *Gut.* 2006 Dec;55(12):1760-7. Epub 2006 Apr 28.

Cookson WO & Moffatt MF. Asthma: an epidemic in the absence of infection? *Science.* 1997 Jan 3;275(5296):41-2.

Cucchiara S, Iebba V, Conte MP & Schippa S. The microbiota in inflammatory bowel disease in different age groups. *Dig Dis.* 2009;27(3):252-8. Epub 2009 Sep 24.

De Filippo C, Cavalieri D, Di Paola M, Ramazzotti M, Poullet JB, Massart S, Collini S, Pieraccini G & Lionetti P. Impact of diet in shaping gut microbiota revealed by a comparative study in children from Europe and rural Africa. *Proc Natl Acad Sci U S A.* 2010 Aug 17;107(33):14691-6. Epub 2010 Aug 2.

De Winter H, Cheroutre H & Kronenberg M. Mucosal immunity and inflammation. II. The yin and yang of T cells in intestinal inflammation: pathogenic and protective roles in a mouse colitis model. *Am. J. Physiol.* 1999 Jun;276(6 Pt 1):G1317-21.

Dethlefsen L & Relman DA. Incomplete recovery and individualized responses of the human distal gut microbiota to repeated antibiotic perturbation. *Proc Natl Acad Sci U S A*. 2011 Mar 15;108 Suppl 1:4554-61. Epub 2010 Sep 16.

Dethlefsen L, McFall-Ngai M & Relman DA. An ecological and evolutionary perspective on human-microbe mutualism and disease. *Nature*. 2007;449:811–818.

Eckburg PB, Bik EM, Bernstein CN, Purdom E, Dethlefsen L, Sargent M, Gill SR, Nelson KE & Relman DA. Diversity of the human intestinal microbial flora. *Science*. 2005 Jun 10;308(5728):1635-8. Epub 2005 Apr 14.

el-Serag HB & Sonnenberg A. Opposing time trends of peptic ulcer and reflux disease. *Gut*. 1998 Sep;43(3):327-33.

Elson CO, Cong Y, Weaver CT, Schoeb TR, McClanahan TK, Fick RB & Kastelein RA. Monoclonal anti-interleukin 23 reverses active colitis in a T cell-mediated model in mice. *Gastroenterology*. 2007 Jun;132(7):2359-70. Epub 2007 Apr 13

Elson CO. Commensal bacteria as targets in Crohn's disease. *Gastroenterology*. 2000 Jul;119(1):254-7.

Falk, PG, Hooper LV, Midtvedt T & Gordon JI. Creating and maintaining the gastrointestinal ecosystem: what we know and need to know from gnotobiology. *Microbiol. Mol. Biol. Rev*. 1998 Dec;62(4):1157-70.

Fasano A & Nataro JP. Intestinal epithelial tight junctions as targets for enteric bacteria-derived toxins. *Adv Drug Deliv Rev*. 2004 Apr 19;56(6):795-807.

Flint HJ, Duncan SH, Scott KP & Louis P. Interactions and competition within the microbial community of the human colon: links between diet and health. *Environ Microbiol*. 2007;9: 1101–1111.

Frank DN, St Amand AL, Feldman RA, Boedeker EC, Harpaz N & Pace NR. Molecular-phylogenetic characterization of microbial community imbalances in human inflammatory bowel diseases. *Proc. Natl Acad. USA*. 2007 Aug 21;104(34):13780-5. Epub 2007 Aug 15.

Furrie E, Macfarlane S, Cummings JH & Macfarlane GT. Systemic antibodies towards mucosal bacteria in ulcerative colitis and Crohn's disease differentially activate the innate immune response. *Gut*. 2004 Jan;53(1):91-8.

Galeazzi M, Gasbarrini G, Ghirardello A, Grandemange S, Hoffman HM, Manna R, Podswiadek M, Punzi L, Sebastiani GD, Touitou I & Doria A. Auto-inflammatory syndromes. *Clin Exp Rheumatol*. 2006 Jan-Feb;24(1 Suppl 40):S79-85.

Gill SR, Pop M, Deboy RT, Eckburg PB, Turnbaugh PJ, Samuel BS, Gordon JI, Relman DA, Fraser-Liggett CM & Nelson KE. Metagenomic analysis of the human distal gut microbiome. *Science*. 2006 Jun 2;312(5778):1355-9.

Gordon JH & Dubos R. The anaerobic bacterial flora of the mouse cecum. *J Exp Med*. 1970 Aug 1;132(2):251-60.

Greiner T & Bäckhed F. Effects of the gut microbiota on obesity and glucose homeostasis. *Trends Endocrinol Metab*. 2011 Apr;22(4):117-23. Epub 2011 Feb 23.

Harris MA, Reddy CA, Carter GR. Anaerobic bacteria from the large intestine of mice. *Appl Environ Microbiol*. 1976 Jun;31(6):907-12.

Hattori M & Taylor TD. The human intestinal microbiome: a new frontier of human biology. *DNA Res*. 2009 Feb;16(1):1-12. Epub 2009 Jan 15.

Hooper LV, Midtvedt T & Gordon JI. How host-microbial interactions shape the nutrient environment of the mammalian intestine. *Annu Rev Nutr.* 2002;22:283–307.

Hooper LV, Wong MH, Thelin A, Hansson L, Falk PG & Gordon JI. Molecular analysis of commensal host-microbial relationships in the intestine. *Science.* 2001 Feb 2;291(5505):881-4.

ISAAC. Worldwide variation in prevalence of symptoms of asthma, allergic rhinoconjunctivitis, and atopic eczema: ISAAC. The International Study of Asthma and Allergies in Childhood (ISAAC) Steering Committee. *Lancet* 1998; 351:1225–32.

Kalliomaki M & Isolauri E. Role of intestinal flora in the development of allergy. *Curr. Opin. Allergy Clin. Immunol.* 2003 Feb;3(1):15-20.

Khachatryan ZA, Ktsoyan ZA, Manukyan GP, Kelly D, Ghazaryan KA & Aminov RI. Predominant role of host genetics in controlling the composition of gut microbiota. *PLoS One.* 2008 Aug 26;3(8):e3064.

Lee YK & Mazmanian SK. Has the microbiota played a critical role in the evolution of the adaptive immune system? *Science.* 2010 Dec 24;330(6012):1768-73.

Leser TD & Mølbak L. Better living through microbial action: the benefits of the mammalian gastrointestinal microbiota on the host. *Environ Microbiol.* 2009 Sep;11(9):2194-206.

Ley RE, Bäckhed F, Turnbaugh P, Lozupone CA, Knight RD & Gordon JI. Obesity alters gut microbial ecology. *Proc Natl Acad Sci U S A.* 2005 Aug 2;102(31):11070-5. Epub 2005 Jul 20.

Ley RE, Peterson DA & Gordon JI. Ecological and evolutionary forces shaping microbial diversity in the human intestine. *Cell.* 2006 Feb 24;124(4):837-48.

Li M, Wang B, Zhang M, Rantalainen M, Wang S, Zhou H, Zhang Y, Shen J, Pang X, Zhang M, Wei H, Chen Y, Lu H, Zuo J, Su M, Qiu Y, Jia W, Xiao C, Smith LM, Yang S, Holmes E, Tang H, Zhao G, Nicholson JK, Li L & Zhao L. Symbiotic gut microbes modulate human metabolic phenotypes. *Proc Natl Acad Sci U S A.* 2008 Feb 12;105(6):2117-22. Epub 2008 Feb 5.

Macpherson A, Khoo UY, Forgacs I, Philpott-Howard J & Bjarnason I. Mucosal antibodies in inflammatory bowel disease are directed against intestinal bacteria. *Gut.* 1996 Mar;38(3):365-75.

Macpherson, AJ & Harris N. L. Interactions between commensal intestinal bacteria and the immune system. *Nature Rev. Immunol.* 2004 Jun;4(6):478-85.

Mahowald MA, Rey FE, Seedorf H, Turnbaugh PJ, Fulton RS, Wollam A, Shah N, Wang C, Magrini V, Wilson RK, Cantarel BL, Coutinho PM, Henrissat B, Crock LW, Russell A, Verberkmoes NC, Hettich RL & Gordon JI. Characterizing a model human gut microbiota composed of members of its two dominant bacterial phyla. *Proc Natl Acad Sci U S A.* 2009 Apr 7;106(14):5859-64. Epub 2009 Mar 24.

Manukyan GP, Ghazaryan KA, Ktsoyan ZA, Khachatryan ZA, Arakelova KA, Kelly D, Grant G & Aminov RI. Elevated systemic antibodies towards commensal gut microbiota in auto-inflammatory condition. *PLoS One.* 2008 Sep 9;3(9):e3172.

Martinon F, Mayor A & Tschopp J. The inflammasomes: guardians of the body. *Annu Rev Immunol.* 2009;27:229-65.

Masoli M, Fabian D, Holt S, & Beasley R. The global burden of asthma: executive summary of the GINA Dissemination Committee report. *Allergy* 2004; 59:469–78.

Mazmanian SK, Round JL & Kasper DL. A microbial symbiosis factor prevents intestinal inflammatory disease. *Nature.* 2008 May 29;453(7195):620-5.

Mielants H, De Vos M, Cuvelier C & Veys EM. The role of gut inflammation in the pathogenesis of spondyloarthropathies. *Acta Clin Belg.* 1996;51(5):340-9.

Mueller S, Saunier K, Hanisch C, Norin E, Alm L, Midtvedt T, Cresci A, Silvi S, Orpianesi C, Verdenelli MC, Clavel T, Koebnick C, Zunft HJ, Doré J & Blaut M. Differences in fecal microbiota in different European study populations in relation to age, gender, and country: a cross-sectional study. *Appl Environ Microbiol.* 2006 Feb;72(2):1027-33.

Nahar S, Kibria KM, Hossain ME, Sultana J, Sarker SA, Engstrand L, Bardhan PK, Rahman M & Endtz HP. Evidence of intra-familial transmission of Helicobacter pylori by PCR-based RAPD fingerprinting in Bangladesh. *Eur. J. Clin. Microbiol. Infect. Dis.* 2009 Jul;28(7):767-73. Epub 2009 Feb 4.

Palmer C, Bik EM, Digiulio DB, Relman, DA & Brown, PO. Development of the human infant intestinal microbiota. *PLoS Biol.* 2007 Jul;5(7):e177. Epub 2007 Jun 26.

Penders J, Thijs C, van den Brandt PA, Kummeling I, Snijders B, Stelma F, Adams H, van Ree R & Stobberingh EE. Gut microbiota composition and development of atopic manifestations in infancy: the KOALA Birth Cohort Study. *Gut.* 2007 May;56(5):661-7. Epub 2006 Oct 17.

Pohl H & Welch HG. The role of overdiagnosis and reclassification in the marked increase of esophageal adenocarcinoma incidence. *J. Natl Cancer Inst.* 2005 Jan 19;97(2):142-6.

Prescott SL, Macaubas C, Smallacombe T, Holt BJ, Sly PD & Holt PG. Development of allergen-specific T-cell memory in atopic and normal children. *Lancet.* 1999 Jan 16;353(9148):196-200.

Pryde SE, Duncan SH, Hold GL, Stewart CS & Flint HJ. The microbiology of butyrate formation in the human colon. *FEMS Microbiol Lett.* 2002;217:133–139.

Rakoff-Nahoum S, Paglino J, Eslami-Varzaneh F, Edberg S & Medzhitov R. Recognition of commensal microflora by tolllike receptors is required for intestinal homeostasis. *Cell.* 2004;118:229–241.

Rescigno M, Lopatin U & Chieppa M. Interactions among dendritic cells, macrophages, and epithelial cells in the gut: implications for immune tolerance. *Curr Opin Immunol.* 2008 Dec;20(6):669-75. Epub 2008 Oct 22.

Robert C & Bernalier-Donadille A. The cellulolytic microflora of the human colon: evidence of microcrystalline cellulosedegrading bacteria in methane excreting subjects. *FEMS Microbiol Ecol.* 2003;46:81–89.

Rodríguez-Reyna TS, Martínez-Reyes C & Yamamoto-Furusho JK. Rheumatic manifestations of inflammatory bowel disease. *World J Gastroenterol.* 2009 Nov 28;15(44):5517-24.

Round JL & Mazmanian SK. The gut microbiota shapes intestinal immune responses during health and disease. *Nat Rev Immunol.* 2009 May;9(5):313-23.

Schippa S, Iebba V, Barbato M, Di Nardo G, Totino V, Checchi MP, Longhi C, Maiella G, Cucchiara S & Conte MP. A distinctive 'microbial signature' in celiac pediatric patients. *BMC Microbiol.* 2010 Jun 17;10:175.

Schloss PD & Handelsman J. Status of the microbial census. *Microbiol Mol Biol Rev.* 2004 Dec;68(4):686-91.

Segain JP, Raingeard de la Blétière D, Bourreille A, Leray V, Gervois N, Rosales C, Ferrier L, Bonnet C, Blottière HM & Galmiche JP. Butyrate inhibits inflammatory responses through NFkappaB inhibition: implications for Crohn's disease. *Gut.* 2000 Sep;47(3):397-403.

Snook JA, de Silva HJ & Jewell DP. The association of autoimmune disorders with inflammatory bowel disease. *Q J Med.* 1989 Sep;72(269):835-40.

Sokol H, Pigneur B, Watterlot L, Lakhdari O, Bermúdez-Humarán LG, Gratadoux JJ, Blugeon S, Bridonneau C, Furet JP, Corthier G, Grangette C, Vasquez N, Pochart P, Trugnan G, Thomas G, Blottière HM, Doré J, Marteau P, Seksik P & Langella P. *Faecalibacterium prausnitzii* is an anti-inflammatory commensal bacterium identified by gut microbiota analysis of Crohn disease patients. *Proc Natl Acad Sci U S A.* 2008 Oct 28;105(43):16731-6. Epub 2008 Oct 20.

Sorrentino D, Ferraccioli GF, De Vita S, Labombarda A, Boiocchi M & Bartoli E. *Helicobacter pylori* infection and autoimmune processes: an emerging field of study. *Ital J Gastroenterol Hepatol.* 1998 Oct;30 Suppl 3:S310-2.

Sousa T, Paterson R, Moore V, Carlsson A, Abrahamsson B & Basit AW. The gastrointestinal microbiota as a site for the biotransformation of drugs. *Int J Pharm.* 2008 Nov 3;363(1-2):1-25. Epub 2008 Jul 16.

Stecher B & Hardt WD. The role of microbiota in infectious disease. *Trends Microbiol.* 2008;16:107–114.

Sullivan A, Edlund C & Nord CE. Effect of antimicrobial agents on the ecological balance of human microflora. *Lancet Infect Dis.* 2001 Sep;1(2):101-14.

Tappenden KA & Deutsch AS. The physiological relevance of the intestinal microbiota - contributions to human health. *J Am Coll Nutr.* 2007;26(Suppl):S679–S683.

Turnbaugh PJ & Gordon JI. The core gut microbiome, energy balance and obesity. *J Physiol.* 2009 Sep 1;587(Pt 17):4153-8. Epub 2009 Jun 2.

Turnbaugh PJ, Hamady M, Yatsunenko T, Cantarel BL, Duncan A, Ley RE, Sogin ML, Jones WJ, Roe BA, Affourtit JP, Egholm M, Henrissat B, Heath AC, Knight R & Gordon JI. A core gut microbiome in obese and lean twins. *Nature.* 2009 Jan 22;457(7228):480-4. Epub 2008 Nov 30.

Turnbaugh PJ, Ley RE, Hamady M, Fraser-Liggett CM, Knight R & Gordon JI. The human microbiome project. *Nature.* 2007 Oct 18;449(7164):804-10.

van der Waaij D, Berghuis-de Vries JM & Lekkerkerkvan der Wees JEC. Colonization resistance of the digestive tract in conventional and antibiotic-treated mice. *J Hyg.* 1971;69:405–411.

Vanhoutte T, Huys G, Brandt E & Swings J. Temporal stability analysis of the microbiota in human feces by denaturing gradient gel electrophoresis using universal and group-specific 16S rRNA gene primers. *FEMS Microbiol Ecol.* 2004 Jun 1;48(3):437-46.

Vaughan EE, Schut F, Heilig HG, Zoetendal EG, de Vos WM & Akkermans AD. A molecular view of the intestinal ecosystem. *Curr Issues Intest Microbiol.* 2000 Mar;1(1):1-12.

Weflen AW, Alto NM & Hecht GA. Tight junctions and enteropathogenic *E. coli.* *Ann N Y Acad Sci.* 2009 May;1165:169-74.

Zaneveld J, Turnbaugh PJ, Lozupone C, Ley RE, Hamady M, Gordon JI & Knight R. Host–bacterial coevolution and the search for new drug targets. *Curr. Opin. Chem. Biol.* 2008 Feb;12(1):109-14. Epub 2008 Mar 5.

Zoetendal EG, Akkermans AD & De Vos WM. Temperature gradient gel electrophoresis analysis of 16S rRNA from human fecal samples reveals stable and host-specific communities of active bacteria. *Appl Environ Microbiol.* 1998 Oct;64(10):3854-9.

9

Immunological Effects of Silica and Related Dysregulation of Autoimmunity

Naoko Kumagai[1], Hiroaki Hayashi[2], Megumi Maeda[1], Yoshie Miura[3],
Hidenori Matsuzaki[1], Suni Lee[1], Yasumitsu Nishimura[1],
Wataru Fujimoto[2] and Takemi Otsuki[1]

[1]*Department of Hygiene,*
[2]*Department of Dermatology,*
[1,2]*Kawasaki Medical School, Kurashiki,*
[3]*Division of Molecular and Clinical Genetics, Department of Molecular Genetics,*
Medical Institute of Bioregulation, Kyushu University, Higashi-ku, Fukuoka,
Japan

1. Introduction

Silicosis is known as environmental and occupational pulmonary fibrosis and the most typical form of pneumoconiosis results from long-term exposure (ten years or more) to relatively low concentrations of silica dust and usually appears ten to thirty years after the first exposure (Hoffman & Wanderer, 2010; Madl, 2008; Rimal, 2005). Patients with this type of silicosis, especially in the early stages, may not have obvious signs or symptoms of disease, but abnormalities may be detected by x-ray. Chronic cough and exertional dyspnea are common clinical findings. Radiographically, chronic simple silicosis reveals a profusion of small (less than 10 mm in diameter) opacities, typically rounded, and predominating in the upper lung zones. Patients with silicosis are particularly susceptible to tuberculosis infection — known as silicotuberculosis (Brown, 2009). It is thought that silica damages pulmonary macrophages, inhibiting their ability to kill mycobacteria. Pulmonary complications of silicosis also include chronic bronchitis and airflow limitation, non-tuberculous *Mycobacterium* infection, fungal lung infection, compensatory emphysema, and pneumothorax (Cohe & Velho, 2002; Rees & Murray, 2007). Lung cancer is also considered to be associated with silicosis and the International Agency for Research on Cancer (IARC) categorized crystalline silica as a causative of lung cancer (Cocco, 2007; IARC, 1997; Pelucchi, 2006). In addition, it is well known that silicosis patients (SILs) often experience complications due to autoimmune diseases (Shanklin & Smalley, 1998; Steenland & Goldsmith, 1995; Uber & McReynolds, 1982) such as rheumatoid arthritis (known as Caplan syndrome) (Caplan, 1959, 1962), systemic lupus erythematosus (SLE) (Bartsch, 1980; Yamazaki 2007), systemic scleroderma (SSc) (Barnadas, 1986; Cowie, 1987 Haustein, 1990; Haustein & Anderegg, 1998; Sluis-Cremer, 1985) and anti-neutrophil cytoplasmic autoantibody (ANCA)-related vasculitis/nephritis (Bartůnková, 2006; Mulloy, 2003; Tervaert, 1998).

Silica-induced dysregulation of autoimmunity has been thought to be caused by the adjuvant effect of silica (Cooper, 2008; Davis, 2001, Parks, 1999). Although this represents one mechanism by which silica might be involved in the development of autoimmune diseases, silica can influence circulating immunocompeting cells and dysregulate the T responder (Tresp) survival and activation status, since several different autoimmune diseases may be associated with silica dust exposure as mentioned above. In addition, silica may affect the regulatory T cell (Treg, CD4+25+FoxP3+), since Treg has been considered the most important subpopulation of T cells for the control of Tresp activation by the recognition of foreign and/or auto-antigens (Baecher-Allan, 2004; Bluestone & Tang, 2005; Schwartz, 2005). If the function or number of Treg is reduced, continuous stimulation of Tresp is thought to be maintained.

Furthermore, recent findings regarding the NOD-like receptor family, pryin domain containing 3 (NLRP3, Nalp3)-inflammasome, have contributed substantially to our understanding of the sequential cellular events occurring when silica is inhaled into the pulmonary region and alveolar macrophages try to treat silica particles as a foreign substance (Cassel, 2008; Dostert, 2008; Hormung, 2008).

At first, initial recognition of silica occurs by cell membrane receptors such as the macrophage receptor with collagenous structure (MARCO), scavenger receptor (SR)-AI and SR-AII (Brown, 2007; Hamilton, 2006; Thakur, 2009). The next stage involves capture of silica by macrophages and entrapment within lysosomes and their activation of the nucleotide-binding domain and leucine-rich repeat containing proteins, the NLRP3 inflammasome, to cleave pro-caspase 1 to an active form (Cassel, 2008; Dostert, 2008; Hormung, 2008). Thereafter, cleavage of pro-interleukin (IL)-1β occurs to an active form for release to form fibrotic nodules and production of reactive oxygen species (ROS) and reactive nitrogen species (RNS) in the macrophages yielded (37-40). As a consequence, the induction of cellular and tissue damages occur due to the production of ROS and RNS and the apoptosis of alveolar macrophages. Various cytokines/chemokines such as IL-1β, tumor necrosis factor (TNF)-α, macrophage inflammatory protein (MIP)-1/2, monocyte-chemoattractant protein-1 (MCP-1) and IL-8 are produced that cause chronic inflammation and proliferation of collagenic fibers (Barrett, 1999; Hamilton, 2008; Hubbard, 2001; Porter, 2002). Silica particles are released from alveolar macrophages and the similar cellular reactions described above by newly-recognizing nearby macrophages will be repeated. Finally, silica particles are transferred to regional lymph nodes. As these cellular and molecular reactions are continuously repeated, pulmonary fibrosis will gradually and progressively appear.

Even though details of these initial biological sequential reactions are recognized, it is still unclear how silica causes dysregulation of autoimmunity. From this viewpoint, we have been investigating the following perspectives:

1. Alteration of Fas and related molecules to affect long-term survival of lymphocytes.
2. Chronic activation of Tresp exposed to silica particles.
3. Alteration of Treg function and/or numbers exposed to silica particles.

In this chapter, we describe and summarize our experimental findings regarding the above three viewpoints, and insights concerning silica-induced dysregulation of autoimmunity will be discussed. Investigation using patient materials such as serum and lymphocytes were approved by the Institutional Ethics Committee of Kawasaki Medical School, Kusaka Hospital or Hinase-Urakami Iin. The specimens were only obtained from patients who gave documented informed consent. All of the patients were Japanese brickyard workers in Bizen City (Okayama prefecture, Japan), and were monitored at either Kusaka Hospital or the Hinase-Urakami Clinic. The silica in materials handled by these workers (e.g., dirt, sand, mud, concrete), and thus presenting the potential risk of being inhaled by these individuals in their work environment, was estimated to reach levels as high as 40–60% (by mass). The subjects were diagnosed with pneumoconiosis according to the ILO 2000 Guideline (ILO, 2004). These patients displayed neither clinical symptoms related to autoimmune diseases (e.g., sclerotic skin, Raynaud's phenomenon, facial erythema, or arthralgia) nor any cancers.

2. Alteration of Fas/CD95 and its related molecules in SILs

The discovery of Fas has led to a remarkable improvement in our understanding of apoptosis and its signal transduction (Matiba, 1997; Nagata, 1996; Nagata & Golstein, 1995). Abnormal regulation of apoptosis, particularly in relation to the Fas/Fas ligand (FasL) pathway, has been thought to play a role in the pathogenesis of autoimmune diseases (Eguchi, 2001; Rudin, 1996; Yonehara, 2002). Mutations of the *fas* gene and the *fas ligand* gene which lead to defects in apoptosis have been found in autoimmune strains of mice (*lpr* mice and *gld* mice, respectively) and human autoimmune lymphoproliferative syndrome (ALPS) in childhood (Nagata, 1998; Nagata & Suda, 1995, Mountz & Edwards, 1992; Steinberg, 1994). Fas/CD95, which is mainly expressed on the cell membrane of lymphocytes, usually exists as membrane-type Fas and forms a Fas-trimer after binding with FasL (Matiba, 1997; Nagata, 1996; Nagata & Golstein, 1995). The signal-transducing death domain located in the intracellular domain of Fas then recruits Fas-associated protein with Death Domain (FADD) and pro-caspase 8 to form the active death-inducing signaling complex (DISC) (Curtin & Cotter, 2003; Yu & Shi, 2008). Thereafter, activated caspase-8 triggers a caspase-cascade involving the activation of CAD/CPAN/DFF40 by removing its inhibitor, ICAD/DFF45, DNA fragmentation, and finally apoptotic cell death (Sabol, 1998; Sakahira, 1998).

The most typical alternatively spliced variant of the wild-type *fas* gene transcript is known as soluble Fas (sFas). Since this variant transcript lacks 63 bp of the transmembrane domain, its product (sFas) can be secreted from cells to suppress membrane Fas-mediated apoptosis by blocking the binding between membrane Fas and the FasL in the extracellular region (Matiba, 1997; Nagata, 1996; Nagata & Golstein, 1995). If there is a high level of sFas in the extracellular regions, lymphocytes in these regions may avoid apoptosis and survive longer. Actually, there have been several studies showing elevated serum levels of sFas in patients with autoimmune diseases (Cheng, 1994; Knipping, 1995; Tokano, 1996).

The following findings were obtained from our series of analyses of specimens from SILs. The detection of autoantibody to Fas and caspase-8, as well as topoisomerase I and desmoglein (Takata-Tomokuni, 2005; A. Ueki, 2001a, 2002; H. Ueki, 2001). Anti-Fas autoantibody detected in SILs was functionally active and caused Fas-mediated apoptosis (takata-Tomokuni, 2005). The level of serum sFas was higher in SILs than healthy volunteers (HVs), although the level of serum soluble FasL did not differ between SILs and HVs (Tomokuni, 1997, 1999). The mean fluorescent intensity (MFI) of membrane Fas was lower with lymphocytes from SILs than those from HVs, although total numbers of Fas-positive lymphocytes (membrane Fas expression) did not differ between the two populations (Otsuki, 2005). The weaker membrane Fas expressers (among lymphocytes) were identified to be weaker *fas* message expressers (Otsuki, 2005). The gene expression levels of extracellular inhibitor competing membrane Fas-FasL binding such as sFas, decoy receptor 3 (DCR3), and other alternatively spliced variants of the *fas* gene were higher in peripheral blood mononuclear cells (PBMC) from SILs than HVs (Otsuki, 2000a, 2000b). The intracellular apoptosis-inhibitory genes including *i-flice, sentrin, survivine* and *icad* showed a lower expression in PBMC from SILs than HDs (Guo, 2001; Otsuki, 2000c).

Although significant mutations of *fas* and *fas ligand* genes were not detected, these results indicated that two populations of lymphocytes may exist in the peripheral blood of SILs. As shown on the right side of Fig. 1, one population is a weaker membrane Fas expresser and these cells may have developed out of an excessive transcription of the alternatively spliced *fas* gene and other variant messages. Therefore, these cells may be resistant to the functional anti-fas autoantibody, secrete higher levels of sFas, DCR3 and spliced variants, and are resistant to Fas-mediated apoptosis (Murakami, 2007, Otsuki, 2005, 2007). As reported previously (Otsuki, 2005), patients with a weaker MFI of membrane Fas often have a higher titer of anti-nuclear antibodies (ANA), and self-recognizing clones in silicosis may be included in the fraction because these clones may survive longer and show resistance to apoptosis.

The other population, shown on the left side of Fig. 1, represents stronger membrane Fas expressers that may be sensitive to Fas-mediated apoptosis including cell death caused by anti-Fas autoantibody, show a reduced expression of intracellular inhibitor genes of Fas-mediated apoptosis, and undergo apoptosis. These cells may be recruited from bone marrow after reaching the final stage of cell death. This recruited fraction would not have encountered silica and would be sensitive to Fas-mediated apoptosis. As a result, cells in this fraction would be continuously undergoing renewal and then apoptosis (Murakami, 2007, Otsuki, 2005, 2007).

The overall findings support the supposition that the long-term surviving subpopulation of T cells may include self-recognizing clones. However, these results provide no evidence that the lymphocytes in SILs are activated continuously. Thus, an investigation that incorporates experimental and patient-oriented studies is required to observe the chronic activation of Tresp by silica.

3. Chronic activation of Tresp by exposure to silica

To investigate the hypothesis that silica chronically activates Tresp, we first examined the *in vitro* activation of Tresp by exposure to silica (Wu, 2005). Freshly isolated PBMCs from HVs were cultured with or without phytohaemagglutinin (PHA), Min-U-silica (25 or 50 μg/ml) or chrysotile A (an asbestos, 50 μg/ml) for ten days. The expression of CD69 was used as the marker for early activation of T cells. Results showed that only silica can upregulate CD69 expression in T cells slowly and gradually in a dose-dependent manner in regard to cell surface expression (as shown in Fig. 2-A) and the message level (Wu, 2005). Although the data is not shown here, it was evident that PHA can stimulate T cells and that CD69 expression was observed at day 1 as the peak and then gradually reduced until day 5 (Wu, 2005). Additionally, chrysotile A was not able to induce CD69 expression (Wu, 2005). In this study, the necessity of the existence of phagocytosed cells in contact with lymphocytes was also found, and soluble factors secreted from phagocytosed cells contributed to approximately half of the induced CD69 expression in T cells (Wu, 2005). These results indicated the importance of the NLRP3 inflammasome in these experimental situations. Moreover, if Tresp in SILs encounter silica at the pulmonary circulation and also regional lymph nodes where silica is accumulated after it is handled by alveolar macrophages, they can be exposed to silica chronically and recurrently. In view of this consideration, the activation of Tresp in circulating peripheral blood Tresp and collateral evidence of Tresp activation were then investigated.

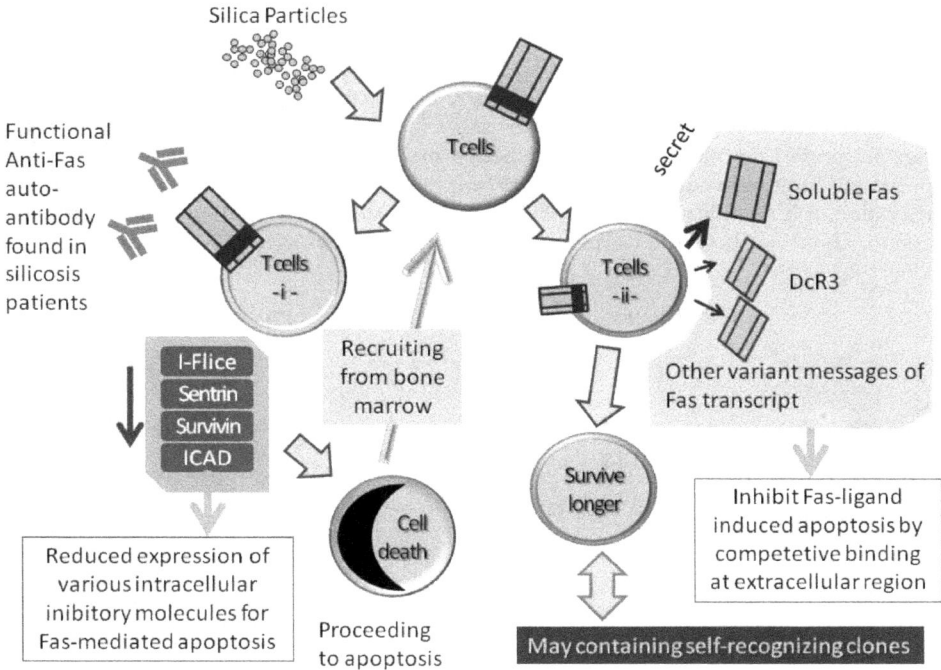

Fig. 1. Schematic model of the dysregulation of Fas and Fas-related molecules found in patients with silicosis. Two groups (temporarily designated T cell - i – and - ii -) may exist among lymphocytes from these patients: a population repeatedly undergoing apoptosis caused by silica and recruited from bone marrow, and another population surviving in the long term by avoiding apoptosis due to self-producing inhibitory molecules such as soluble Fas that may include self-recognizing clones.

With the recent recognition of Treg, most of the peripheral CD4+25+ T cells, particularly the higher expresser of CD25, are considered as Treg (Baecher-Allan, 2004; Bluestone & Tang, 2005; Schwartz, 2005). However, activated Tresp also express CD25 on their surface. Although Treg is defined in regard to the nuclear forkhead box P3 (FoxP3) gene as the master gene of Treg to manifest Treg function in order to inhibit the Tresp activation response against auto, foreign, cancerous and transplanted antigens (Baecher-Allan, 2004; Bluestone & Tang, 2005; Schwartz, 2005), observation of FoxP3 expression by flow cytometry requires the permeabilization of cell surface and nuclear membranes. This procedure is not suitable for subsequent biological examinations using sorted cells. Thus, in the following experiments, CD4+25+ cells were sorted to examine gene expression and the inhibitory function of the fraction.

As the marker for activation, we again used CD69 as an early activation marker and programmed cell death-1 (PD-1) genes (Saresella, 2008; Wang, 2009). Peripheral blood CD4+25- and CD4+25+ cells derived from HVs or SILs were collected by flow cytometry and relative gene expressions of CD69 and PD-1 were analyzed by real-time RT-PCR in comparison to glyceraldehyde-3-phosphate dehydrogenase (GAPDH) expression (Hayashi, 2010). As shown in Fig. 2-B, the CD4+25- fraction from both HVs and SILs revealed a higher expression of CD69 than CD25+ cells. In addition, CD69 expression in the CD25- fraction of SILs was significantly higher than that of HVs. Furthermore, as shown in Fig. 2-C, the expression of PD-1 was higher in the CD25- and CD25+ fractions of SILs than HVs. These findings supported the view that Tresp in SILs were chronically and recurrently activated and possessed long-term survival. Since CD69 expression was limited in the early stage of T cell activation, it is significant that the CD25+ fraction from both populations showed lower expression. However, both the CD25- and CD25+ fractions showed a higher expression of

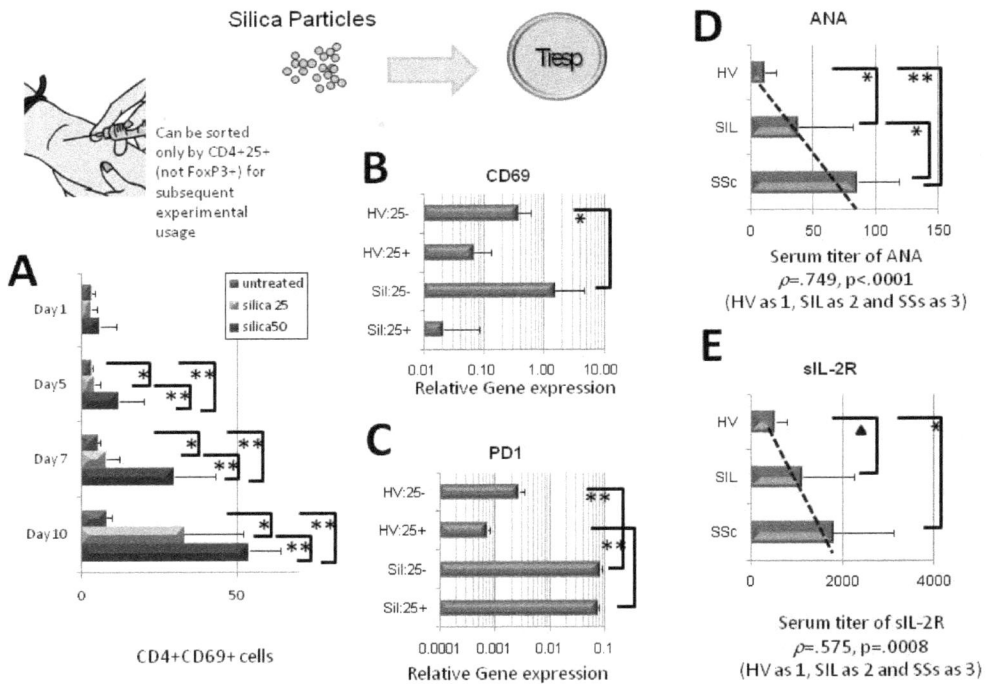

Fig. 2. Various examinations to recognize the effects of silica exposure on responder T cells (Tresp). ＊ : p<0.05, ＊＊<0.01 and ▲ : 0.05<p<0.1. [A] Peripheral blood mononuclear cells from healthy volunteers (HVs) were incubated with or without silica particles (25 or 50 µg/ml) for ten days. CD69 expression in CD4+ cells was analyzed by flow cytometry. [B] and [C] Peripheral blood CD4+25- and CD4+25+ cell fractions derived from HVs and silicosis patients (SILs) were sorted by flow cytometry, extracted total RNAs from individual fractions, and synthesized cDNA. Real-time RT-PCR analyses were employed to compare the gene expression of CD69 and PD-1, respectively. [D] and [E] Serum levels of the ANA titer and soluble IL-2 receptor (sIL-2R), respectively, were measured by ELISA methods and compared among HVs, SILs and patients with systemic sclerosis (SSc). In addition, after a numbered disease status set to 1 for HVs, 2 for SILs and 3 for SSc, correlations between disease status number and titers of ANA or sIL-2R were analyzed.

PD-1 (Hayashi, 2010). This may suggest that silica can activate both Tresp and Treg, and that the CD25+ fraction in SILs may include chronically activated Tresp in which surface CD25 expression occurred continuously due to recurrent stimulation by silica (Hayashi, 2010).

To investigate another marker of Tresp activation, we measured the serum soluble IL-2 receptor (sIL-2R) in SILs and compared results with those obtained from HVs and patients with SSc, since sIL-2R is known to arise in the serum of apparently healthy individuals who subclinically possess neoplastic (i.e., certain lymphoid malignancies such as T cell leukemia and early cell leukemia), autoimmune or inflammatory diseases (Carlson, 1992; Nelson & Willerford, 1998; Pizzolo, 1991; Rubin & Nelson, 1990; Zerler, 1991). The high-affinity IL-2R is a multichain receptor which possesses at least three IL-2 binding chains: IL-2Rα/CD25 (55 kDa), IL-2Rβ/CD122 (75 kDa) and IL-2Rγ/CD132 (64 kDa). sIL-2R is the naturally occurring soluble form of IL-2Rα. For this analysis, the serum titer of anti-nuclear antigens (ANA) was measured in HVs, SILs and SSc using the Enzyme-Linked ImmunoSorbent Assay (ELISA)-based MESACUP ANA TEST (MBL Co. Ltd., Nagoya, Japan), which includes several recombinant proteins such as RNP, SS-A/Ro, SS-B/La, Scl-70, Jo-1 and Ribosomal P *in vitro* transcribed U1 RA and CENP-B protein, and purified antigen (Sm, SS-A/Ro, Scl-70m Histone and DNA) (Hayashi, 2009). As shown in Fig. 2-D, the ANA titer in SSc was the highest among the three groups, and significantly higher than that of HVs or SILs, whereas the ANA titer in SILs was also significantly higher than that of HVs. In addition, if disease status was numbered and set to 1 for HV, 2 for SIL and 3 for SSc, a significant positive correlation was obtained between the serum titer of ANA and disease status. Even our patients did not manifest any clinical symptoms for autoimmune diseases, and SILs subclinically tended to present a dysregulation of autoimmunity. Following these findings, serum sIL-2R was also analyzed in a manner similar to that used for the serum ANA titer. As shown in Fig. 2-E, SSc patients showed significantly higher serum sIL-2R than HVs or SILs, and the level shown by SILs tended to be higher than that shown by HVs. In addition, a significant positive correlation was detected between serum sIL-2R and disease status. These results suggest that sIL-2R may be used to detect immunological alteration in SILs, and that Tresp in SILs is activated chronically to an unknown higher level of sIL-2R (Hayashi, 2009).

4. Chronic activation of Treg by exposure to silica

As we have investigated Tresp activation in SILs as described above, the next point of interest was the function and activation of Treg. It has been revealed that CD4+25+ Treg contribute to maintaining self-tolerance by down-regulating the immune response to self and non-self antigens in an antigen-non-specific manner, presumably at the T cell activation stage (Baecher-Allan, 2004; Bluestone & Tang, 2005; Schwartz, 2005). Elimination and/or reduction of CD4+25+ T cells relieves this general suppression, thereby enhancing immune responses to non-self Ags and eliciting autoimmune responses to certain self-antigens. Recent studies have shown that CD4+25+ Treg specifically express transcription factor Foxp3 (Baecher-Allan, 2004; Bluestone & Tang, 2005; Schwartz, 2005). Genetic anomalies in Foxp3 cause autoimmune and inflammatory diseases in rodents and humans by affecting the development and function of CD4+CD25+ Treg (Baecher-Allan, 2004; Bluestone & Tang, 2005; Schwartz, 2005). Clinically, a deficiency in Treg function or decrease in the proportion of Treg has been shown to influence the pathogenesis of collagen or autoimmune diseases such as multiple sclerosis (O'Connor & Anderton, 2008), rheumatoid arthritis (Toh &

Miossec, 2007), systemic lupus erythematosus (Mudd, 2006), and pemphigus vulgaris (Yokoyama & Amagai, 2010). These findings at the cellular and molecular levels provide firm evidence that CD4+25+Foxp3+ Treg cells are an indispensable cellular constituent of the normal immune system, and that these cells play crucial roles in establishing and maintaining immunologic self-tolerance and immune homeostasis.

As mentioned above, CD25 molecules are also expressed on non-Treg subsets such as antigen-activated responder/effector T cells. Therefore, Foxp3 has been utilized as a useful marker to identify CD25+ regulatory T cells from CD25+ activated Tresp, although several distinguishable markers such as CD127 and PD-1 have been utilized to distinguish Treg from activated CD4+CD25+ Tresp (Liu, 2006; Hartigan-O'Connor, 2007; Saresella, 2008; Wang, 2009).

As described above, since the peripheral blood CD4+25+ fraction showed higher PD-1 expression (Fig. 2-C) and several findings demonstrate the chronic and recurrent activation of Tresp in SILs, the peripheral CD4+25+ fraction in SILs may be contaminated by these activated Tresp expressing CD25 on the base of Treg (Hayashi, 2010).

Thus, we first analyzed the function of the Treg fraction (actually, the peripheral CD4+25+ fraction sorted by flow cytometry in which Treg is mainly included and there is no availability of FoxP3-sorted cells for biological use as mentioned above) (Wu, 2006). As shown in Fig. 3-A, the inhibitory function of the CD4+25+ sorted fraction from SILs was lower than that of HVs when this fraction was added to the mixed lymphocyte culture (MLR) (Tresp was stimulated by irradiated allo-PBMCs) with the ratio 1:$^1/_4$ or 1:$^1/_2$, and tended to be lower when added with the ratio 1:$^1/_8$ or 1:1. There may be a reduced number of true Treg in the CD4+25+ fraction from SILs or an impaired function of true Treg (wu, 2006). Taken together with the results of chronic and recurrent activation of Tresp in SILs (Hayashi, 2010; Wu, 2005), these findings support the possibility that the CD4+25+ fraction in SILs may include activated Tresp due to silica exposure. To examine this possibility, Treg-specific gene expression such as FoxP3 and cytotoxic T-lymphocyte antigen 4 (CTLA-4) was analyzed in CD4+25- and CD4+25+ fractions derived from HVs and SILs. As shown in Fig. 3-B and 3-C, the CD4+25+ fraction from SILs lost the dominant expression levels of both genes. These results suggested the CD4+25+ fraction in SILs was contaminated with chronically activated Tresp by exposure to silica (Hayashi, 2010; Wu, 2006). As expected and shown in Fig. 3-D, the percentage of the CD4+25+ fraction in peripheral lymphocytes was significantly smaller in HVs than SILs. Although the CD4+FoxP3+ fraction did not differ between HVs and SILs, the CD25+FoxP3- population was higher in SILs than HVs (Hayashi, 2010; Wu, 2006). These analyses indicated that the CD4+25+ fractions in SILs were contaminated by chronically activated Tresp due to exposure to silica (Hayashi, 2010; Wu, 2006). Although this may explain the results of reduced inhibitory function of the CD4+25+ fraction from SILs, there may be another possibility regarding the number of true Treg in SILs. Even the percentage of the CD4+FoxP3+ fraction did not differ between SILs and HVs, and a certain loss of Treg may occur, otherwise the reduced inhibitory function may not be fully explained.

We again take an interest with the Fas/CD95 molecule. As Tresp upregulated its CD25 expression due to chronic exposure to silica, Treg may have excess expression of Fas/CD95 because it has been shown that Treg expresses Fas/CD95 and is more sensitive to Fas-mediated apoptosis than Tresp (Fritzsching, 2005, 2006). To investigate this possibility, peripheral blood mononuclear cells from HVs and SILs were stained with CD4, CD25,

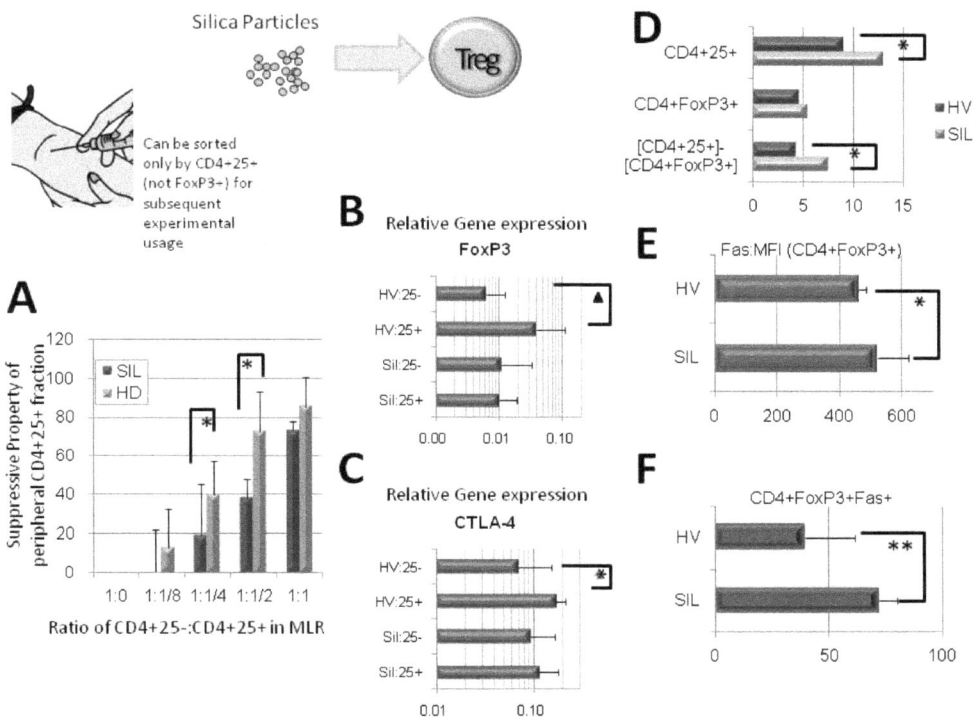

Fig. 3. Various examinations to recognize the effects of silica exposure on regulatory T cells (Treg). ＊ : p<0.05, ＊＊ <0.01 and ▲ : 0.05<p<0.1. [A] The CD4+25- and CD4+25+ fractions from healthy volunteers (HVs) and silicosis patients (SILs) were collected by flow cytometry. CD4+25- cells with or without various ratios of CD4+25+ cells, such as 1:0, 1:¹/₈, 1:¹/₄, 1:¹/₂ and 1:1, were applied to a mixed lymphocyte reaction (MLR). Allogenic irradiated peripheral blood mononuclear cells were used as a stimulator. Graphs express suppressive properties of added CD4+25+ fractions. The degree to which the added CD4+25+ fraction reduced Cd4+25- DNA synthesis was measured by the ³H-thymidine incorporation assay. [B] and [C] Peripheral blood CD4+25- and CD4+25+ cell fractions derived from HVs and SILs were sorted by flow cytometry, extracted total RNAs from individual fractions, and synthesized cDNA. Real-time RT-PCR analyses were employed to compare the gene expression of FoxP3 and CTLA-4, respectively. [D] Peripheral blood CD4+25+ and CD4+FoxP2+ populations were compared between HVs and SILs. [E] and [F] Peripheral blood CD4+FoxP3+ cells derived from HVs and SILs were compared in regard to CD95/Fas expression by means of fluorescent intensity and positive cell percentage, respectively.

CD95/Fas and FoxP3, and CD95/Fas expression (MFI) and positive cell frequency were analyzed in the CD4+FoxP3+ cell fraction. As shown in Fig. 3-E (MFI) and 3-F (positive cell frequency), Treg from SILs showed significantly higher expression levels of CD95/Fas than those from HVs. In addition, CD4+25+ cells from SILs were significantly more sensitive against Fas-mediated apoptosis inducing monoclonal antibody (CH-11) than those from HVs (data not shown), and proceeded faster to apoptosis as previously reported (Hayashi,

2010). All of these findings indicate that Treg may lose its true Treg ability due to chronic activation of Treg by recurrent exposure to silica mediated by excess expression of Fas/CD95 on the Treg cell surface.

5. Silica-induced dysfunction of the Treg fraction in SILs

Our results and those of our previous findings suggest that silica can reconstitute the peripheral CD4+CD25+ fraction to facilitate a decline in the number and function of Treg by the activation of both Tresp and Treg cells (Hayashi, 2010; Maeda, 2010), as outlined in Fig. 4.

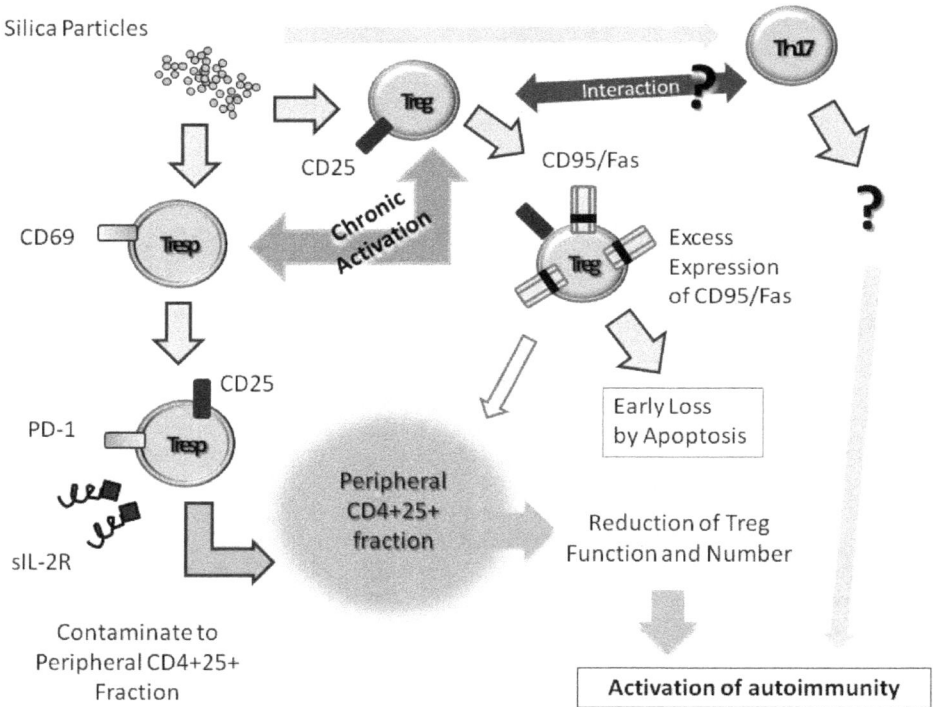

Fig. 4. Schematic representation of the immunological effects of silica exposure on alteration of autoimmunity. Silica chronically activates CD4+FoxP3 T cells (Treg), resulting in the induction of higher Fas expression. This up-regulated Fas marks Treg for Fas-mediated apoptosis. However, silica induces the change of CD4+FoxP3- T cells (Tresp) to CD4+25+FoxP3- activated Tresp. This population contaminates the peripheral CD4+25+ fraction in which Treg should be located. This imbalance between a decreased Treg and increased activated Tresp results in a dysfunction of the so-called CD4+25+ Treg fraction, which may trigger the occurrence of autoimmune diseases such as SSc. However, the roles and alterations of Th17 in silica-exposed patients are unknown and should be clarified through further research in order to obtain a better understanding of the immunological effects of silica on the human immune system.

Many issues remain to be resolved, such as delineating the complications of SSc in SILs (Barnadas, 1986; Cowie, 1987 Haustein, 1990; Haustein & Anderegg, 1998; Sluis-Cremer, 1985), or those complications associated with malignant tumors such as mesothelioma and lung cancer in patients exposed to the mineral silicate asbestos (Greillier, 2008; Toyokuni, 2009; Miura, 2008). Regarding the relationship between tumor immunity and Treg function, it may be that Treg enhances cell numbers or function to reduce tumor immunity (Chattopadhyay, 2005; Danese & Rutella, 2007; Kretschmer, 2006). If this is the case, future investigations will need to determine whether silica and asbestos possess opposite effects on Treg. Furthermore, specific parameters will need to be examined such as the degree of silica exposure, the progression of respiratory diseases (Otsuki, 1999), and identification of a possible individual factor such as the HLA type (A. Ueki, 2001b) that leads to the development of autoimmune complications in SILs.

In addition, the recent discovery of T helper type 17 cells (Th17) has contributed to the recognition of the occurrence of autoimmunity (Afzali, 2007; Awasthi & Kuchroo, 2009; Harrington, 2006; Jin, 2008; Louten, 2009; Stockinger, 2007). Research on the biology of Th17 cells suggests a critical role for Th17 in the development of inflammatory and autoimmune diseases. Furthermore, Th17 has been shown to interact with Treg cells (Afzali, 2007; Awasthi & Kuchroo, 2009; Harrington, 2006; Jin, 2008; Louten, 2009; Stockinger, 2007). TGF-β not only regulates the generation of Foxp3+ Treg cells, but together with IL-6 initiates Th17 differentiation. A reciprocal relationship between Th17 and Treg development has been proposed, since the generation of Foxp3+ Treg cells and Th17 cells both require TGF-β signaling. If the frequencies of Th17 and Treg were regulated by each other, silica-induced early loss of Treg may have an inverse effect by increasing the Th17 population, and represents another way to induce dysregulation of autoimmunity in SILs. Although we have just begun to investigate the status of Th17 in SILs, this is another important and critical issue to be resolved for a better understanding of environmental disturbance of autoimmunity such as that involving silica-induced autoimmune diseases (Shanklin & Smalley, 1998; Steenland & Goldsmith, 1995; Uber & McReynolds, 1982).

In the future, a comprehensive understanding of the immunological effects of silica may lead to the discovery of preventive and therapeutic molecular targets for autoimmune diseases, and will help to clarify the pathophysiological mechanisms involved in the development of dysregulation of autoimmunity.

6. Acknowledgments

The authors specially thank Dr. Masayasu Kusaka (Kusaka Hospital, 1122 Nishikatagami, Bizen, 705-0121, Japan) and Dr. Kozo Urakami (Hinase Urakami Iin, 243-4 Hinase, Hinase-cho, Bizen, 701-3204, Japan) for their particular contribution to the organization of patients. We also thank Ms. Tamayo Hatayama, Yoshiko Yamashita, Minako Kato, Tomoko Sueishi, Keiko Kimura, Misao Kuroki, Naomi Miyahara and Shoko Yamamoto for their technical help. This study was supported in part by Special Coordination Funds for Promoting Science and Technology (H18-1-3-3-1, Comprehensive approach on asbestos-related diseases), KAKENHI grants (18390186, 19659153 and 20390178), Kawasaki Medical School Project Grants (18-601, 19-603T, 20-410I, 20-603, 21-606 and 22-A7), a Sumitomo Foundation Grant (053027), a Yasuda Memorial Foundation Grant (H18), funding from the Takeda Science Foundation (I-2008) and Young Investigator Activating Grant in Japanese Society of Hygiene (H189).

7. References

Afzali, B., Lombardi, G., Lechler, R.I. and Lord, G.M. (2007) The role of T helper 17 (Th17) and regulatory T cells (Treg) in human organ transplantation and autoimmune disease. *Clin Exp Immunol.* 148, 32-46, ISSN:0009-9104

Awasthi, A. and Kuchroo, V.K. (2009) Th17 cells: from precursors to players in inflammation and infection. *Int Immunol.* 21, 489-498, ISSN:0953-8178

Baecher-Allan, C., Viglietta, V. and Hafler, D.A. (2004) Human CD4+CD25+ regulatory T cells. *Semin Immunol.* 16, 89-98, ISSN:1044-5323

Barnadas, M.A., Tuneu, A., Rajmil, H.O., Abud, O. and de Moragas, J.M. (1986) Impotence in silicosis-associated scleroderma. *J Am Acad Dermatol.* 15, 1294-1296, ISSN:0190-9622

Barrett, E.G., Johnston, C., Oberdörster, G. and Finkelstein, J.N. (1999) Silica-induced chemokine expression in alveolar type II cells is mediated by TNF-alpha-induced oxidant stress. *Am J Physiol Lung Cell Mol Physiol.* 276, L979-988, ISSN:1040-0605

Bartsch, P., Salmon, J. and Mahieu, P. (1980) Asbestosis and systemic lupus erythematosus. *Int Arch Allergy Appl Immunol.* 61, 28-31, ISSN:0020-5915

Bartůnková, J., Pelclová, D., Fenclová, Z., Sedivá, A., Lebedová, J., Tesar, V., Hladíková, M. and Klusácková, P. (2006) Exposure to silica and risk of ANCA-associated vasculitis. *Am J Ind Med.* 49, 569-576, ISSN:0271-3586

Bluestone, J.A. and Tang, Q. (2005) How do CD4+CD25+ regulatory T cells control autoimmunity? *Curr Opin Immunol.* 17, 638-642, ISSN:0952-7915

Brown, J.M., Swindle, E.J., Kushnir-Sukhov, N.M., Holian, A. and Metcalfe. D.D. (2007) Silica-directed mast cell activation is enhanced by scavenger receptors. Am J Respir Cell Mol Biol. 36, 43-52, ISSN:0145-5680

Brown, T. (2009) Silica exposure, smoking, silicosis and lung cancer--complex interactions. *Occup Med (Lond).* 59, 89-95, ISSN:0962-7480

Caplan, A. (1959) Rheumatoid disease and pneumoconiosis (Caplan's syndrome). *Proc R Soc Med.* 52, 1111-1113, ISSN:0035-9157

Caplan, A., Payne, R.B. and Withey, J.L. (1962) A broader concept of Caplan's syndrome related to rheumatoid factors. *Thorax.* 17, 205-212, ISSN:0040-6376

Carlson, I.H. (1992) New markers in serum for lymphocyte activation for predicting allograft rejection. Neopterin and soluble interleukin-2 receptor. *Clin Lab Med.* 12, 99-111, ISSN:0272-2712

Cassel, S.L., Eisenbarth, S.C., Iyer, S.S., Sadler, J.J., Colegio, O.R., Tephly, L.A., Carter, A.B., Rothman, P.B., Flavell, R.A. and Sutterwala, F.S. (2008) The Nalp3 inflammasome is essential for the development of silicosis. *Proc Natl Acad Sci U S A.* 105, 9035-9040, ISSN:0027-8424

Chattopadhyay, S., Chakraborty, N.G. and Mukherji, B. (2005) Regulatory T cells and tumor immunity. *Cancer Immunol Immunother.* 54, 1153-1161, ISSN:0340-7004

Cheng, J., Zhou, T., Liu, C., Shapiro, J.P., Brauer, M.J., Kiefer, M.C., Barr, P.J. and Mountz, J.D. (1994) Protection from Fas-mediated apoptosis by a soluble form of the Fas molecule. *Science.* 263, 1759-1762, ISSN:0036-8075

Cocco, P., Dosemeci, M. and Rice, C. (2007) Lung cancer among silica-exposed workers: the quest for truth between chance and necessity. *Med Lav.* 98, 3-17, ISSN:0025-7818

Cohen, R. and Velho, V. (20062 Update on respiratory disease from coal mine and silica dust. *Clin Chest Med.* 23, 811-826, ISSN:0272-5231

Cooper, G.S., Gilbert, K.M., Greidinger, E.L., James, J.A., Pfau, J.C., Reinlib, L., Richardson, B.C. and Rose, N.R. (2008) Recent advances and opportunities in research on lupus: environmental influences and mechanisms of disease. *Environ Health Perspect.* 116, 695-702, ISSN:0091-6765

Cowie, R.L. (1987) Silica-dust-exposed mine workers with scleroderma (systemic sclerosis). *Chest.* 92, 260-262, ISSN:0012-3692

Curtin, J.F. and Cotter, T.G. (2003) Live and let die: regulatory mechanisms in Fas-mediated apoptosis. *Cell Signal.* 15, 983-992, ISSN:0898-6568

Danese, S. and Rutella, S. (2007) The Janus face of CD4+CD25+ regulatory T cells in cancer and autoimmunity. *Curr Med Chem.* 14, 649-666, ISSN:0929-8673

Davis, G.S., Holmes, C.E., Pfeiffer, L.M. and Hemenway, D.R. (2001) Lymphocytes, lymphokines, and silicosis. *J Environ Pathol Toxicol Oncol.* 20S1, 53-65, ISSN:0731-8898

Dostert, C., Pétrilli, V., Van Bruggen, R., Steele, C., Mossman, B.T. and Tschopp, J. (2008) Innate immune activation through Nalp3 inflammasome sensing of asbestos and silica. *Science.* 320, 674-677, ISSN:0036-8075

Eguchi, K. (2001) Apoptosis in autoimmune diseases. *Intern Med.* 40, 275-284, ISSN:0918-2918

Fritzsching, B., Oberle, N., Eberhardt, N., Quick, S., Haas, J., Wildemann, B., Krammer, P.H. and Suri-Payer, E. (2005) In contrast to effector T cells, CD4+CD25+FoxP3+ regulatory T cells are highly susceptible to CD95 ligand- but not to TCR-mediated cell death. *J Immunol.* 175, 32-36, ISSN:0022-1767

Fritzsching, B., Oberle, N., Pauly, E., Geffers, R., Buer, J., Poschl, J., Krammer, P., Linderkamp, O. and Suri-Payer, E. (2006) Naive regulatory T cells: a novel subpopulation defined by resistance toward CD95L-mediated cell death. *Blood.* 108, 3371-3378, ISSN:0006-4971

Greillier, L. and Astoul, P. (2008) Mesothelioma and asbestos-related pleural diseases. Respiration. 76, 1-15, ISSN:0025-7931

Guo, Z-Q., Otsuki, T., Shimizu, T., Tachiyama, S., Sakaguchi, H., Isozaki, Y., Tomokuni, T., Hyodoh, F., Kusaka, M. and Ueki, A. (2001) Reduced expression of survivin gene in PBMC from silicosis patients. *Kwasaki Med J.* 27, 75-81, ISSN:0386-5924

Hamilton, R.F. Jr., Thakur, S.A., Mayfair, J.K. and Holian, A. (2006) MARCO mediates silica uptake and toxicity in alveolar macrophages from C57BL/6 mice. *J Biol Chem.* 281, 34218-23426, ISSN:0021-9258

Hamilton, R.F. Jr., Thakur, S.A. and Holian, A. (2008) Silica binding and toxicity in alveolar macrophages. *Free Radic Biol Med.* 44, 1246-1258, ISSN:0891-5849

Hartigan-O'Connor, D.J., Poon, C., Sinclair, E. amd McCune, J.M. (20079 Human CD4+ regulatory T cells express lower levels of the IL-7 receptor alpha chain (CD127), allowing consistent identification and sorting of live cells. *J Immunol Methods.* 319, 41-52, ISSN:0022-1759

Harrington, L.E., Mangan, P.R. and Weaver, C.T. (2006) Expanding the effector CD4 T-cell repertoire: the Th17 lineage. *Curr Opin Immunol.* 18, 349-356, ISSN:0952-7915

Hayashi, H., Maeda, M., Murakami, S., Kumagai, N., Chen, Y., Hatayama, T., Katoh, M., Miyahara, N., Yamamoto, S., Yoshida, Y., Nishimura, Y., Kusaka, M., Fujimoto, W. and Otsuki, T. (2009) Soluble interleukin-2 receptor as an indicator of immunological disturbance found in silicosis patients. *Int J Immunopathol Pharmacol.* 22, 53-62, ISSN:0394-6320

Hayashi, H., Miura, Y., Maeda, M., Murakami, S., Kumagai, N., Nishimura, M., Kusaka, M., Uragami, K., Fujimoto, W. and Otsuki, T. (2010) Reductive alteration of the regulatory function of the CD4+CD25+ T cell fraction in silicosis patients. *Int J Immunopathol Pharmacol.* 23, 1099-1109, ISSN:0394-6320

Haustein, U.F., Ziegler, V., Herrmann, K., Mehlhorn, J. and Schmidt, C. (1990) Silica-induced scleroderma. *J Am Acad Dermatol.* 22, 444-448, ISSN:0190-9622

Haustein, U.F and Anderegg, U. (1998) Silica induced scleroderma--clinical and experimental aspects. *J Rheumatol.* 25, 1917-1926, ISSN:0315-162X

Hoffman, H.M. and Wanderer, A.A. (2010) Inflammasome and IL-1β-mediated disorders. *Curr Allergy Asthma Rep.* 10, 229-235, ISSN:1529-7322

Hornung, V., Bauernfeind, F., Halle, A., Samstad, E.O., Kono, H., Rock, K.L., Fitzgerald, K.A. and Latz, E. (2008) Silica crystals and aluminum salts activate the NALP3 inflammasome through phagosomal destabilization. *Nat Immunol.* 9, 847-856, ISSN:1529-2908

Hubbard, A.K., Thibodeau, M. and Giardina, C. (2001) Cellular and molecular mechanisms regulating silica-induced adhesion molecule expression in mice. *J Environ Pathol Toxicol Oncol.* 20S1, 45-51, ISSN:0731-8898

IARC, IARC (ed) (1997) *Silica, Some Silicates, Coal Dust and para-Aramid Fibrils. IARC Monograph on the Evaluation of Carcinogenic Risks to Humans, IARC Monographs, Vol 68,* IARC Publisher, ISBN-13/9789283212683, ISBN-10/9283212681, Geneva , Switzerland

ILO, ILO (ed) (2002) Guidelines for the Use of the ILO International Classification of Radiographs of Pneumoconioses: *Revised Edition 2000,* ILO publisher, ISBN : 9789221108320, Geneva, Switzerland

Jin, D., Zhang, L., Zheng, J. and Zhao, Y. (2008) The inflammatory Th 17 subset in immunity against self and non-self antigens. *Autoimmunity.* 41, 154-162, ISSN:0891-6934

Knipping, E., Krammer, P.H., Onel, K.B., Lehman, T.J., Mysler, E. and Elkon, K.B. (1995) Levels of soluble Fas/APO-1/CD95 in systemic lupus erythematosus and juvenile rheumatoid arthritis. *Arthritis Rheum.* 38, 1735-1737, ISSN:0004-3591

Kretschmer, K., Apostolou, I., Jaeckel, E., Khazaie, K. and von Boehmer, H. (20069 Making regulatory T cells with defined antigen specificity: role in autoimmunity and cancer. *Immunol Rev.* 212, 163-169, ISSN:0105-2896

Liu, W., Putnam, A.L., Xu-Yu, Z., Szot, G.L., Lee, M.R., Zhu, S., Gottlieb, P.A., Kapranov, P., Gingeras, T.R., Fazekas de St Groth, B., Clayberger, C., Soper, D.M., Ziegler, S.F. and Bluestone, J.A. (2006) CD127 expression inversely correlates with FoxP3 and suppressive function of human CD4+ T reg cells. *J Exp Med.* 203, 1701-1711, ISSN:0022-1007

Louten, J., Boniface, K. and de Waal Malefyt, R. (2009) Development and function of TH17 cells in health and disease. *J Allergy Clin Immunol.* 123, 1004-10011, ISSN:0091-6749

Madl, A.K., Donovan, E.P., Gaffney, S.H., McKinley, M.A., Moody, E.C., Henshaw, J.L. and Paustenbach, D.J. (2008) State-of-the-science review of the occupational health hazards of crystalline silica in abrasive blasting operations and related requirements for respiratory protection. *J Toxicol Environ Health B Crit Rev.* 11, 548-608, ISSN:1093-7404

Maeda, M., Nishimura, Y., Kumagai, N., Hayashi, H., Hatayama, T., Katoh, M., Miyahara, N., Yamamoto, S., Hirastuka, J. and Otsuki, T. (2010) Dysregulation of the immune system caused by silica and asbestos. *J Immunotoxicol.* 7, 268-278, ISSN:1547-691X

Matiba, B., Mariani, S.M. and Krammer, P.H. (1997) The CD95 system and the death of a lymphocyte. *Semin Immunol.* 9, 59-68, ISSN:1044-5323

Miura, Y., Nishimura, Y., Maeda, M., Murakami, S., Hayashi, H., Fukuoka, K., Kishimoto, T., Nakano, T. and Otsuki, T. (2008) Immunological alterations found in mesothelioma patients and their experimental evidences. *Environ Health Prev Med.* 13, 55-59, ISSN:1342-078X

Mountz, J.D. and Edwards, C.K. 3rd. (19929 Murine models of autoimmunity: T-cell and B-cell defects. Curr Opin Rheumatol. 4, 612-620, ISSN:1040-8711

Mudd, P.A., Teague, B.N. and Farris, A.D. (2006) Regulatory T cells and systemic lupus erythematosus. *Scand J Immunol.* 64, 211-218, ISSN:0300-9475

Mulloy, K.B. (2003) Silica exposure and systemic vasculitis. Environ Health Perspect. 111, 1933-1938, ISSN:0091-6765

Murakami, S., Nishimura, Y., Maeda, M., Kumagai, N., Hayashi, H., Chen, Y., Kusaka, K., Kishimoto, T. and Otsuki, T. (2009) Cytokine alteration and speculated immunological pathophysiology in silicosis and asbestos-related diseases. *Environ Health Prev Med.* 14, 216-222, ISSN:1342-078X

Nagata, S. and Golstein, P. (1995) The Fas death factor. Science. 267, 1449-1456, ISSN:0036-8075

Nagata, S. and Suda, T. (1995) Fas and Fas ligand: lpr and gld mutations. *Immunol Today.* 16, 39-43, ISSN:0167-5699

Nagata, S. (1996) Fas-mediated apoptosis. *Adv Exp Med Biol.* 406, 119-124, ISSN:0065-2598

Nagata, S. (1998) Human autoimmune lymphoproliferative syndrome, a defect in the apoptosis-inducing Fas receptor: a lesson from the mouse model. *J Hum Genet.* 43, 2-8, ISSN:1434-5161

Parks, C.G., Conrad, K. and Cooper, G.S. (1999) Occupational exposure to crystalline silica and autoimmune disease. Environ Health Perspect. 107S5, 793-802, ISSN:0091-6765

Nelson, B.H. and Willerford, D.M. (1998) Biology of the interleukin-2 receptor. *Adv Immunol.* 70, 1-81, ISSN:0065-2776

O'Connor, R.A. and Anderton, S.M. (2008) Foxp3+ regulatory T cells in the control of experimental CNS autoimmune disease. *J Neuroimmunol.* 193, 1-11, ISSN:0165-5728

Otsuki, T., Ichihara, K., Tomokuni, A., Sakaguchi, H., Aikoh, T., Matsuki, T., Isozaki, Y., Hyodoh, F., Kusaka, M., Kita, S. and Ueki, A. (1999) Evaluation of cases with silicosis using the parameters related to Fas-mediated apoptosis. *Int J Mol Med.* 4, 407-411, ISSN:1107-3756

Otsuki, T., Tomokuni, A., Sakaguchi, H., Aikoh, T., Matsuki, T., Isozaki, Y., Hyodoh, F., Ueki, H., Kusaka, M., Kita, S. and Ueki, A. (2000a) Over-expression of the decoy receptor 3 (DcR3) gene in peripheral blood mononuclear cells (PBMC) derived from silicosis patients. *Clin Exp Immunol.* 119, 323-327, ISSN:0009-9104

Otsuki, T., Sakaguchi, H., Tomokuni, A., Aikoh, T., Matsuki, T., Isozaki, Y., Hyodoh, F., Kawakami, Y., Kusaka, M., Kita, S. and Ueki, A. (2000b) Detection of alternatively spliced variant messages of Fas gene and mutational screening of Fas and Fas ligand coding regions in peripheral blood mononuclear cells derived from silicosis patients. *Immunol Lett.* 72, 137-143, ISSN:0165-2478

Otsuki, T., Tomokuni, A., Sakaguchi, H., Hyodoh, F., Kusaka, M. and Ueki, A. (2000c) Reduced expression of the inhibitory genes for Fas-mediated apoptosis in silicosis patients. *J Occup Health*.42, 163-168, ISSN:1341-9145

Otsuki, T., Miura, Y., Nishimura, Y., Hyodoh, F., Takata, A., Kusaka, M., Katsuyama, H., Tomita, M., Ueki, A. and Kishimoto, T. (2006) Alterations of Fas and Fas-related molecules in patients with silicosis. *Exp Biol Med (Maywood)*. 231, 522-533, ISSN:1535-3702

Otsuki, T., Maeda, M., Murakami, S., Hayashi, H., Miura, Y., Kusaka, M., Nakano, T., Fukuoka, K., Kishimoto, T., Hyodoh, F., Ueki. A. and Nishimura, Y. (2007) Immunological effects of silica and asbestos. *Cell Mol Immunol*. 4, 261-268, ISSN:1672-7681

Pelucchi, C., Pira, E., Piolatto, G., Coggiola, M., Carta, P. and La Vecchia, C.(2006) Occupational silica exposure and lung cancer risk: a review of epidemiological studies 1996-2005. *Ann Oncol*. 17, 1039-1050, ISSN:0923-7534

Pizzolo, G. (1991) The soluble interleukin-2 receptor as a new biological marker in diseases. *Allergol Immunopathol (Madr)*. 19, 176-180, ISSN:0301-0546

Porter, D.W., Millecchia, L., Robinson, V.A., Hubbs, A., Willard, P., Pack, D., Ramsey, D., McLaurin, J., Khan, A., Landsittel, D., Teass, A. and Castranova, V. (2002) Enhanced nitric oxide and reactive oxygen species production and damage after inhalation of silica. *Am J Physiol Lung Cell Mol Physiol*. 283, L485-493, ISSN:1040-0605

Rees, D. and Murray, J. (2007) Silica, silicosis and tuberculosis. *Int J Tuberc Lung Dis*. 11, 474-484, ISSN:1027-3719

Rimal, B., Greenberg, A.K. and Rom, W.N. (2005) Basic pathogenetic mechanisms in silicosis: current understanding. *Curr Opin Pulm Med*. 11, 169-173, ISSN:1070-5287

Rubin, L.A. and Nelson, D.L. (1990) The soluble interleukin-2 receptor: biology, function, and clinical application. *Ann Intern Med*. 113, 619-627, ISSN:0003-4819

Rudin, C.M., Van Dongen, J. and Thompson, C.B. (1996) Apoptotic signaling in lymphocytes. *Curr Opin Hematol*. 3, 35-40, ISSN:1065-6251

Sabol, S.L., Li, R., Lee, T.Y. and Abdul-Khalek, R. (1998) Inhibition of apoptosis-associated DNA fragmentation activity in nonapoptotic cells: the role of DNA fragmentation factor-45 (DFF45/ICAD). *Biochem Biophys Res Commun*. 253, 151-158, ISSN:0006-291X

Sakahira, H., Enari, M. and Nagata, S. (1998) Cleavage of CAD inhibitor in CAD activation and DNA degradation during apoptosis. *Nature*. 391, 96-99, ISSN:0028-0836

Saresella, M., Marventano, I., Longhi, R., Lissoni, F., Trabattoni, D., Mendozzi, L., Caputo, D., and Clerici, M. (2008) CD4+CD25+FoxP3+PD1- regulatory T cells in acute and stable relapsing-remitting multiple sclerosis and their modulation by therapy. *FASEB J*. 22, 3500-3508, ISSN:0892-6638

Schwartz, R.H. (2005) Natural regulatory T cells and self-tolerance. *Nat Immunol*. 6, 327-330, ISSN:1529-2908

Shanklin, D.R. and Smalley, D.L. (1998) The immunopathology of siliconosis. History, clinical presentation, and relation to silicosis and the chemistry of silicon and silicone. *Immunol Res*. 18, 125-173, ISSN:0257-277X

Sluis-Cremer, G.K., Hessel, P.A., Nizdo, E.H., Churchill, A.R. and Zeiss, E.A. (1985) Silica, silicosis, and progressive systemic sclerosis. *Br J Ind Med.* 42, 838-843, ISSN:0007-1072

Steenland, K. and Goldsmith, D.F. (1995) Silica exposure and autoimmune diseases. *Am J Ind Med.* 28, 603-608, ISSN:0271-3586

Steinberg, A.D. (1994) MRL-lpr/lpr disease: theories meet Fas. *Semin Immunol.* 6, 55-69, ISSN:1044-5323

Stockinger, B., Veldhoen, M. and Martin, B. (2007) Th17 T cells: linking innate and adaptive immunity. *Semin Immunol.* 19, 353-361, ISSN:1044-5323

Takata-Tomokuni, A., Ueki, A., Shiwa, M., Isozaki, Y., Hatayama, T., Katsuyama, H., Hyodoh, F., Fujimoto, W., Ueki, H., Kusaka, M., Arikuni, H. and Otsuki, T. (2005) Detection, epitope-mapping and function of anti-Fas autoantibody in patients with silicosis. *Immunology.* 116, 21-29, ISSN:0019-2805

Tervaert, J.W., Stegeman, C.A. and Kallenberg, C.G. (1998) Silicon exposure and vasculitis. *Curr Opin Rheumatol.* 10, 12-17, ISSN:1040-8711

Thakur, S.A., Beamer, C.A., Migliaccio, C.T. and Holian, A. (2009) Critical role of MARCO in crystalline silica-induced pulmonary inflammation. *Toxicol Sci.* 108, 462-471, ISSN:1096-6080

Tokano, Y., Miyake, S., Kayagaki, N., Nozawa, K., Morimoto, S., Azuma, M., Yagita, H., Takasaki, Y., Okumura, K. and Hashimoto, H. (1996) Soluble Fas molecule in the serum of patients with systemic lupus erythematosus. *J Clin Immunol.* 16, 261-265, ISSN:0271-9142

Toh, M.L. and Miossec, P. (2007) The role of T cells in rheumatoid arthritis: new subsets and new targets. *Curr Opin Rheumatol.* 19, 284-288, ISSN:1040-8711

Tomokuni, A., Aikoh, T., Matsuki, T., Isozaki, Y., Otsuki, T., Kita, S., Ueki, H., Kusaka, M., Kishimoto, T. and Ueki, A. (1997) Elevated soluble Fas/APO-1 (CD95) levels in silicosis patients without clinical symptoms of autoimmune diseases or malignant tumours. *Clin Exp Immunol.* 110, 303-309, ISSN:0009-9104

Tomokuni, A., Otsuki, T., Isozaki, Y., Kita, S., Ueki, H., Kusaka, M., Kishimoto, T. and Ueki, A. (1999) Serum levels of soluble Fas ligand in patients with silicosis. *Clin Exp Immunol.* 118, 441-444, ISSN:0009-9104

Toyokuni, S. (2009) Mechanisms of asbestos-induced carcinogenesis. *Nagoya J Med Sci.* 71, 1-10, ISSN:0027-7622

Uber, C.L. and McReynolds, R.A. (1982) Immunotoxicology of silica. *Crit Rev Toxicol.* 10, 303-319, ISSN:1040-8444

Ueki, A., Isozaki, Y., Tomokuni, A., Otsuki, T., Hydoh, F., Sakaguchi, H., Tanaka, S. and Kusaka, M. (2001) Is the anti-topoisomerase I autoantibody response associated with a distinct amino acid sequence in the HLA-DQbeta1 domain? *Arthritis Rheum.* 44, 491-492, ISSN:0004-3591

Ueki, A., Isozaki, Y., Tomokuni, A., Hatayama, T., Ueki, H., Kusaka, M., Shiwa, M., Arikuni, H., Takeshita, T. and Morimoto, K. (2002) Intramolecular epitope spreading among anti-caspase-8 autoantibodies in patients with silicosis, systemic sclerosis and systemic lupus erythematosus, as well as in healthy individuals. *Clin Exp Immunol.* 129, 556-561, ISSN:0009-9104

Ueki, A., Isozaki, Y., Tomokuni, A., Tanaka, S., Otsuki, T., Kishimoto, T., Kusaka, M., Aikoh, T., Sakaguchi, H. and Hydoh, F. (2001) Autoantibodies detectable in the sera of silicosis patients. The relationship between the anti-topoisomerase I antibody response and HLA-DQB1*0402 allele in Japanese silicosis patients. *Sci Total Environ.* 270, 141-148.

Ueki, H., Kohda, M., Nobutoh, T., Yamaguchi, M., Omori, K., Miyashita, Y., Hashimoto, T., Komai, A., Tomokuni, A. and Ueki, A. (2001) Antidesmoglein autoantibodies in silicosis patients with no bullous diseases. *Dermatology.* 202, 16-21, ISSN:0742-3217

Wang, W., Lau, R., Yu, D., Zhu, W., Korman, A, and Weber, J. (2009) PD1 blockade reverses the suppression of melanoma antigen-specific CTL by CD4+ CD25(Hi) regulatory T cells. *Int Immunol.* 21, 1065-1077, ISSN:0953-8178

Wu, P., Hyodoh, F., Hatayama, T., Sakaguchi, H., Hatada, S., Miura, Y., Takata-Tomokuni. A., Katsuyama, H. and Otsuki, T. (2005) Induction of CD69 antigen expression in peripheral blood mononuclear cells on exposure to silica, but not by asbestos/chrysotile-A. *Immunol Lett.* 98, 145-152, ISSN:0165-2478

Wu, P., Miura, Y., Hyodoh, F., Nishimura, Y., Hatayama, T., Hatada, S., Sakaguchi, H., Kusaka, M., Katsuyama, H., Tomita, M. and Otsuki, T. (2006) Reduced function of CD4+25+ regulatory T cell fraction in silicosis patients. *Int J Immunopathol Pharmacol.* 19, 357-368, ISSN:0394-6320

Yamazaki, S., Yoshiike, F., Hirai, K., Kakegawa, T., Ikeda, M., Nagata, A., Saito, G., Nishimura, H., Hosaka, N. and Ehara, T. (2007) Silica-associated systemic lupus erythematosus in an elderly man. *Intern Med.* 46, 1867-1871, ISSN:0918-2918

Yokoyama, T. and Amagai, M. (2010) Immune dysregulation of pemphigus in humans and mice. *J Dermatol.* 37, 205-213, ISSN:0385-2407

Yonehara, S. (2002) Death receptor Fas and autoimmune disease: from the original generation to therapeutic application of agonistic anti-Fas monoclonal antibody. *Cytokine Growth Factor Rev.* 13, 393-402, ISSN:1359-6101

Yu, J.W. and Shi, Y. (2008) FLIP and the death effector domain family. *Oncogene.* 27, 6216-6227, ISSN:0950-9232

Zerler, B. (1991) The soluble interleukin-2 receptor as a marker for human neoplasia and immune status. *Cancer Cells.* 3, 471-479, ISSN:1042-2196

Part 2

Pathogenetic Aspects
of Organ Specific Autoimmune Diseases

10

Immunogenetics of Type 1 Diabetes

Rajni Rani
National Institute of Immunology, New Delhi,
India

1. Introduction

Type 1 diabetes (T1D), also known as Insulin dependent diabetes mellitus (IDDM) is an incurable multi-factorial autoimmune disorder. The disease is characterized by the loss of insulin producing beta cells of the pancreas resulting in abnormal metabolism of glucose which may lead to ketoacidosis and several other complications like retinopathy, nephropathy and even cardio-vascular diseases and pre-mature deaths (Pociot & Mcdermott, 2002). World-wide disease affects 1 in 300-400 children (Todd, 1995). Population based data from South India shows the incidence of T1D for four year period to be 10.5/100,000/ year (Ramachandran et al., 1996). Similar prevalence of type 1 diabetes has been observed in North India. A study from district of Karnal in North India reported the prevalence to be 10.20/100,000 population, with a higher prevalence in urban (26.6/100,000) as compared to rural areas (4.27/100,000) (Kalra et al. 2010). T1D develops as a result of complex interaction of many genetic and environmental factors leading to autoimmune destruction of the insulin producing pancreatic beta cells. While 20 genomic intervals have been implicated for the manifestation of the disease (Pociot & Mcdermott, 2002), role of an intricate network of the products of these genes cannot be ruled out. However, unravelling different factors involved and how they interact in integrated networks is like solving a jig-saw puzzle which is the aim of our studies. Basic problem with T1D patients is that by the time they first report to the physician, most of their pancreatic beta cells are already destroyed which leaves the clinicain with no option but to give daily insulin injections. So, there is a need to identify the prediabetics before the onset of the disease and device ways to inhibit autoimmunity in them. Following sections will show the work done in our laboratory to understand the intricate networks in which the genes involved in immune responses interact and their implications.

2. Role of Major Histocompatibility Complex (IDDM1)

The Major Histocompatibility Complex (MHC) region on chromosome 6p21.31 has been shown to have major role in predisposition to get type 1 diabetes. It is also called IDDM1.

2.1 Genes and proteins of the Major Histocompatibility Complex (MHC)

The human MHC, Human Leukocyte Antigen (HLA) system is the most polymorphic system of the human genome with more than 5000 alleles. The alleles of HLA loci are co-dominant i.e. both the alleles at a particular locus are equally expressed. The genes of HLA code for glycoprotein molecules which are expressed on nucleated cells and are responsible for the recognition of non-self from self. The function of MHC molecules is to present exogenous and endogenous antigens in the form of peptides to the T cells for subsequent immune response to take place. The gene map of the MHC region of man on chromosome 6p21.3 shows that it spans about 4 megabases (3,838,986 bp to be precise). It is the most gene-dense region of the human genome with 224 genes of which 128 are known to be expressed. 40% of the expressed genes in this region have immune related functions (Horton et al., 2004).

There are two types of MHC molecules : MHC Class-I and Class-II which differ from each other in their constituents as well as their functions.

2.1.1 MHC class-I genes and proteins

MHC class-I genes are expressed on all nucleated cells in the form of cell surface glycoproteins. Function of MHC class-I molecules is to present antigenic peptides to $CD8^+$ cytotoxic T cells (CTLs). The classical class-I genes in humans are HLA-A, HLA-B and HLA-C. All these genes are very polymorphic with 1519 alleles for HLA-A locus, 2069 alleles for B-locus and 1016 alleles for C-locus and these numbers are increasing with the discovery of new alleles everyday.

The MHC class-I molecule is a hetero-dimer of a heavy alpha chain (about 40-45 KDa) and the light chain, beta 2 microglobulin (β_2m) of 12 KDa (Bjorkman et al., 1987). While the genes for the heavy chains i.e. the alpha chains are encoded on chromosome 6, the gene for β_2m is encoded on human chromosome 15. The alpha chain of the MHC class-I molecule has three domains alpha 1 (α1), alpha 2 (α2)and alpha 3 (α3). Alpha 1 (α1) and alpha 2 (α2) domains are the most polymorphic domains since they constitute the peptide binding groove of the MHC molecule. The genes encoding MHC class-I alpha chain have 8 exons with second and the third exons of the alpha chain gene being most polymorphic since they code for the α1 and α2 domains. The peptides that are presented by the MHC molecules have allele specific motifs, which means that certain peptides can be presented by certain MHC molecules. The affinity of the peptide to bind to the peptide binding groove is determined by the anchors present on the peptide binding groove where the peptides go and bind through hydrogen bonds. Specific motifs on the peptides determine which peptides would bind to which MHC molecule (Falk et al., 1991, Garrett et al., 1989).

2.1.2 MHC class-II genes and proteins

MHC class-II glycoproteins in humans are HLA-DR, -DP and –DQ. The MHC class-II molecule is a heterodimer of two polypeptide chains: an alpha (25-33 KDa) and a beta chain (24-29KDa) (Brown et al., 1993, De Vries & Van Rood, 1985). Unlike MHC class-I, both alpha and beta chains of the class-II molecule are encoded on chromosome 6. DRB1 gene encodes DR beta chain while DRA1 encodes DR alpha chain with 966 DRB1 alleles and 3 DRA1 alleles. Similarly DQB1 and DPB1 encode beta chains of DQ and DP molecules with 144 and 145 alleles respectively and DQA1 and DPA1 encode the alpha chains of DQ and DP molecules with 35 and 28 alleles respectively (Robinson et al., 2009).

While HLA class-I molecules are expressed on all nucleated cells, HLA class-II molecules are expressed on antigen presenting cells like macrophages, dendritic cells, B cells, thymic epithelium and activated T cells (Holling et al., 2004). The function of MHC class-II molecules is to present antigenic peptides to the $CD4^+$ T helper cells (Th cells) which in turn initiate a cascade of immunological events resulting in activation of $CD8^+$ cytotoxic T cells

(Horton et al., 2004). When a non-self antigen is presented to CD4+ T helper cells, they get activated and secrete certain cytokines like Interferon gamma and TNF-alpha in case of Th1 cells and IL-4, IL-5 and/or IL-6 in case of Th2 cells. While the cytokines secreted by Th1 cells activate the cytotoxic T cells which have already seen the antigen in the context of HLA class-I, Th2 cytokines activate the B cells to become plasma cells which make the antibodies against antigen they have seen. Thus an immune response takes place which varies in strength depending on the host factors and the peptides being presented.

There are about 50,000-100,000 MHC molecules on each cell. Most MHC molecules are occupied by self peptides and the T cells are tolerized against them during thymic education so that auto-immune responses do not take place, however, some times something goes awry and there is a break in the tolerance resulting in recognition of self as non-self by the immune system resulting in an auto-immune response. This could be due to low expression of some antigens in the thymus which may result in self-reactive T cells to reach the peripheral circulation. Or it could be due to escape of self-reactive T cells from clonal deletion during T cell development.

2.2 MHC and Type 1 diabetes

Despite so much polymorphism, significant increase of one or more alleles of HLA in a disease population as compared to healthy controls, suggests functional implications due to their role in antigen presentation. We observed a significant increase of $DRB1*03:01$ (p<10^{-6}, Odds Ratio (OR) =11.0), $DRB1*04:01$ (p<0.01, OR=6.4) and $DRB1*04:05$ (p<0.03, OR=5) in the patients (Figure 1a) using high resolution typing method of polymerase chain reaction followed by hybridization with sequence specific oligonucleotide probes(PCR-SSOP) (Rani et al., 2004, Rani et al., 1999).

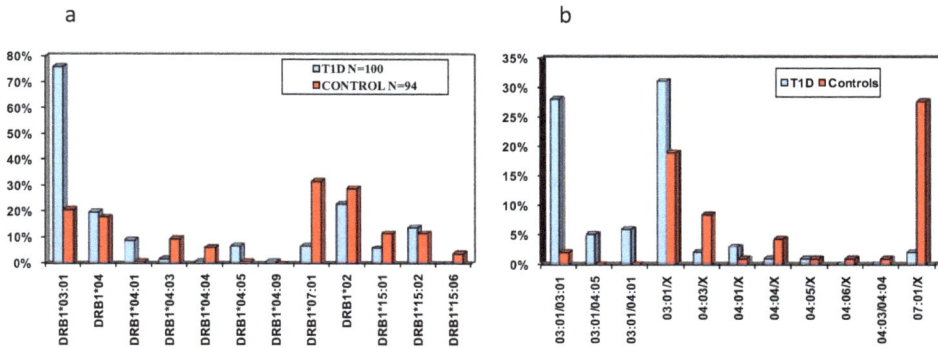

Rani et al., Tissue Antigens : 64:145-155, 2004

Fig. 1. Distribution of *HLA-DRB1* alleles significantly increased in Type 1 diabetes. **a.** *DRB1*03:01, DRB1*04:01, DRB1*04:05* showing significant increase and *DRB1*04:03, DRB1*04:04 and DRB1*07:01* showing significant reduction in T1D patients as compared to healthy controls. **b.** shows the homozygosity and heterozygosity of predisposing and protective alleles significantly increased or reduced in the T1D patients. Homozygous *DRB1*03:01/03:01,* heterozygous *DRB1*03:01/04:05, DRB1*03:01/04:01* and *DRB1*03:01/X* were significantly increased and *DRB1*04:03/X* and *DRB1*07:01 X* were significantly reduced in the T1D patients as compared to controls.

Our results were in concordance with earlier studies in North Indians (Gupta et al., 1991, Kanga et al., 2004, Mehra et al., 2002, Sanjeevi et al., 1999, Witt et al., 2002). However, we also observed DRB1*07:01(p<7x10⁻⁶, OR= 0.16), DRB1*04:03 (p< 0.02, OR=0.25) and DRB1*04:04 (p< 0.05, OR= 0.2) to be significantly decreased in the patients as compared to controls. We did not find any significant reduction of HLA-DR2 haplotype DRB1*15:01-DQB1*06:02 which has been shown to confer strong protection from T1D in most ethnic groups (Baisch et al., 1990, Pugliese et al., 1995), probably because this haplotype has been found with a low frequency of only 1.06% in North Indians (Rani et al., 1998). On the other hand, we observed a marginally reduced frequency of DRB1*15:06 in patients as compared to controls, which did not remain significant when p was corrected for the number of alleles tested for DRB1 locus (Rani et al., 2004).

Figure 1b shows the homozygosity and heterozygosity of DRB1*03:01 and DRB1*04 alleles significantly increased in T1D. Homozygous DRB1*03:01 (p<10⁻⁷, OR=14.54), heterozygous DRB1*03:01/*04:05 (p<0.03, OR =10.9) and DRB1*03:01/*04:01 (p<0.01, OR = 13) were significantly increased in the patients as compared to controls who lacked this heterozygous combination. Heterozygous 03:01/X (i.e. any other allele) (p<0.04, OR = 1.89) was also significantly increased in the patients as compared to controls. Heterozygous DRB1*04:03/X (p<0.04, OR = 0.22) and DRB1*07:01/X (p < 10⁻⁷, OR = 0.066) were significantly reduced in the T1D patients as compared to controls suggesting their protective role. Significant protection has been shown to be associated with DRB1*04:03 allele in a Belgian study of diabetes (Van Der Auwera et al., 1995). DRB1*03:01, DRB1*04:01 and DRB1*04:05 have also been shown to be associated with T1D patients in Sardinians, black population from Zimbabwe, Lithuanians, Czecks, Lebanese, Brazilians and African Americans (Alves et al., 2009, Cucca et al., 1995, Ei Wafai et al., , Fernandez-Vina et al., 1993, Garcia-Pacheco et al., 1992, Skrodeniene et al., , Tait et al., 1995, Weber et al.).

Cucca et al suggested that amino acid position β74 and β86 in DR beta chain are the key residues in the P4 and P1 pockets of the peptide binding groove of HLA-DR molecules (Cucca et al., 2001). A combined presence of Asp, Glu and Val in positions β57 (P9), β74 (P4) and β86 (P1) in protective DRB1*04:03 has been shown to be different from high risk DRB1*04:05 which has Ser, Ala and Gly at these positions. However, in the North Indians we observed DRB1*03:01 to be at highest risk and this allele has Asp, Arg, and Val in the three positions (Figure 2). A less predisposing allele in North Indians, DRB1*04:01 has Asp, Ala, Gly and the protective DRB1*04:04 and DRB1*07:01 have Asp, Ala, Val and Val, Gln and Gly in the three positions respectively. Thus, Asp, Arg and Val in DRB1*03:01 is entirely different from Val, Gln, and Gly in DRB1*07:01 which seems to be important in our study since all the four DR4 alleles are present in less than 10% of the patients or control samples. In essence, these data suggest that it is probably not β74 and β86 alone, rather an integration of all the pockets of the peptide binding groove that determines which peptide of an auto-antigen would bind to the MHC molecule and result in auto-aggression based on the thymic education.

We also studied the alleles of DQB1 locus. DQB1*02:01 which is linked to DRB1*03:01 was significantly increased (p<1x10⁻⁸, OR=5.08) in patients (Figure 3a). However DQB1*03:02 and DQB1*03:07, alleles linked with DRB1*04:01, DRB1*04:03, DRB1*04:04 and DRB1*04:05 were not significantly increased in the patients because two of these alleles DRB1*04:01 and DRB1*04:05 were increased in the patients and the other two DR4 alleles DRB1*04:03 and DRB1*04:04 were significantly reduced in the patients. DQB1*03:01 (p<6x10⁻⁴, OR=0.27) and

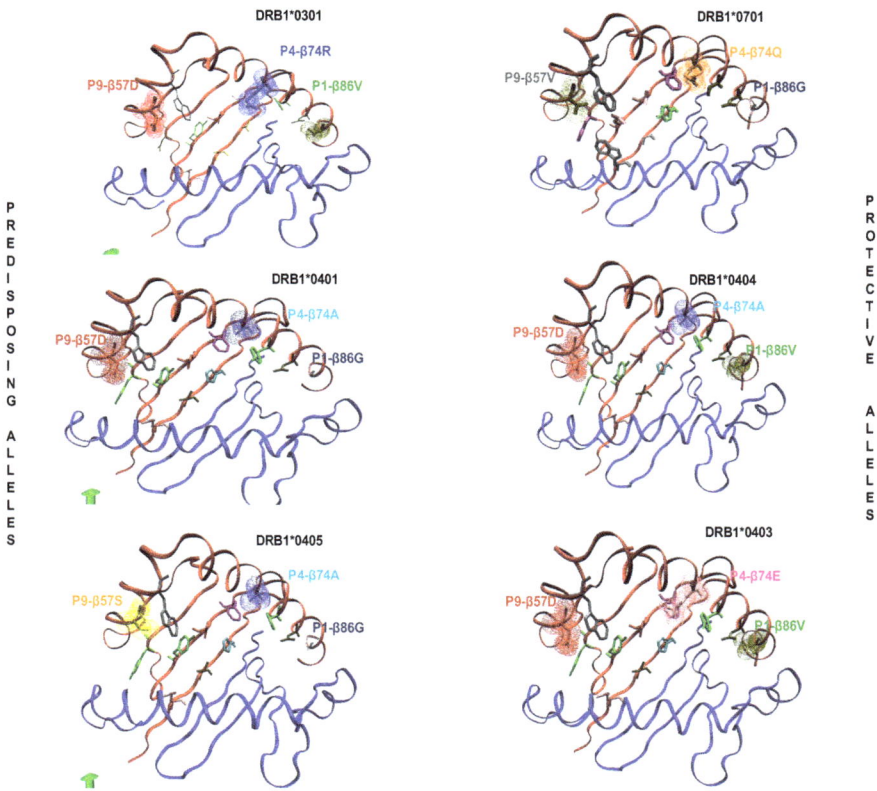

Fig. 2. Peptide binding groove of the predisposing and protective HLA-DRB1 alleles showing positions β57 (P9), β74 (P4) and β86 (P1) for predisposing *DRB1*03:01, DRB1*04:01* and *DRB1*04:05* and protective *DRB1*07:01, DRB1*04:04* and *DRB1*04:03* alleles.

*DQB1*05:03* (6x10⁻⁴, OR=0.28) were significantly reduced in the patients. Homozygosity of *DQB1*02:01* was significantly (p<1x10⁻⁵, OR=5.4) increased in the patients (Figure 3b). *DQB1*03:02* which was not significantly increased in the patients, showed a significant increase in heterozygous combination with *DQB1*0201* (p<2x10⁻⁵, OR=34.16). In fact none of the controls had *DQB1*0201/*0302* heterozygous combination. In a Swedish study, *DQA1*0301/DQB1*0302* and heterozygous combinations of *DQA1*0301/DQB1*0302* and *DQA1*0201/DQB1*0501* have been shown to confer the highest susceptibility (Sanjeevi et al., 1995).

Some critical residues within the peptide binding sites of HLA-DQ beta chain have been proposed to play a crucial role in conferring predisposition to and protection from the diseases (Nepom & Kwok, 1998, Sheehy, 1992, Todd et al., 1987). Several studies have suggested that aspartic acid at DQβ residue 57 confers protection while DQB1 alleles with alanine at that position (*DQB1*02:01* and *DQB1*03:02*) and DQA1 with arginine at position 52 (R⁵²) confer susceptibility (Badenhoop et al., 1995, Chauffert et al., 1995, Todd et al., 1987). However, an individual can be either homozygous or heterozygous for alleles carrying

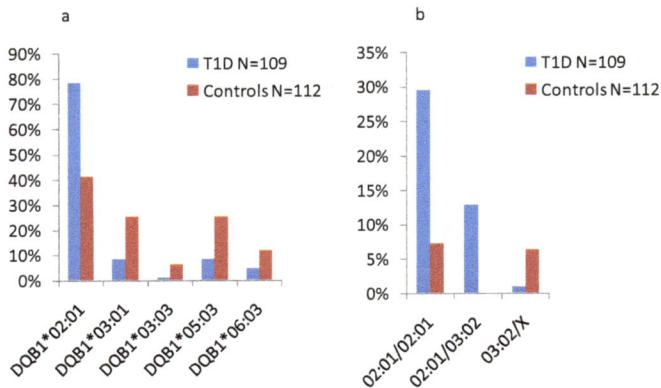

Rani et al., Tissue Antigens : 64:145-155, 2004

Fig. 3. Distribution of *HLA-DQB1* alleles in T1D patients and controls. **a** shows *DQB1*02:01* was significantly increased and *DQB1*03:01* and *DQB1*05:03* were significantly reduced in T1D patients as compared to controls. **b**. Homozygous and heterozygous DQB1 alleles in T1D. Homozygous *DQB1*02:01/*02:01* and heterozygous *DQB1*02:01/*03:02* were significantly increased and *DQB1*03:02/X* were significantly reduced in T1D patients as compared to controls (Rani et al., 2004).

Asp[57] in DQB1 or Arg[52] in DQA1. Our in-depth investigation revealed that when DR3 homozygosity was considered along with codon 57 of *DQB1* and codon 52 of *DQA1*, the only combination that was significantly increased in the patients group as compared to the controls was *DRB1*03:01,03:01-DQB1*XX-DQA1*RR*, suggesting that *DRB1*03:01* association is primary since the *DQB1* and *DQA1* alleles which are in linkage disequilibrium with *DRB1*03:01* have non-Asp57 (DQB1*X) and Arg52 (DQA1*R), respectively(Rani et al., 1999).

3. Insulin linked polymorphic region in T1D (IDDM2)

Insulin linked polymorphic region *(IDDM2)* consists of a highly polymorphic stretch of 14-15 base pair repeats of DNA lying 365 bp upstream of the initiation of transcription of the *insulin (INS)* gene. *IDDM2* has been shown to have a role in transcription of insulin in thymus. Several forms of IDDM2 have been reported based on the number of repeats (Bell et al., 1981, Kennedy et al., 1995). These *INS-variable number of tandem repeats (VNTR)* are divided into three different classes based on their sizes: *class-I* (26-63 repeats), *Class II* (about 85 repeats) and *class III* (141-209 repeats) (Bell et al., 1982, Bennett et al., 1995, Rotwein et al., 1986). T1D is associated with class I homozygosity (Bell et al., 1981, Bennett et al., 1995, Kennedy et al., 1995, Lucassen et al., 1993). We studied *INS-VNTR Class-I* and *Class-III* alleles based on typing for *Insulin gene 1127 Pst I* site (3′end) by PCR-RFLP as described by Pugliese et al (Pugliese et al., 1997)

Table 1 shows the frequencies of *Insulin VNTR* in T1D patients and healthy controls. While the frequency of *class-I VNTR* was increased significantly in the patients, *class-III VNTR* was decreased in them as compared to the controls. However, when the genotypes were studied, *class I* homozygosity was considerably increased in the patients as compared to controls, giving an Odds ratio of 7.8. *Class I, III* heterozygosity was significantly reduced in the patients (Rani et al., 2004).

INS-VNTR	DIABETES		CONTROLS		p value	OR
	No.	%	No.	%		
Class I	108	98.2	85	89.47	0.008	6.35
Class III	64	58.2	87	91.57	2 X 10^{-8}	0.13
Genotypes						
Class I, I	46	41.8	8	8.42	2X10^{-8}	7.8
Class I, III	62	56.4	77	81.05	10^{-5}	0.301
Class III, III	2	1.8	10	10.52	0.008	0.157

Table 1. INS-VNTR allele frequencies and Genotype frequencies in T1D patients and controls.

3.1 Simultaneous presence of predisposing *HLA-DRB1* and *INS-VNTR* alleles

MHC and *VNTR* are encoded on two different chromosomes. However, they may have integrated roles in manifestation of T1D due to the functional implications of these genes. So, we studied if simultaneous presence of the predisposing alleles of the two genes had any role to play in manifestation of T1D.

Our investigation revealed that homozygous *Class-I INS-VNTR* along with homozygous or heterozygous *DRB1*03:01* were significantly increased in the T1D patients (p<1x10^{-8}) with a Relative Risk of 70.81 (Rani et al., 2004). In fact, none of the controls had homozygous *Class-I INS-VNTR* along with *DRB1*03:01* in homozygous or heterozygous state. This combination gives a positive predictive value (PPV) of 100% with a specificity of 100% and sensitivity of 32.63% since only 32.63% of the patients showed this combination. Since *DRB1*03:01* homozygosity is significantly increased in the patients, homozygous *DRB1*03:01* and heterozygous *DRB1*03:01* only with *DRB1*04:01* and *DRB1*04:05* along with heterozygous *I, III-INS-VNTR* may also be considered as predisposing since it gives a relative risk of 10.55 (Rani et al., 2004).

If we add all these predisposing combinations i.e. simultaneous presence of homozygous or heterozygous *HLA-DRB1*03:01* along with homozygous (Class-I, I) or heterozygous (I, III) VNTR class-I and III, 50.53% of the patients as compared to only 1.4% of the controls had these combinations giving a relative risk of 48.67. This combination gives a PPV of 97.96% with a specificity of 98.6% and sensitivity of 50.5% since only 50.5% of the patients showed this combination. Thus, our results showed that: (1) homozygous or heterozygous *DRB1*03:01* along with homozygous Class-I INS-VNTR and (2) homozygous *DRB*03:01* and heterozygous *DRB1*03:01* only with *DRB1*04:01* or *DRB1*04:05* with heterozygous *Class-I/III* INS-VNTR may be used to predict a pre-diabetic before the onset of the disease in North Indian high risk group (Rani et al., 2004). However, typing a larger cohort may be required to confirm such a major increase in risk.

Pathogenesis of T1D is extremely complex. Significant association with *HLA-DRB1*03:01* and *INS-VNTR Class-I* may have functional implications. Increase in frequency of particular MHC allele suggests that these molecules may be preferentially presenting certain auto-peptides to the T cells resulting in subsequent autoimmune responses. Studies on *INS-VNTR*, however, have shown that *class-III* alleles are associated with 2 to 3 fold higher mRNA levels of insulin than *Class-I* in thymii of fetuses, suggesting poor expression of thymic INS expression   resulting in poor thymic education for insulin in people with homozygous *Class-I,I* and *class-I,III VNTRs* resulting in break of tolerance in predisposed individuals. However, higher expression of insulin in the thymii of individuals with homozygous *class-III, III* may be able to facilitate immune tolerance induction, as a mechanism for dominant protective effect of *Class-III* alleles (Pugliese et al., 1997, Vafiadis et al., 1997).

Our results are contrary to that of Veijola et al. (Veijola et al., 1995) on Finnish children who showed that both 5' and 3' INS loci showed an association with T1D in *non-DR3/non-DR4* patients (Veijola et al., 1995). However, in our studies only 9.47% of the non-DR3/DR4 patients were homozygous for *Class-I INS-VNTR* as compared to 4.2% controls and this difference was not significant statistically. Julier et al. (Julier et al., 1991), on the other hand, had reported that the risk contributed by the INS region was increased in *DR4*-positive patients. Again, in our study only 6.32% of the patients as compared to 1.39% of controls had *INS-VNTR class-I* homozygosity with *DRB1*04:01* and *DRB1*04:05* alleles and this difference was not significant statistically.

4. Cytokine genes

Cytokines are the coordinators of the immune system that interact in integrated networks and functions of one cytokine may be modulated or substituted by another (Bidwell et al., 1999). A cascade of cytokines are involved in pro-inflammatory auto-immune responses in T1D. Single nucleotide polymorphisms (SNPs) in different pro-inflammatory and anti-inflammatory cytokine genes at certain defined regions have been shown to be associated with differential amount of their production (Asderakis et al., 2001, Awad et al., 1998, Bittar et al., 2006, Burzotta et al., 2001, Fishman et al., 1998, Louis et al., 1998, Pociot et al., 1993). Pro-inflammatory cytokines and their integrated influences are known to regulate complex immune responses during autoimmune destruction of tissues (Rabinovitch, 1994). Hence it is necessary that they are studied and analysed in context of each other and not in isolation from each other. We had reported for the first time the integration and interaction of *TNF-α* gene with other cytokine genes and *HLA-DRB1* and *B* loci alleles (Kumar et al., 2007).

We studied the cytokine gene polymorphism using XIIIth International Histocompatibility Workshop's (IHWC, Heidelberg kit) and One lambda's cytokine typing kits (Canoga Park, CA, USA) based on Polymerase Chain reaction (PCR) with sequence specific primers (PCR-SSP). PCR-SSPs were done for *IFN-γ (A^{+874}T)* (14), *TNF-α (G^{-308}A)* (15), *IL-6 (G^{-174}C)* (9), *IL-10 (A^{-1082}G, T^{-819}C, C^{-592}A)* (16), and *TGFβ1 (T^{cdn10}C, G^{cdn25}C)* (11). T→C substitution in nucleotide 29, codon 10 of the first exon of TGFβ1, changes the amino acid Leu → Pro. Similarly G→ C substitution in nucleotide 74, codon 25 of first exon of *TGFβ1*, changes the amino acid Arg → Pro. However, since we are studying the SNPs in the two codons, we will refer to the SNPs in codons 10 and 25 hereafter. and not the resultant amino acids to avoid any confusion and to maintain consistency with the other SNPs.

Our results showed that the high producing genotype of *TNF-α-308GA* and *AA* were significantly increased and low producing genotype *GG* was significantly reduced in T1D patients as compared to controls (p < 7 x10^{-6}). None of the other cytokine genes showed any significant difference between the patients and controls.

4.1 Simultaneous presence of TNF-α genotypes with IFN-γ, IL-6, IL-10 and TGF-β1 genotypes and haplotypes

TNF-α, IFN-γ, IL-10, IL-6 and *TGF-β1* genes are localized on different chromosomes. *TNF-α* is encoded on chromosome 6p21.3, *IFN-γ* is encoded on 12q14, *IL-10* is encoded on 1q31-q32, *IL-6* is encoded on 7p21 and *TGF-β1* is encoded on 19q13.2. However, the products of these genes interact in integrated networks. Since only *TNF-α* showed a significant association with T1D, we studied whether simultaneous presence of *TNF-α* genotypes with different genotypes of the other cytokines in an individual could suggest an interaction between these cytokine genes.

Other cytokines Genotype / haplotype	TNF-α GA/AA				TNF-α GG			
	T1D No. (%)	Controls No. (%)	p	OR (95% CI)	T1D No. (%)	Controls No. (%)	p	OR (95% CI)
IFN-γ Int +874	N=235	N=128			N=235	N=128		
AA (L)	41 (17.4)	9 (7.0)	0.003@	2.79 (1. 25-6.42)	46 (19.6)	44 (34.4)	0.001@	0.465 (0.28-0.77)
TA+TT (H)	56 (23.8)	15 (11.07)	0.003@	2.39 (1.24-4.66)	92 (39.1)	60 (46. 9)	0.188	0.729 (0.461-1.15)
IL-6 -174	N=235	N=127$			N=235	N=127$		
CC (L)	11 (4.7)	1 (0.78)	0.03#	4.3 (1. 21-14.56)	14 (5.95)	8 (6.29)	0.531	0.919 (0.357-2.53)
GG+GC (H)	86 (36.6)	23 (18.1)	0.0001@	2.61 (1.5-4.56)	124 (52.75)	95 (74.8)	0.000004@	0.76 (0.227-0.621)
*IL-10 Haplotypes**	N=235	N=128			N=235	N=128		
Low secretor	45 (19.2)	16 (12.7)	0.068	1.65 (0.86-3.22)	77 (32.76)	57 (44.5)	0.03#	0. 607 (0. 38-0.96)
High Secretor	52 (22.1)	8 (6. 25)	0.0001@	4.26 (1.9-10.1)	61 (25.95)	47 (36.7)	0.04#	0.6 (0.37-0.98)
*TGF-β1 Haplotypes**	N=235	N=128			N=235	N=128		
Low secretor	8 (3.4)	1 (0.8)	0.11	3.17 (0.87-12.11)	7 (2.98)	3 (2.3)	0.506	1.17 (0.443-3.23)
High Secretor	89 (37.8)	23 (18.0)	0.00004@	2.8 (1.6-4.86)	131 (55.7)	101 (78.9)	0.000006@	0. 336 (0.198-0.568)

N=Total number of samples studied, $Number of control samples studied for IL-6 were 127, one sample could not be typed due to PCR failure. TNF-α GA/AA have been combined as high secretor genotypes.
# Corrected p value (pc) not significant, @ Corrected p value (pc) significant,
*IL-10 : halpotype combinations -1082/-819/-590 : GCC,GCC; GCC,ACC; GCC,ATA= high secretors; ACC,ACC; ACC,ATA = Low secretors.
TGF- β1 halpotype combinations Cdn10/Cdn25 : TG,TG; TG,CG; TG,CC; CG,CG =High secretors, CG,CC, CC,CC = Low secretors.

Table 2. Simultaneous presence of *TNF-α* genotypes with *IFN-γ, IL-6, IL-10* and *TGF-β1* genotypes and haplotypes (Kumar et al., 2007).

Table 2 shows the simultaneous presence of high and low secreting genotypes of *TNF-α*, along with *IFN-γ, IL-6, IL-10* and *TGF-β1* genotypes and haplotypes. When *IFN-γ* was studied by itself, it did not show any significant difference between patients and controls. However, when studied in the context of *TNF-α -308G/A*, both low and high secretor genotypes, *IFN-γ (+874AA* and *TA+TT* respectively) along with high secretor genotypes of *TNF-α -308 GA+AA* were significantly increased in patients as compared to controls, suggesting its effect is rather neutral. However, low producer genotypes of *TNF-α -308GG* along with low producer genotype of *IFN-γ +874 AA* seems to be protective. Interestingly, 66. 7% of the patients who had low producer genotype of *TNF-α -308GG* had high producer genotype of *IFN-γ +874 TA+TT*. Hence, in the absence of high secretor genotype of *TNF-α*, *IFN-γ* may have a role in autoimmune destruction of pancreatic beta cells. *IFN-γ* acts singularly as well as synergistically with other inflammatory stimuli to induce NO production which can be cytotoxic and thus has been implicated in pathogenesis of certain autoimmune and inflammatory diseases (Mccartney-Francis et al., 1993).

Similarly, promoter SNPs of *IL-6 -174G/C* did not show any significant difference between patients and controls, but when studied in the context of *TNF-α -308G/A*, high producer genotypes, *IL-6 -174 GG+GC* (Fishman et al., 1998) were increased in patients with *TNF-α - 308 GA+AA*. Kristiansen and Mandrup-Poulsen (Kristiansen & Mandrup-Poulsen, 2005) have shown that IL-6 promotes islet inflammation but is unable to promote β-cell destruction for which other pro-inflammatory cytokines are needed. The other pro-inflammatory cytokine playing a role in destruction β-cells in the present scenario could be

HLA-B-DRB1-haplotypes	Patients N=210		Controls N=91.		p	OR (95% C.I.)
	No*	%	No*	%		
B*8-DRB1*03	69	32.85	3	3.3	10^{-8}	14.35 (4.19 -37.93)
B*8- Non DRB1*03	2	0.95	1	1.1	0.662	0.865 (0.498-1.5)
B*50 – DRB1*03	41	19.5	3	3.3	6×10^{-5}	7.11 (2.04-21.47)
B*50 – Non-DRB1*03	6	2.86	4	4.4	0.355	0.639 (0.155-2.77)
B*58 – DRB1*03	36	17.1	5	5.5	0.003	3.55 (1.27-10.72)
B*58 – Non DRB1*03	3	1.4	8	8.8	0.003	0.165 (0.06-0.433)
NonB8/B50/58-DRB1*03	35	16.7	6	6.6	0.01	2.83 (1.09-7.82)
NonB8/B50/B58/non DRB1*03	38	18.1	59	64.8	10^{-8}	0.12 (0.06-0.216)

* No. of patients / Controls with the haplotypes shown in the first column.

Table 3. Comparison of HLA-B-DRB1 haplotypes showing significant association, between patients and controls (Kumar et al., 2007)

TNF- α in patients with *GA* and *AA* genotypes and IFN-γ in patients with *TNF-α GG* genotype. High producer genotype *IL-6 -174 GG+GC* along with low producer genotype of *TNF-α -308GG* seems to be protective.

Different haplotypes of *IL-10* based on SNPs in the promoter region have been shown to be associated with quantity of IL-10 production in-vitro (Asderakis et al., 2001, Stanilova et al., 2006). The frequency of low producer haplotype of *IL-10 ATA* (haplotype with positions -1082/-819/-590) has been shown to be increased in the adult onset patients in Japan, with no significant differences between T1D patients and controls (Ide et al., 2002). Reynier et al (Reynier et al., 2006) did not see any significant association of *IL-10-1082G/A* with T1D in French population. However, they did observe a significant association of *IL-10 -1082* polymorphism to be associated with GAD and IA-2 antibody at clinical onset. In our study also, we did not observe any significant difference between TID patients and controls when *IL-10* was studied by itself. However, simultaneous presence of high producer genotypes of *TNF-α -308 GA+AA* and high producer haplotypes of *IL-10* in the patients may have a role in recruitment of islet specific CD8+ T cells and thus may have a role in insulitis through ICAM-1 dependent pathway. In non-obese diabetic (NOD) mice (animal model for human Type 1 diabetes) pancreatic IL-10 has been shown to hyper-induce ICAM-1 expression on vascular endothelium. However, in the absence of ICAM-1, insulitis and diabetes could be prevented, thus providing evidence that IL-10 is sufficient to drive pathogenic autoimmune responses and accelerated diabetes via an ICAM-1 dependent pathway (Balasa et al., 2000). Presence of IL-10 during early stages of IDDM has also been shown to favor the generation of effector CD8+ T cells leading to accelerated diabetes in NOD mice (Balasa et al., 2000). Treatment of young mice with anti-TNF-α and anti-IL-10 mAb has also been shown to prevent diabetes and insulitis (Lee et al., 1996, Yang et al., 1994).

Similarly, when *TGF-β1* was studied by itself, no significant difference was observed between patients and controls. A significant increase of high producer haplotypes of *TGF-β1* with *TNF-α -308 GA+AA* and a significant decrease of high producer haplotypes of *TGF-β1* with *TNF-α -308GG* in T1D patients as compared to controls was observed. These results show that different cytokines work in concert with each other and may alter or modulate their functions depending on the milieu. TGF-β1 has been shown to be an extremely potent chemotactic factor in-vitro which influences monocyte recruitment and accumulation via increased expression of α and β integrins (Wahl et al., 1993). It has been shown to rapidly and transiently up-regulate α-4 integrin dependent adhesion of leukocyte cell lines and peripheral blood lymphocytes (Bartolome et al., 2003). α-4 integrin, in turn, has been shown to play a prominent role in the spontaneous development of insulitis and diabetes in NOD mice (Yang et al., 1997). Increased levels of TGF-β1 have been associated with destruction of pancreatic beta cells and pathogenesis of diabetic complications (Korpinen et al., 2001). Hence, in the presence of high secretors of *TNF-α*, the high secretor genotypes of *TGF-β1* may have a role both in destruction of pancreatic beta cells as well as in migration of CD4+ and CD8+ T cells into the pancreas (Insulitis) through α-4 integrin, which act against pancreatic beta cells along with Nitric oxide mediated cytotoxicity. Under these circumstances, TGF-β1 may not be able to arrest the pro-inflammatory functions of TNF-α and IFN-γ.

So, our data provides circumstantial evidence justifying the presence of high secretor genotypes of *TNF-α -308GA* and *AA* along with high secretor genotypes of *IL-6, IL-10* and *TGF-β1* and provide an immunogenetic basis for the autoimmune responses in T1D. The data suggest that the beta cell destruction in T1D may be mediated by both CD4+ T helper cells and CD8+ cytotoxic T cells recruited through Integrins and ICAM-1 dependent pathways in the pancreas for which cytokine genes seem to play a pivotal role.

4.2 TNF- α and HLA genes

TNF-α gene is very closely linked to the MHC. Deng et al (Deng et al., 1996) observed that the TNF-α associations in Caucasians and Chinese of Taiwan, may be due to its being in linkage disequilibrium with DR3-DQB1*0201 haplotype. We too had observed DRB1*03:01, DRB1*04:01 and DRB1*04:05 to be associated with T1D in North Indians (Rani et al., 2004). Hence, we wanted to study if the TNF-α association was independent of these alleles or due to linkage disequilibrium (LD) between TNF-α -308A and the predisposing DRB1 alleles. Interestingly, the LD analysis showed that both TNF-α -308A as well as TNF-α -308G alleles are in LD with DRB1*03:01, the most predisposing HLA-DRB1 allele, suggesting that the effect of TNF-α -308A is not because of its being in LD with HLA-DRB1*03:01, the predisposing MHC allele.

Since TNF-α locus is very closely linked to HLA-B locus, we also studied the alleles of B-locus for a possibility of TNF-α -308A allele being in LD with one of the B-locus alleles . Surprisingly we observed LD between TNF-α -308G with B*08 and TNF-α -308A allele with HLA B*50:01 and B*58:01. All the three B-locus alleles B*08:01, B*50:01 and B*58:01 were in linkage disequilibrium with DRB1*03:01 (Table 3). Because of HLA-B*08 being in LD with TNF-α -308G, B*08:01-DRB1*03:01 haplotype was also in LD with TNF-α -308G (Table 4).

HLA-B-TNF-α-DRB1- haplotypes	Number of haplotypes observed 2N=418	Haplotype frequencies	D_{abc}#
B*8- TNF-α -308A-DRB1*03	19	0.045	-0.013
B*8- TNF-α -308G-DRB1*03	75	0.179	0.015
B*50- TNF-α -308A-DRB1*03	42	0.1	0.0329
B*50- TNF-α -308G-DRB1*03	32	0.076	-0.0023
B*58- TNF-α -308A-DRB1*03	33	0.079	0.0141
B*58- TNF-α -308G-DRB1*03	28	0.067	-0.0032

Table 4. Linkage disequilibrium analysis of HLA-B- TNF-a -DRB1 haplotypes prevalent in T1D patients from North India (Kumar et al., 2007).

However, B*50:01-DRB1*03:01 and B*58:01-DRB1*03:01 haplotypes were in LD with TNF-α -308A allele. We observed 48.8 % of the patients had B*08/non-B*08/non-B*50:01/non-B*58:01-TNF-α-308G-DRB1*03:01 haplotypes as compared to 34 % with B*50:01/ B*58:01-TNF-α -308A-DRB1*03:01 haplotypes. With this in-depth analysis, it becomes clear that the effect of TNF-α -308A allele is not because of its being in LD with DRB1*03:01, B*08:01, B*50:01 or B*58:01, but due its functional implications and its integrated effect with other cytokines. In conclusion, while the MHC may be involved in auto-antigen presentation, TNF- alpha and other cytokines play an integrated role in destruction of the pancreatic beta cells though enrichment and recruitment of autoantigen specific CD4+ and CD8+ T cells which have immunogenetic bases (Figure 6).

5. Vitamin D receptor

Vitamin D Receptor (VDR) is a ligand dependent transcription factor that belongs to the super family of the Nuclear Hormone Receptors (Evans, 1988). The ligand for VDR is

Vitamin D3 i.e., 1,25-(OH)$_2$D$_3$ which mediates its biological actions through VDR. When 1,25-(OH)$_2$D$_3$ binds to VDR, it induces conformational changes in VDR promoting its hetero-dimerization with Retinoid X Receptor (RXR), followed by translocation of this complex into the nucleus. The RXR-VDR heterodimer in turn binds to the vitamin D$_3$ responsive elements (VDRE) in promoter regions of vitamin D responsive genes (Boonstra et al., 2001). This results in the regulatory function of Vitamin D3. In the absence of classical responsive elements, 1,25-(OH)$_2$D$_3$ may controls the expression of some genes like cytokine genes by targeting inducible transcription factors like NFAT in IL-2 in a sequence specific manner (Takeuchi et al., 1998). 1,25-(OH)$_2$D$_3$ has been shown to have an important immuno-modulatory role since it represses transcription of Th1 cytokines like *IL-2* (Alroy et al., 1995, Bhalla et al., 1984), *IFN-γ* (Cippitelli & Santoni, 1998) and *IL-12* (D'ambrosio et al., 1998) and up regulates the production of Th2 cytokines IL-4 and TGF-β1 (Cantorna et al., 1998). It has been shown to enhance the development of TH2 cells via a direct effect on naive CD4$^+$ cells (Boonstra et al., 2001). Besides, 1,25-(OH)$_2$D$_3$ has also been shown to modulate the expression of *HLA* class-II alleles on monocytes and human bone cells (Rigby et al., 1990, Skjodt et al., 1990)

Studies have shown that administration of Vitamin D3 in NOD mice, before the onset of Insulitis, can effectively prevent the disease progression. However, when administered after the establishment of insulitis, vitamin D3 was not as effective. Similarly, in humans too, vitamin D supplementation in early childhood has been shown to reduce the incidence of T1D (Hypponen et al., 2001, Jones et al., 1998). Since 1,25-(OH)$_2$D$_3$ mediatesi its effect through VDR, we studied the *VDR* gene polymorphisms and their interaction with the most predisposing *MHC* alleles to investigate their role, if any, in the pathophysiology of T1D.

The VDR SNPs studied include the T>C SNP in exon2 initiation codon detected with *FokI* restriction enzyme (Gross et al., 1996), the A>G SNP detected with *BsmI* (Morrison et al., 1992) and G>T SNP detected with *ApaI* (Faraco et al., 1989) located in Intron 8, and a silent C>T SNP (Durrin et al., 1999) detected with *TaqI*, located in Exon 9. These SNPS were studied using PCR amplification and restriction digestion by the aforesaid enzymes as described earlier (Faraco et al., 1989, Hustmyer et al., 1993). We also studied the interaction between *VDR* alleles and predisposing *HLA* alleles using LD based statistics (Zhao et al., 2006) and subsequently sequenced the promoter region of the predisposing *MHC* allele to detect the VDRE sequence which has been shown to modulate the expression of the HLA alleles (Ramagopalan et al., 2009), suggesting the functional implications of the statistically significant interaction (Israni et al., 2009). We further provided documentary evidence that expression of HLA class-II molecules was being modulated by vitamin D3.

5.1 VDR *FokI*, *BsmI*, *ApaI* and *TaqI* genotypes and haplotypes in T1D patients

While there were no significant differences in the genotypes of *ApaI* and *TaqI* in patients and controls. *FokI* 'ff' was significantly increased in the patient group as compared to controls and *BsmI* 'bb' was significantly decreased in the patient group. However, these differences did not remain significant after Boneferroni's correction (Israni et al., 2009).

Haplotype analysis was carried out for the four restriction sites studied in the VDR gene in patients and controls using SHEsis program (http://202.120.7.14/analysis/myAnalysis.php) (Shi & He, 2005). Additionally, Famhap (http://famhap.meb.uni-bonn.de) was used to confim the frequencies of the haplotypes. Haplotype *FBAt* and *fBAT* were significantly increased in T1D patients and *fBAt* was significantly reduced in them as compared to controls.

5.2 Gene to gene interaction of *VDR* haplotypes with predisposing *HLA* alleles

Simulateneous presence of different VDR haplotypes along with the predisposing *HLA* alleles was studied in patients. Interestingly, simultaneous presence of haplotypes *FBAT* and *FbaT* along with the predisposing *DRB1* alleles was significantly increased while the same haplotypes were protective when associated with non-predisposing alleles of *DRB1*. Similar results were obtained with other haplotypes like *FBAt, fBAT and fbaT* in association with the predisposing *HLA-DRB1* alleles (Israni et al., 2009).

To study the interaction between two unlinked loci i.e., *VDR* and the predisposing *HLA-DRB1* alleles, we used LD based statistics as described by Zhao et al (Zhao et al., 2006). The analysis revealed that *F* and *T* alleles in the exons 2 and 9 for *FokI* and *TaqI* restriction sites respectively showed significant interactions with predisposing *HLA-DRB1* allele *DRB1*03:01* (Israni et al., 2009).

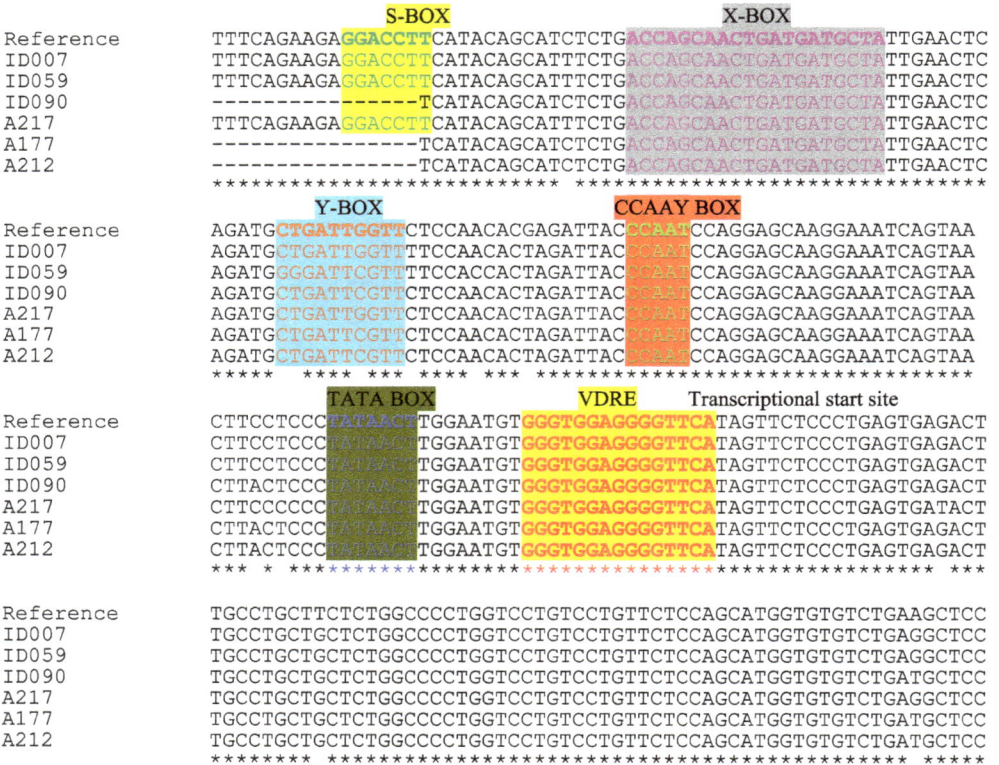

```
                         S-BOX                                X-BOX
Reference     TTTCAGAAGAGGACCTTCATACAGCATCTCTGACCAGCAACTGATGATGCTATTGAACTC
ID007         TTTCAGAAGAGGACCTTCATACAGCATTTCTGACCAGCAACTGATGATGCTATTGAACTC
ID059         TTTCAGAAGAGGACCTTCATACAGCATTTCTGACCAGCAACTGATGATGCTATTGAACTC
ID090         --------------TCATACAGCATCTCTGACCAGCAACTGATGATGCTATTGAACTC
A217          TTTCAGAAGAGGACCTTCATACAGCATTTCTGACCAGCAACTGATGATGCTATTGAACTC
A177          ---------------TCATACAGCATCTCTGACCAGCAACTGATGATGCTATTGAACTC
A212          ---------------TCATACAGCATCTCTGACCAGCAACTGATGATGCTATTGAACTC
              *********************** *  *************************************
                     Y-BOX                         CCAAY BOX
Reference     AGATGCTGATTGGTTCTCCAACACGAGATTACCCAATCCAGGAGCAAGGAAATCAGTAA
ID007         AGATGCTGATTGGTTTTCCAACACTAGATTACCCAATCCAGGAGCAAGGAAATCAGTAA
ID059         AGATGGGGATTCGTTTTCCACCACTAGATTACCCAATCCAGGAGCAAGGAAATCAGTAA
ID090         AGATGCTGATTCGTTCTCCAACACTAGATTACCCAATCCAGGAGCAAGGAAATCAGTAA
A217          AGATGCTGATTGGTTCTCCAACACTAGATTACCCAATCCAGGAGCAAGGAAATCAGTAA
A177          AGATGCTGATTCGTTCTCCAACACTAGATTACCCAATCCAGGAGCAAGGAAATCAGTAA
A212          AGATGCTGATTCGTTCTCCAACACTAGATTACCCAATCCAGGAGCAAGGAAATCAGTAA
              *****  ****  ***  ****  ***  **************************
                     TATA BOX                  VDRE        Transcriptional start site
Reference     CTTCCTCCCTATAACTTGGAATGTGGGTGGAGGGGTTCATAGTTCTCCCTGAGTGAGACT
ID007         CTTCCTCCCTATAACTTGGAATGTGGGTGGAGGGGTTCATAGTTCTCCCTGAGTGAGACT
ID059         CTTCCTCCCTATAACTTGGAATGTGGGTGGAGGGGTTCATAGTTCTCCCTGAGTGAGACT
ID090         CTTCCTCCCTATAACTTGGAATGTGGGTGGAGGGGTTCATAGTTCTCCCTGAGTGAGACT
A217          CTTCCCCCCTATAACTTGGAATGTGGGTGGAGGGGTTCATAGTTCTCCCTGAGTGATACT
A177          CTTACTCCCTATAACTTGGAATGTGGGTGGAGGGGTTCATAGTTCTCCCTGAGTGAGACT
A212          CTTACTCCCTATAACTTGGAATGTGGGTGGAGGGGTTCATAGTTCTCCCTGAGTGAGACT
              *** *  *************************************************** ***

Reference     TGCCTGCTTCTCTGGCCCCTGGTCCTGTCCTGTTCTCCAGCATGGTGTGTCTGAAGCTCC
ID007         TGCCTGCTGCTCTGGCCCCTGGTCCTGTCCTGTTCTCCAGCATGGTGTGTCTGAGGCTCC
ID059         TGCCTGCTGCTCTGGCCCCTGGTCCTGTCCTGTTCTCCAGCATGGTGTGTCTGAGGCTCC
ID090         TGCCTGCTGCTCTGGCCCCTGGTCCTGTCCTGTTCTCCAGCATGGTGTGTCTGATGCTCC
A217          TGCCTGCTGCTCTGGCCCCTGGTCCTGTCCTGTTCTCCAGCATGGTGTGTCTGAGGCTCC
A177          TGCCTGCTGCTCTGGCCCCTGGTCCTGTCCTGTTCTCCAGCATGGTGTGTCTGATGCTCC
A212          TGCCTGCTGCTCTGGCCCCTGGTCCTGTCCTGTTCTCCAGCATGGTGTGTCTGATGCTCC
              ********* ************************************************ *****
```

Fig. 4. *HLA- DRB1*03:01* promoter sequence from 3 subjects suffering from T1D and 3 normal healthy individuals homozygous for *DRB1*03:01*. Important regulatory elements like S-box, X-box, Y-box, CCAAY-box, TATA-box and VDRE are highlighted. Star (*) in the last row shows homology and dots (.) shows nucleotide substitution in one or more samples at that particular site and dashes(-) represent gaps inserted to maximize the homology. (Israni et al., 2009).

5.3 Sequence analysis of HLA DRB1*0301 promoter region

Amongst the predisposing *HLA-DRB1* alleles, majority of the patients (85.9%) had *DRB1*03:01*. Thus, we sought to look for the VDRE in the promoter region of the allele. The promoter regions of 3 T1D subjects and 3 healthy controls homozygous for *HLA-DRB1*03:01* were amplified and sequenced to determine the VDRE variants in the North Indian population. Sequences were aligned using ClustalW2, and the presence of a VDRE was confirmed in-silico using JASPAR_CORE version 3.0 database using default conditions (Sandelin et al., 2004). Figure 4 shows the *HLA- DRB1*03:01* promoter sequences showing the localization of vitamin D response element (VDRE) in the promoter region of HLA-*DRB1*0301* from the 6 subjects.

Interestingly, the alignment showed exactly the same sequence of VDRE in the promoter region of *HLA-DRB1*03:01* which has been shown to influence the expression of *HLA* allele *DRB1*15:01* by Ramagopalan et al (Ramagopalan et al., 2009) suggesting the bases for interaction of VDR with *HLA-DRB1*03:01*

5.4 Altered expression of *HLA-DRB1*03:0*1 by 1,25-(OH)$_2$D$_3$ (Calcitriol)
5.4.1 Flow cytometry

To study if vitamin D3 administartion would alter the expression of MHC class-II, we stimulated *HLA-DRB1*03:01* homozygous B-lymphoblastoid cell (B-LCL) line VAVY (International Histocompatibility Workshop cell line Number IHW09023) with 100nM of calcitriol (Sigma) for 24 hours and stained with anti-HLA DR-PE antibody (BD Biosciences) and acquired on BD-LSR to study the expression of HLA-DR on stimulated and unstimulated B-LCL The data was analysed using WinMDI 2.9 software. The results showed significantly higher expression of HLA-DR in the B-LCL stimulated with calcitriol as compared to the unstimulated one (Figure 5A and B).

5.4.2 Real time PCR

We also studied the levels of transcripts for *HLA-DRB1* in B-LCL VAVY after 24 hour stimulation with calcitriol and compared it to unstimulated B-LCL using real time PCR. The data shows 1.89 fold increase in the *HLA-DRB1* transcripts from B-LCL stimulated with calcitriol as compared to the unstimulated one. These results were confirmed on perpheral blood mononuclear cells (PBMCs) derived from a normal healthy control homozygous for *HLA-DRB1*03:01*.

Our results showed enhanced expression of HLA-DR on the B-LCLs stimulated with calcitriol as compared to the unstimulated one confirming that indeed the interaction of VDR with *HLA-DRB1*03:01* is occurring through the VDRE present in the promoter region of the gene. Based on the earlier studies and the present data one can speculate that in the absence of required amount of Vitamin D in early life in the predisposed individuals with *HLA-DRB1*03:01*, the expression of the allele may be impaired in the thymus (Ramagopalan et al., 2009) resulting in escape from thymic deletion of autoreactive T cells leading to T1D manifestations.

6. Conclusions

Our studies show that simultaneous presence of *DRB1*03:01* along with homozygous *INS-VNTR* class-I was significantly increased ($p < 10^{-8}$) in T1D patients, giving a relative risk of 70.81 (Rani et al., 2004). *INS-VNTR* class-I has been shown to be associated with lower

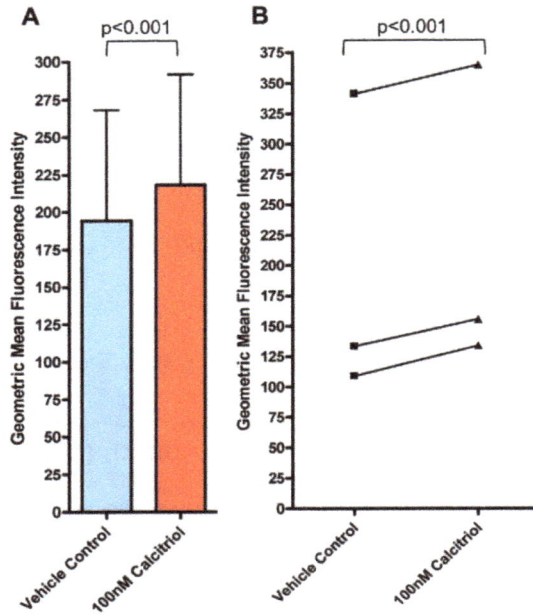

Fig. 5. Flow cytometric analysis of HLA-DR expression. A: Histogram of HLA-DR-PE staining of B-LCL-VAVY cells treated with and without 100nM calcitriol. The figure shows enhanced expression of HLA-DR in stimulated B-LCL as compared to unstimulated one. B: VAVY cells show a significant increase in surface HLA-DR expression as determined by the geometric mean flurescence intensity of antibody staining (Israni et al., 2009).

expression of Insulin in thymii of fetuses as compared to Class-III alleles (Pugliese et al., 1997, Vafiadis et al., 1997) which may be responsible for poor thymic education for insulin resulting in autoimmunity against pancreatic beta cells. Our studies provide additional evidence based on the statistically significant interaction between the predisposing HLA allele and high producer alleles of VDR which may be detrimental for the manifestation of T1D in the absence of 1,25-(OH)$_2$D$_3$ in early childhood and/or in-utero and this interaction is mediated by VDRE present in the promoter region of DRB1*03:01(Israni et al., 2009). With poor thymic education for insulin and HLA-DRB1*03:01 protein, environmental factors like viral infections, vitamin D deficiency and some milk proteins may be involved in initiation of the autoimmune responses against the pancreatic beta cells. While HLA class-II molecules may be involved in auto-antigen presentation to T helper cells, higher producing genotypes of pro-inflammatory cytokines like IFN-gamma and TNF-alpha may be involved in enhancing the cell mediated immune responses through proliferation of CD4+ and CD8+ T cells, while higher producing genotypes of IL-10 and TGF-beta may have a role in recruitment of these autoreactive T cells in the pancreas through ICAM-1 and Integerin dependent pathways. Final destruction of pancreatic beta cells may occur through CD4+ and CD8+ T cells and nitric oxide production since IFN-γ may act singularly as well as synergistically with other inflammatory stimuli to induce NO production which can be cytotoxic and thus may have a role in pathogenesis of T1D (Figure 6). Future studies should focus on developing approaches to inhibit autoimmunity before the onset of the disease.

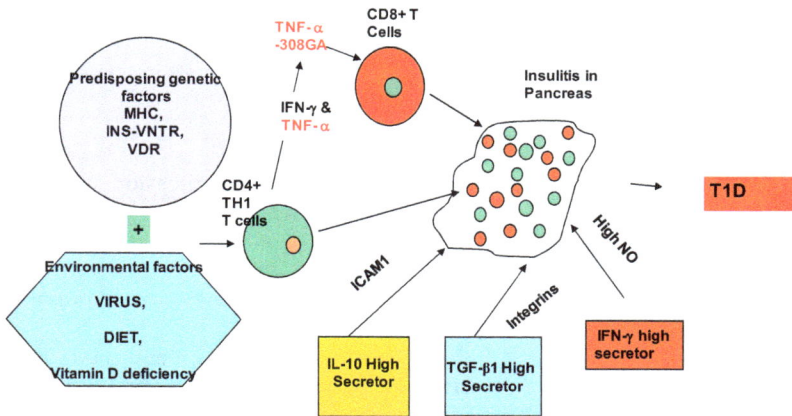

Fig. 6. Conclusions of our studies. Predisposing genetic factors like MHC, INS-VNTR and VDR may be involved in poor thymic education for insulin and *HLA-DRB1*03:01* protein resulting in recognition of self proteins as non-self by T cells . These genetic factors along with environmental factors like viral infections, vitamin D deficiency and some milk proteins may be involved in initiation of the autoimmune responses against the pancreatic beta cells. While HLA class-II molecules may be involved in auto-antigen presentation to T helper cells, higher producing genotypes of pro-inflammatory cytokines like *IFN-γ* and *TNF-α* may be involved in the cell mediated immune responses. Higher producing genotypes of *IL-10* and *TGF-beta,* may have a role in recruitment of the autoreactive CD4+ and CD8+ T cells in the pancreas through ICAM-1 and Integerin dependent pathways respectively. Final destruction of pancreatic beta cells may occur through CD4+ and CD8+ T cells and nitric oxide production since IFN-γ may act singularly as well as synergistically with other inflammatory stimuli to induce NO production which can be cytotoxic and thus may have a role in pathogenesis of T1D.

7. Acknowledgment

The studies were funded in part by grants from Department of Science and Technology (DST), Department of Biotechnology (DBT), Ministry of Science and Technology, Government of India and partly by Core funds of National Institute of Immunology, New Delhi, India. The patient sample for this work came from All India Institute of Medical Sciences (AIIMS), New Delhi and I would like to acknowledge Dr. Ravinder Goswami, the endocrinologist from AIIMS for the same. I would like to acknowledge the students and project fellows who have been involved in doing this work: Avinash Kumar, Rashmi Kumar, Shruti Agarwal, Neetu Israni, Shailendra Kumar Singh. I am thankful to Dr. Alberto Pugliese for valuable suggestions and INS-VNTR protocol. I would like to thank Dr. Joannis Mytilineos and the technical staff of Heidelberg University for the cytokine typing kit supplied for cytokine gene polymorphism component of XIIIth International Histocompatibility Workshop. We are thankful to Yong Yong Shi for providing the SHEsis program (http://202.120.7.14/analysis/myAnalysis.php) for haplotype analysis. We are thankful to the Fred Hutchinson Cancer Research Center IHWG Cell and Gene Bank for providing *HLA-DRB1*03:01* homozygous lymphoblastoid Cell lines for studies showing effect of vitamin D on HLA-DR expression. Mr. Kapoor Chand's technical support is acknowledged. Help of Dr. Narendra Kumar, Georgia Institute of Technology, USA, in making the ribbon diagrams for HLA-DRB1 peptide binding pockets is acknowledged.

8. References

Alroy, I., Towers, T.L. & Freedman, L.P. (1995). Transcriptional repression of the interleukin-2 gene by vitamin D3: direct inhibition of NFATp/AP-1 complex formation by a nuclear hormone receptor. *Mol Cell Biol*, 15, 10,(Oct, 1995) 5789-99.

Alves, C., Toralles, M.B. & Carvalho, G.C. (2009). HLA class II polymorphism in patients with type 1 diabetes mellitus from a Brazilian racially admixtured population. *Ethn Dis*, 19, 4,(Autumn, 2009) 420-4.

Asderakis, A., Sankaran, D., Dyer, P., Johnson, R.W., Pravica, V., Sinnott, P.J., Roberts, I. & Hutchinson, I.V. (2001). Association of polymorphisms in the human interferon-gamma and interleukin-10 gene with acute and chronic kidney transplant outcome: the cytokine effect on transplantation. *Transplantation*, 71, 5,(Mar 15, 2001) 674-7.

Awad, M.R., El-Gamel, A., Hasleton, P., Turner, D.M., Sinnott, P.J. & Hutchinson, I.V. (1998). Genotypic variation in the transforming growth factor-beta1 gene: association with transforming growth factor-beta1 production, fibrotic lung disease, and graft fibrosis after lung transplantation. *Transplantation*, 66, 8,(Oct 27, 1998) 1014-20.

Badenhoop, K., Walfish, P.G., Rau, H., Fischer, S., Nicolay, A., Bogner, U., Schleusener, H. & Usadel, K.H. (1995). Susceptibility and resistance alleles of human leukocyte antigen (HLA) DQA1 and HLA DQB1 are shared in endocrine autoimmune disease. *J Clin Endocrinol Metab*, 80, 7,(Jul, 1995) 2112-7.

Baisch, J.M., Weeks, T., Giles, R., Hoover, M., Stastny, P. & Capra, J.D. (1990). Analysis of HLA-DQ genotypes and susceptibility in insulin-dependent diabetes mellitus. *N Engl J Med*, 322, 26,(Jun 28, 1990) 1836-41.

Balasa, B., La Cava, A., Van Gunst, K., Mocnik, L., Balakrishna, D., Nguyen, N., Tucker, L. & Sarvetnick, N. (2000). A mechanism for IL-10-mediated diabetes in the nonobese diabetic (NOD) mouse: ICAM-1 deficiency blocks accelerated diabetes. *J Immunol*, 165, 12,(Dec 15, 2000) 7330-7.

Bartolome, R.A., Sanz-Rodriguez, F., Robledo, M.M., Hidalgo, A. & Teixido, J. (2003). Rapid up-regulation of alpha4 integrin-mediated leukocyte adhesion by transforming growth factor-beta1. *Mol Biol Cell*, 14, 1,(Jan, 2003) 54-66.

Bell, G.I., Karam, J.H. & Rutter, W.J. (1981). Polymorphic DNA region adjacent to the 5' end of the human insulin gene. *Proc Natl Acad Sci U S A*, 78, 9,(Sep, 1981) 5759-63.

Bell, G.I., Selby, M.J. & Rutter, W.J. (1982). The highly polymorphic region near the human insulin gene is composed of simple tandemly repeating sequences. *Nature*, 295, 5844,(Jan 7, 1982) 31-5.

Bennett, S.T., Lucassen, A.M., Gough, S.C., Powell, E.E., Undlien, D.E., Pritchard, L.E., Merriman, M.E., Kawaguchi, Y., Dronsfield, M.J., Pociot, F. & et al. (1995). Susceptibility to human type 1 diabetes at IDDM2 is determined by tandem repeat variation at the insulin gene minisatellite locus. *Nat Genet*, 9, 3,(Mar, 1995) 284-92.

Bhalla, A.K., Amento, E.P., Serog, B. & Glimcher, L.H. (1984). 1,25-Dihydroxyvitamin D3 inhibits antigen-induced T cell activation. *J Immunol*, 133, 4,(Oct, 1984) 1748-54.

Bidwell, J., Keen, L., Gallagher, G., Kimberly, R., Huizinga, T., McDermott, M.F., Oksenberg, J., McNicholl, J., Pociot, F., Hardt, C. & D'Alfonso, S. (1999). Cytokine gene polymorphism in human disease: on-line databases. *Genes Immun*, 1, 1,(Sep, 1999) 3-19.

Bittar, M.N., Carey, J.A., Barnard, J.B., Pravica, V., Deiraniya, A.K., Yonan, N. & Hutchinson, I.V. (2006). Tumor necrosis factor alpha influences the inflammatory response after coronary surgery. *Ann Thorac Surg*, 81, 1,(Jan, 2006) 132-7.

Bjorkman, P.J., Saper, M.A., Samraoui, B., Bennett, W.S., Strominger, J.L. & Wiley, D.C. (1987). Structure of the human class I histocompatibility antigen, HLA-A2. *Nature*, 329, 6139,(Oct 8-14, 1987) 506-12.

Boonstra, A., Barrat, F.J., Crain, C., Heath, V.L., Savelkoul, H.F. & O'Garra, A. (2001). 1alpha,25-Dihydroxyvitamin d3 has a direct effect on naive CD4(+) T cells to enhance the development of Th2 cells. *J Immunol*, 167, 9,(Nov 1, 2001) 4974-80.

Brown, J.H., Jardetzky, T.S., Gorga, J.C., Stern, L.J., Urban, R.G., Strominger, J.L. & Wiley, D.C. (1993). Three-dimensional structure of the human class II histocompatibility antigen HLA-DR1. *Nature*, 364, 6432,(Jul 1, 1993) 33-9.

Burzotta, F., Iacoviello, L., Di Castelnuovo, A., Glieca, F., Luciani, N., Zamparelli, R., Schiavello, R., Donati, M.B., Maseri, A., Possati, G. & Andreotti, F. (2001). Relation of the -174 G/C polymorphism of interleukin-6 to interleukin-6 plasma levels and to length of hospitalization after surgical coronary revascularization. *Am J Cardiol*, 88, 10,(Nov 15, 2001) 1125-8.

Cantorna, M.T., Woodward, W.D., Hayes, C.E. & DeLuca, H.F. (1998). 1,25-dihydroxyvitamin D3 is a positive regulator for the two anti-encephalitogenic cytokines TGF-beta 1 and IL-4. *J Immunol*, 160, 11,(Jun 1, 1998) 5314-9.

Chauffert, M., Cisse, A., Chevenne, D., Parfait, B., Michel, S. & Trivin, F. (1995). HLA-DQ beta 1 typing and non-Asp57 alleles in the aborigine population of Senegal. *Diabetes Care*, 18, 5,(May, 1995) 677-80.

Cippitelli, M. & Santoni, A. (1998). Vitamin D3: a transcriptional modulator of the interferon-gamma gene. *Eur J Immunol*, 28, 10,(Oct, 1998) 3017-30.

Cucca, F., Lampis, R., Congia, M., Angius, E., Nutland, S., Bain, S.C., Barnett, A.H. & Todd, J.A. (2001). A correlation between the relative predisposition of MHC class II alleles to type 1 diabetes and the structure of their proteins. *Hum Mol Genet*, 10, 19,(Sep 15, 2001) 2025-37.

Cucca, F., Lampis, R., Frau, F., Macis, D., Angius, E., Masile, P., Chessa, M., Frongia, P., Silvetti, M., Cao, A., De Virgiliis, S. & Congia, M. (1995). The distribution of DR4 haplotypes in Sardinia suggests a primary association of type I diabetes with DRB1 and DQB1 loci. *Hum Immunol*, 43, 4,(Aug, 1995) 301-8.

D'Ambrosio, D., Cippitelli, M., Cocciolo, M.G., Mazzeo, D., Di Lucia, P., Lang, R., Sinigaglia, F. & Panina-Bordignon, P. (1998). Inhibition of IL-12 production by 1,25-dihydroxyvitamin D3. Involvement of NF-kappaB downregulation in transcriptional repression of the p40 gene. *J Clin Invest*, 101, 1,(Jan 1, 1998) 252-62.

de Vries, R.R. & van Rood, J.J. (1985). Immunobiology of HLA class-I and class-II molecules. Introduction. *Prog Allergy*, 36, 1985) 1-9.

Deng, G.Y., Maclaren, N.K., Huang, H.S., Zhang, L.P. & She, J.X. (1996). No primary association between the 308 polymorphism in the tumor necrosis factor alpha promoter region and insulin-dependent diabetes mellitus. *Hum Immunol*, 45, 2,(Feb, 1996) 137-42.

Durrin, L.K., Haile, R.W., Ingles, S.A. & Coetzee, G.A. (1999). Vitamin D receptor 3'-untranslated region polymorphisms: lack of effect on mRNA stability. *Biochim Biophys Acta*, 1453, 3,(Mar 30, 1999) 311-20.

Ei Wafai, R.J., Chmaisse, H.N., Makki, R.F. & Fakhoury, H. Association of HLA class II alleles and CTLA-4 polymorphism with type 1 diabetes. *Saudi J Kidney Dis Transpl*, 22, 2,(Mar, 273-81.

Evans, R.M. (1988). The steroid and thyroid hormone receptor superfamily. *Science*, 240, 4854,(May 13, 1988) 889-95.

Falk, K., Rotzschke, O., Stevanovic, S., Jung, G. & Rammensee, H.G. (1991). Allele-specific motifs revealed by sequencing of self-peptides eluted from MHC molecules. *Nature*, 351, 6324,(May 23, 1991) 290-6.

Faraco, J.H., Morrison, N.A., Baker, A., Shine, J. & Frossard, P.M. (1989). ApaI dimorphism at the human vitamin D receptor gene locus. *Nucleic Acids Res*, 17, 5,(Mar 11, 1989) 2150.

Fernandez-Vina, M., Ramirez, L.C., Raskin, P. & Stastny, P. (1993). Genes for insulin-dependent diabetes mellitus (IDDM) in the major histocompatibility complex (MHC) of African-Americans. *Tissue Antigens*, 41, 2,(Feb, 1993) 57-64.

Fishman, D., Faulds, G., Jeffery, R., Mohamed-Ali, V., Yudkin, J.S., Humphries, S. & Woo, P. (1998). The effect of novel polymorphisms in the interleukin-6 (IL-6) gene on IL-6 transcription and plasma IL-6 levels, and an association with systemic-onset juvenile chronic arthritis. *J Clin Invest*, 102, 7,(Oct 1, 1998) 1369-76.

Garcia-Pacheco, J.M., Herbut, B., Cutbush, S., Hitman, G.A., Zhonglin, W., Magzoub, M., Bottazzo, G.F., Kiere, C., West, G., Mvere, D. & et al. (1992). Distribution of HLA-DQA1, -DQB1 and DRB1 alleles in black IDDM patients and controls from Zimbabwe. *Tissue Antigens*, 40, 3,(Sep, 1992) 145-9.

Garrett, T.P., Saper, M.A., Bjorkman, P.J., Strominger, J.L. & Wiley, D.C. (1989). Specificity pockets for the side chains of peptide antigens in HLA-Aw68. *Nature*, 342, 6250,(Dec 7, 1989) 692-6.

Gross, C., Eccleshall, T.R., Malloy, P.J., Villa, M.L., Marcus, R. & Feldman, D. (1996). The presence of a polymorphism at the translation initiation site of the vitamin D receptor gene is associated with low bone mineral density in postmenopausal Mexican-American women. *J Bone Miner Res*, 11, 12,(Dec, 1996) 1850-5.

Gupta, M.M., Raghunath, D., Kher, S.K. & Radhakrishnan, A.P. (1991). Human leucocyte antigen and insulin dependent diabetes mellitus. *J Assoc Physicians India*, 39, 7,(Jul, 1991) 540-3.

Holling, T.M., Schooten, E. & van Den Elsen, P.J. (2004). Function and regulation of MHC class II molecules in T-lymphocytes: of mice and men. *Hum Immunol*, 65, 4,(Apr, 2004) 282-90.

Horton, R., Wilming, L., Rand, V., Lovering, R.C., Bruford, E.A., Khodiyar, V.K., Lush, M.J., Povey, S., Talbot, C.C., Jr., Wright, M.W., Wain, H.M., Trowsdale, J., Ziegler, A. & Beck, S. (2004). Gene map of the extended human MHC. *Nat Rev Genet*, 5, 12,(Dec, 2004) 889-99.

Hustmyer, F.G., DeLuca, H.F. & Peacock, M. (1993). ApaI, BsmI, EcoRV and TaqI polymorphisms at the human vitamin D receptor gene locus in Caucasians, blacks and Asians. *Hum Mol Genet*, 2, 4,(Apr, 1993) 487.

Hypponen, E., Laara, E., Reunanen, A., Jarvelin, M.R. & Virtanen, S.M. (2001). Intake of vitamin D and risk of type 1 diabetes: a birth-cohort study. *Lancet*, 358, 9292,(Nov 3, 2001) 1500-3.

Ide, A., Kawasaki, E., Abiru, N., Sun, F., Takahashi, R., Kuwahara, H., Fujita, N., Kita, A., Oshima, K., Sakamaki, H., Uotani, S., Yamasaki, H., Yamaguchi, Y. & Eguchi, K. (2002). Genetic association between interleukin-10 gene promoter region polymorphisms and type 1 diabetes age-at-onset. *Hum Immunol*, 63, 8,(Aug, 2002) 690-5.

Israni, N., Goswami, R., Kumar, A. & Rani, R. (2009). Interaction of vitamin D receptor with HLA DRB1 0301 in type 1 diabetes patients from North India. *PLoS One*, 4, 12,(2009) e8023.

Jones, G., Strugnell, S.A. & DeLuca, H.F. (1998). Current understanding of the molecular actions of vitamin D. *Physiol Rev*, 78, 4,(Oct, 1998) 1193-231.

Julier, C., Hyer, R.N., Davies, J., Merlin, F., Soularue, P., Briant, L., Cathelineau, G., Deschamps, I., Rotter, J.I., Froguel, P. & et al. (1991). Insulin-IGF2 region on chromosome 11p encodes a gene implicated in HLA-DR4-dependent diabetes susceptibility. *Nature*, 354, 6349,(Nov 14, 1991) 155-9.

Kalra, S., Kalra, B. & Sharma, A. (2010) Prevalence of type 1 diabetes mellitus in Karnal district, Haryana state, India. *Diabetol Metab Syndr*, 2, 14.

Kanga, U., Vaidyanathan, B., Jaini, R., Menon, P.S. & Mehra, N.K. (2004). HLA haplotypes associated with type 1 diabetes mellitus in North Indian children. *Hum Immunol*, 65, 1,(Jan, 2004) 47-53.

Kennedy, G.C., German, M.S. & Rutter, W.J. (1995). The minisatellite in the diabetes susceptibility locus IDDM2 regulates insulin transcription. *Nat Genet*, 9, 3,(Mar, 1995) 293-8.

Korpinen, E., Groop, P.H., Fagerudd, J.A., Teppo, A.M., Akerblom, H.K. & Vaarala, O. (2001). Increased secretion of TGF-beta1 by peripheral blood mononuclear cells from patients with Type 1 diabetes mellitus with diabetic nephropathy. *Diabet Med*, 18, 2,(Feb, 2001) 121-5.

Kristiansen, O.P. & Mandrup-Poulsen, T. (2005). Interleukin-6 and diabetes: the good, the bad, or the indifferent? *Diabetes*, 54 Suppl 2, Dec, 2005) S114-24.

Kumar, R., Goswami, R., Agarwal, S., Israni, N., Singh, S.K. & Rani, R. (2007). Association and interaction of the TNF-alpha gene with other pro- and anti-inflammatory cytokine genes and HLA genes in patients with type 1 diabetes from North India. *Tissue Antigens*, 69, 6,(Jun, 2007) 557-67.

Lee, M.S., Mueller, R., Wicker, L.S., Peterson, L.B. & Sarvetnick, N. (1996). IL-10 is necessary and sufficient for autoimmune diabetes in conjunction with NOD MHC homozygosity. *J Exp Med*, 183, 6,(Jun 1, 1996) 2663-8.

Louis, E., Franchimont, D., Piron, A., Gevaert, Y., Schaaf-Lafontaine, N., Roland, S., Mahieu, P., Malaise, M., De Groote, D., Louis, R. & Belaiche, J. (1998). Tumour necrosis factor (TNF) gene polymorphism influences TNF-alpha production in lipopolysaccharide (LPS)-stimulated whole blood cell culture in healthy humans. *Clin Exp Immunol*, 113, 3,(Sep, 1998) 401-6.

Lucassen, A.M., Julier, C., Beressi, J.P., Boitard, C., Froguel, P., Lathrop, M. & Bell, J.I. (1993). Susceptibility to insulin dependent diabetes mellitus maps to a 4.1 kb segment of DNA spanning the insulin gene and associated VNTR. *Nat Genet*, 4, 3,(Jul, 1993) 305-10.

McCartney-Francis, N., Allen, J.B., Mizel, D.E., Albina, J.E., Xie, Q.W., Nathan, C.F. & Wahl, S.M. (1993). Suppression of arthritis by an inhibitor of nitric oxide synthase. *J Exp Med*, 178, 2,(Aug 1, 1993) 749-54.

Mehra, N.K., Kaur, G., Kanga, U. & Tandon, N. (2002). Immunogenetics of autoimmune diseases in Asian Indians. *Ann N Y Acad Sci*, 958, Apr, 2002) 333-6.

Morrison, N.A., Yeoman, R., Kelly, P.J. & Eisman, J.A. (1992). Contribution of trans-acting factor alleles to normal physiological variability: vitamin D receptor gene polymorphism and circulating osteocalcin. *Proc Natl Acad Sci U S A*, 89, 15,(Aug 1, 1992) 6665-9.

Nepom, G.T. & Kwok, W.W. (1998). Molecular basis for HLA-DQ associations with IDDM. *Diabetes*, 47, 8,(Aug, 1998) 1177-84.

Pociot, F., Briant, L., Jongeneel, C.V., Molvig, J., Worsaae, H., Abbal, M., Thomsen, M., Nerup, J. & Cambon-Thomsen, A. (1993). Association of tumor necrosis factor (TNF) and class II major histocompatibility complex alleles with the secretion of TNF-alpha and TNF-beta by human mononuclear cells: a possible link to insulin-dependent diabetes mellitus. *Eur J Immunol*, 23, 1,(Jan, 1993) 224-31.

Pociot, F. & McDermott, M.F. (2002). Genetics of type 1 diabetes mellitus. *Genes Immun*, 3, 5,(Aug, 2002) 235-49.

Pugliese, A., Gianani, R., Moromisato, R., Awdeh, Z.L., Alper, C.A., Erlich, H.A., Jackson, R.A. & Eisenbarth, G.S. (1995). HLA-DQB1*0602 is associated with dominant protection from diabetes even among islet cell antibody-positive first-degree relatives of patients with IDDM. *Diabetes*, 44, 6,(Jun, 1995) 608-13.

Pugliese, A., Zeller, M., Fernandez, A., Jr., Zalcberg, L.J., Bartlett, R.J., Ricordi, C., Pietropaolo, M., Eisenbarth, G.S., Bennett, S.T. & Patel, D.D. (1997). The insulin gene is transcribed in the human thymus and transcription levels correlated with allelic variation at the INS VNTR-IDDM2 susceptibility locus for type 1 diabetes. *Nat Genet*, 15, 3,(Mar, 1997) 293-7.

Rabinovitch, A. (1994). Immunoregulatory and cytokine imbalances in the pathogenesis of IDDM. Therapeutic intervention by immunostimulation? *Diabetes*, 43, 5,(May, 1994) 613-21.

Ramachandran, A., Snehalatha, C. & Krishnaswamy, C.V. (1996). Incidence of IDDM in children in urban population in southern India. Madras IDDM Registry Group Madras, South India. *Diabetes Res Clin Pract*, 34, 2,(Oct, 1996) 79-82.

Ramagopalan, S.V., Maugeri, N.J., Handunnetthi, L., Lincoln, M.R., Orton, S.M., Dyment, D.A., Deluca, G.C., Herrera, B.M., Chao, M.J., Sadovnick, A.D., Ebers, G.C. & Knight, J.C. (2009). Expression of the multiple sclerosis-associated MHC class II Allele HLA-DRB1*1501 is regulated by vitamin D. *PLoS Genet*, 5, 2,(Feb, 2009) e1000369.

Rani, R., Fernandez-Vina, M.A. & Stastny, P. (1998). Associations between HLA class II alleles in a North Indian population. *Tissue Antigens*, 52, 1,(Jul, 1998) 37-43.

Rani, R., Sood, A. & Goswami, R. (2004). Molecular basis of predisposition to develop type 1 diabetes mellitus in North Indians. *Tissue Antigens*, 64, 2,(Aug, 2004) 145-55.

Rani, R., Sood, A., Lazaro, A.M. & Stastny, P. (1999). Associations of MHC class II alleles with insulin-dependent diabetes mellitus (IDDM) in patients from North India. *Hum Immunol*, 60, 6,(Jun, 1999) 524-31.

Reynier, F., Cazalis, M.A., Lecoq, A., Paye, M., Rosa, A., Durand, A., Jhumka, U., Mougin, B., Miossec, P., Bendelac, N., Nicolino, M. & Thivolet, C. (2006). Lack of association of IL-10 promoter gene variants with type 1 diabetes in a French population. *Hum Immunol*, 67, 4-5,(Apr-May, 2006) 311-7.

Rigby, W.F., Waugh, M. & Graziano, R.F. (1990). Regulation of human monocyte HLA-DR and CD4 antigen expression, and antigen presentation by 1,25-dihydroxyvitamin D3. *Blood*, 76, 1,(Jul 1, 1990) 189-97.

Robinson, J., Waller, M.J., Fail, S.C., McWilliam, H., Lopez, R., Parham, P. & Marsh, S.G. (2009). The IMGT/HLA database. *Nucleic Acids Res*, 37, Database issue,(Jan, 2009) D1013-7.

Rotwein, P., Yokoyama, S., Didier, D.K. & Chirgwin, J.M. (1986). Genetic analysis of the hypervariable region flanking the human insulin gene. *Am J Hum Genet*, 39, 3,(Sep, 1986) 291-9.

Sandelin, A., Alkema, W., Engstrom, P., Wasserman, W.W. & Lenhard, B. (2004). JASPAR: an open-access database for eukaryotic transcription factor binding profiles 10.1093/nar/gkh012. *Nucl. Acids Res.*, 32, suppl_1,(January 1, 2004, 2004) D91-94.

Sanjeevi, C.B., Kanungo, A., Shtauvere, A., Samal, K.C. & Tripathi, B.B. (1999). Association of HLA class II alleles with different subgroups of diabetes mellitus in Eastern India identify different associations with IDDM and malnutrition-related diabetes. *Tissue Antigens*, 54, 1,(Jul, 1999) 83-7.

Sanjeevi, C.B., Landin-Olsson, M., Kockum, I., Dahlquist, G. & Lernmark, A. (1995). Effects of the second HLA-DQ haplotype on the association with childhood insulin-dependent diabetes mellitus. *Tissue Antigens*, 45, 2,(Feb, 1995) 148-52.

Sheehy, M.J. (1992). HLA and insulin-dependent diabetes. A protective perspective. *Diabetes*, 41, 2,(Feb, 1992) 123-9.

Shi, Y.Y. & He, L. (2005). SHEsis, a powerful software platform for analyses of linkage disequilibrium, haplotype construction, and genetic association at polymorphism loci. *Cell Res*, 15, 2,(Feb, 2005) 97-8.

Skjodt, H., Hughes, D.E., Dobson, P.R. & Russell, R.G. (1990). Constitutive and inducible expression of HLA class II determinants by human osteoblast-like cells in vitro. *J Clin Invest*, 85, 5,(May, 1990) 1421-6.

Skrodeniene, E., Marciulionyte, D., Padaiga, Z., Jasinskiene, E., Sadauskaite-Kuehne, V., Sanjeevi, C.B. & Ludvigsson, J. HLA class II alleles and haplotypes in Lithuanian children with type 1 diabetes and healthy children (HLA and type 1 diabetes). *Medicina (Kaunas)*, 46, 8,(505-10.

Stanilova, S.A., Miteva, L.D., Karakolev, Z.T. & Stefanov, C.S. (2006). Interleukin-10-1082 promoter polymorphism in association with cytokine production and sepsis susceptibility. *Intensive Care Med*, 32, 2,(Feb, 2006) 260-6.

Tait, B.D., Drummond, B.P., Varney, M.D. & Harrison, L.C. (1995). HLA-DRB1*0401 is associated with susceptibility to insulin-dependent diabetes mellitus independently of the DQB1 locus. *Eur J Immunogenet*, 22, 4,(Aug, 1995) 289-97.

Takeuchi, A., Reddy, G.S., Kobayashi, T., Okano, T., Park, J. & Sharma, S. (1998). Nuclear factor of activated T cells (NFAT) as a molecular target for 1alpha,25-dihydroxyvitamin D3-mediated effects. *J Immunol*, 160, 1,(Jan 1, 1998) 209-18.

Todd, J.A. (1995). Genetic analysis of type 1 diabetes using whole genome approaches. *Proc Natl Acad Sci U S A*, 92, 19,(Sep 12, 1995) 8560-5.

Todd, J.A., Bell, J.I. & McDevitt, H.O. (1987). HLA-DQ beta gene contributes to susceptibility and resistance to insulin-dependent diabetes mellitus. *Nature*, 329, 6140,(Oct 15-21, 1987) 599-604.

Vafiadis, P., Bennett, S.T., Todd, J.A., Nadeau, J., Grabs, R., Goodyer, C.G., Wickramasinghe, S., Colle, E. & Polychronakos, C. (1997). Insulin expression in human thymus is modulated by INS VNTR alleles at the IDDM2 locus. *Nat Genet*, 15, 3,(Mar, 1997) 289-92.

Van der Auwera, B., Van Waeyenberge, C., Schuit, F., Heimberg, H., Vandewalle, C., Gorus, F. & Flament, J. (1995). DRB1*0403 protects against IDDM in Caucasians with the high-risk heterozygous DQA1*0301-DQB1*0302/DQA1*0501-DQB1*0201 genotype. Belgian Diabetes Registry. *Diabetes*, 44, 5,(May, 1995) 527-30.

Veijola, R., Vahasalo, P., Tuomilehto-Wolf, E., Reijonen, H., Kulmala, P., Ilonen, J., Akerblom, H.K. & Knip, M. (1995). Human leukocyte antigen identity and DQ risk alleles in autoantibody-positive siblings of children with IDDM are associated with reduced early insulin response. Childhood Diabetes in Finland (DiMe) Study Group. *Diabetes*, 44, 9,(Sep, 1995) 1021-8.

Wahl, S.M., Allen, J.B., Weeks, B.S., Wong, H.L. & Klotman, P.E. (1993). Transforming growth factor beta enhances integrin expression and type IV collagenase secretion in human monocytes. *Proc Natl Acad Sci U S A*, 90, 10,(May 15, 1993) 4577-81.

Weber, P., Meluzinova, H., Kubesova, H., Ambrosova, P., Polcarova, V., Cejkova, P. & Cerna, M. Type 1 diabetes and LADA--occurrence of HLA-DRB1 *03 and DRB1 *04 alleles in two age different groups of diabetics. *Adv Gerontol*, 23, 2,(243-8.

Witt, C.S., Price, P., Kaur, G., Cheong, K., Kanga, U., Sayer, D., Christiansen, F. & Mehra, N.K. (2002). Common HLA-B8-DR3 haplotype in Northern India is different from that found in Europe. *Tissue Antigens*, 60, 6,(Dec, 2002) 474-80.

Yang, X.D., Sytwu, H.K., McDevitt, H.O. & Michie, S.A. (1997). Involvement of beta 7 integrin and mucosal addressin cell adhesion molecule-1 (MAdCAM-1) in the development of diabetes in obese diabetic mice. *Diabetes*, 46, 10,(Oct, 1997) 1542-7.

Yang, X.D., Tisch, R., Singer, S.M., Cao, Z.A., Liblau, R.S., Schreiber, R.D. & McDevitt, H.O. (1994). Effect of tumor necrosis factor alpha on insulin-dependent diabetes mellitus in NOD mice. I. The early development of autoimmunity and the diabetogenic process. *J Exp Med*, 180, 3,(Sep 1, 1994) 995-1004.

Zhao, J., Jin, L. & Xiong, M. (2006). Test for interaction between two unlinked loci. *Am J Hum Genet*, 79, 5,(Nov, 2006) 831-45.

11

Tolerance and Autoimmunity in Type 1 Diabetes

Valentina Di Caro[1,2], Nick Giannoukakis[1] and Massimo Trucco[1]
[1]Division of Immunogenetics, Department of Pediatrics,
School of Medicine, University of Pittsburgh,
[2]Rimed Foundation,
[1]USA
[2]Italy

1. Introduction

A functional immune system is able to distinguish between foreign antigens expressed by pathogens and self-antigens expressed by the body. The absence of a pathological response to self-antigens (e.g. tolerance) is dependent on a number of events that occur both centrally and peripherally. Central tolerance is induced at sites of lymphocyte development such as thymus and bone marrow for T cell and B cell respectively. On the other hand, peripheral tolerance occurs at sites of antigen recognition and processing, and includes secondary lymphoid as well as non-lymphoid tissues. Failure of central and/or peripheral tolerance can lead to increased development and expansion of pathogenic effector T cells and subsequent initiation and progression of autoimmunity.

Type 1 Diabetes (T1D) is an autoimmune disease due to a chronic inflammation in the pancreas that leads to the destruction of insulin-producing β-cells. The β-cells are selectively destroyed via both direct and indirect mechanisms by different immune cell types. Studies in animal models and humans have demonstrated that T cells play a major role in β-cell death. However, other cell types are present in the pancreatic infiltrate and in the pancreatic lymph node, where the initial presentation of islet antigen by dendritic cells (DC) to islet antigen specific T cells occurs. Besides different DC subsets, B cells and natural killer (NK) cells also contribute, with different roles, to β-cell destruction. This suggests a strong crosstalk between the immune cells that are involved in pathogenesis and those involved in immune regulation.

Herein, we will describe the autoimmune processes that result in clinical manifestation of this disease and we will discuss the immunologic basis supporting possible new therapeutic interventions.

2. The breakdown of self-tolerance in Type 1 Diabetes

T1D is the most common autoimmune disorder in childhood but the disease may become manifest at any age, even in adults. In the past decade, the incidence of T1D has increased considerably among children under the age of 15 years in most developed countries and, if the present trend continues, the current incidence is predicted to double in European children younger than 5 years, by 2020 (Patterson et al., 2009).

Despite a plethora of data in rodent models of the disease, the etiology and pathogenesis of T1D in humans is largely unknown. The onset of the disease and clinical/diagnostic signs are preceded by a long non-clinical phase during which an aggressive autoimmune reaction is proposed to be taking place. Clinical T1D is the result of end-stage insulitis, and it has been estimated that at the time of diagnosis only 10–20% of the β-cells are still functioning. Studies in the non-obese diabetic (NOD) mouse, a mouse model that spontaneously develops autoimmune diabetes, have highlighted the critical role of adaptive immune responses in the pathogenesis of the disease. Initial β-cell death occurs physiologically in NOD mice, at 2-3 weeks of age, during tissue remodeling and β-cell metabolic changes or it could occur by injury mediated, for example, by viral infections (Turley et al., 2003). Such β-cell death leads to activation of DC, priming and expansion of specific β-cell-autoreactive T cells, initially in the pancreatic draining lymph nodes and subsequently in the pancreas itself. Ultimately, this chronic process ends with enough β-cell mass destruction to need insulin therapy.

It is now well established that a specific genetic constitution is required to develop diabetes. The most important genes contributing to disease susceptibility in humans are located in the HLA class II locus on chromosome 6. Additionally ten other genes or genetic regions have been associated with T1D (Morel et al., 1988; Todd et al., 2007). Nevertheless a relatively small proportion, less than 10%, of individuals with HLA-conferred diabetes susceptibility progress to clinical disease. This implies that additional factors, very likely environmental, are needed to trigger and drive β-cell destruction in genetically predisposed individuals.

Several models illustrate hypotheses on the outcome of the interplay between genetic and environmental factors. The linear β-cell decline hypothesis originally postulated by Eisenbarth remains the most widely referenced benchmark model for T1D (Eisenbarth, 1986). According to this model, genetically susceptible individuals at some point in time encounter certain environmental agents that trigger islet autoimmunity leading to a linear decay in β-cell mass, development of autoantibodies, hyperglycemia, and eventually complete loss of C-peptide. While this view provides an explanation for the sequence of events observed during the course of T1D, it does not integrate factors contributing to the variability along the time axis during the prediabetic phase. Some authors argue that disease progression in T1D is not a linear process, but rather proceeds at variable steps in patients (Chatenoud & Bluestone, 2007). As mentioned before, there is an effect of specific genetic polymorphisms on disease susceptibility but, on the other hand, predisposing DNA sequence variations may by themselves never lead to T1D, or require some degree of environmental insult (viral infection) to culminate in hyperglycemia. Today a more detailed version of the nonlinear model depicting T1D as a "relapsing-remitting" disease has been proposed (Bonifacio et al., 1999; von Herrath et al., 2007; van Belle et al., 2011). Specifically, this model posits that a disequilibrium between autoreactive effector T cells and T regulatory cells could develop over time and eventually lead to a decline in β-cell mass. Whereas the net balance shifts to islet autoimmunity, this effect is temporarily counteracted by the β-cells' proliferative response, perhaps resulting in a late transient phase of reduced insulin requirement called the "honeymoon phase". In an attempt to fit the role of infectious agents into this temporal T1D model, Von Herrath and colleagues introduced the "fertile field" hypothesis (von Herrath et al., 2003). The fertile field is described as a time window that follows viral infection. It can vary depending on the type, anatomical location, and duration of the virus-induced inflammatory response. This fertile field would allow autoreactive T cells to expand and lead to full-blown autoimmunity and clinical T1D (Figure 1).

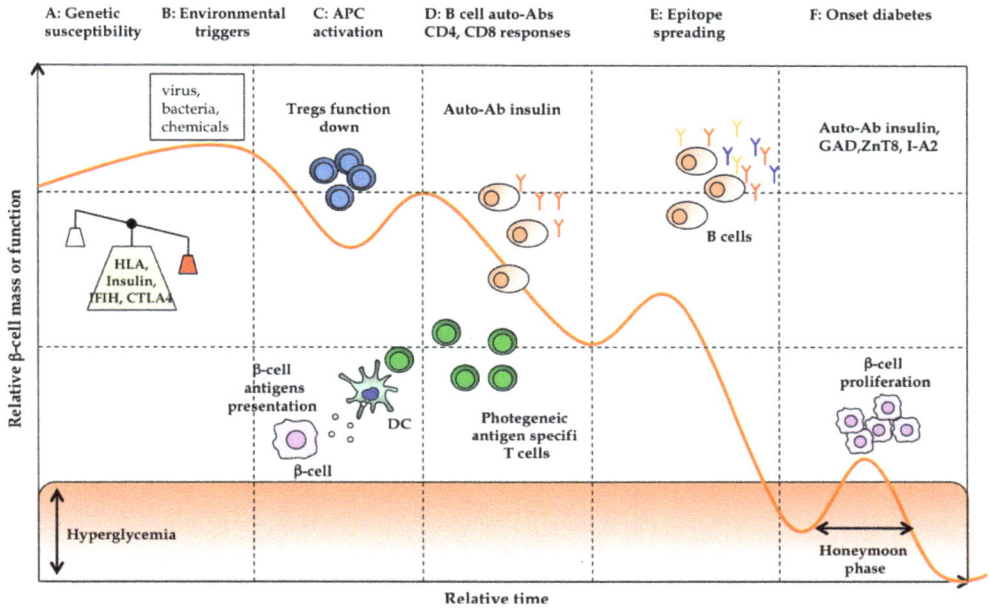

Fig. 1. How T1D might arise. The figure represents the β-cell mass or function (represented by the orange line) as well as the different immunological phases (columns with alphabetized tabs on top) that occur in the pancreas and peripherally. Once the orange line of β-cell function falls into the red zone, the individual is clinically diagnosed with T1D. Initially, a concurrence of genetic susceptibility and an environmental trigger sets an individual up for developing diabetes by causing β-cell death. In the pancreas, β-cell upregulate IFN and subsequently MHC class I. This exposes β-cell to attack by pathogenic antigen specific T cells. Consequently, the released β-cell antigens are picked up by resident APC and transferred to the pancreas-draining lymph nodes. Meanwhile in the periphery, a proinflammatory environment favors effector T cell responses over Treg function. β-cell antigens presented in this proinflammatory context and with CD4 help initiate conversion of B cells into plasma cells and the appearance of insulin autoantibodies . Also, autoreactive CD8 T cells are stimulated to proliferate and migrate into the pancreas. The stress induced by this second wave of β-cell killing causes some β-cell to stop insulin production. The killing also causes the release of new β-cell antigens that are picked up by APCs, including migrated B cells, which get shuttled to the pancreatic lymph node. This engages new antigen-specific clones of CD4 and CD8 T cells and B cells in a process called epitope spreading. Surprisingly, the autoimmune inflammation can also stimulate some β-cell proliferation so that the β-cell mass temporarily increases. The fluctuation between destructive autoreactive responses and β-cell proliferation may create a cyclical relapse-remitting profile of β-cell mass (orange line). Eventually, the autoreactive response wins though, and T1D is diagnosed when only 10 –30% of functional β-cell remains. The remission after clinically diagnosed diabetes is termed the honeymoon phase, a temporary state of relative self-sufficient insulin production.

3. Humoral β-cell autoimmunity

Human and murine T1D studies have shown that the appearance of autoantibodies is the first detectable pre-clinical sign of emerging β-cell autoimmunity. There are four disease-related autoantibodies that have been shown to predict clinical T1D (Knip et al., 2002). These include classical islet cell antibodies (ICA), insulin autoantibodies (IAA), and autoantibodies to the 65 kD isoform of glutamic acid decarboxylase (GADA) and the protein tyrosine phosphatase-related IA-2 molecule (IA–2A). Insulin is the first antigenic target detectable during the early progression of diabetes (Nakayama et al., 2005), although most autoantibodies are targeted against the β-cells themselves and other β-cell secreted proteins (Atkinson & Eisenbarth, 2001). Recently, ZnT8, a pancreatic β-cell specific zinc transporter, has been identified as a candidate autoantigen associated with T1D (Wenzlau et al., 2007). During the progression of T1D, a process of autoantigen epitope spreading occurs. Epitope spreading provides an explanation of how the immune system is capable of recognizing increasing numbers of autoantigens in correlation with increased T1D disease severity (von Herrath et al., 2007). Epitope spreading begins with the immune system recognizing and mounting an immune response against a single antigen, which is recognized via a single epitope. Over time, new antigens can be recognized, and previously recognized antigens can be differentially processed by antigen presenting cells to generate multiple epitopes for a single antigen (Morran et al., 2010).

The number and titer of detectable autoantibodies, rather than the specificity of the autoantibody, is unequivocally related to the risk of progression to overt T1D both in family studies and also in surveys based on general population cohorts. In family studies positivity for three to four autoantibodies is associated with a risk of developing clinical T1D in the range of 60–100% over the next 5–10 years (Barinas-Mitchell et al., 2004; Pietropaolo et al., 2005; Barker, 2006).

Islet specific autoantibodies are, however, considered more diagnostic than causative in T1D. It is generally accepted that the destruction of the β-cells is mediated by cellular immune responses. This is supported by the following facts: (a) T cells are present in insulitis; (b) disease progression is delayed by immunosuppressive drugs directed specifically against T cells; and (c) circulating autoreactive T cells can be detected in patients at clinical presentation of T1D (Roep, 2003).

4. Immune cell crosstalk in Type 1 Diabetes

4.1 T and B lymphocytes

Studies in NOD mice have shown that autoreactive T cells are released into the circulation because of faulty presentation of self-antigens by disease-susceptible MHC molecules that prevent negative selection in the thymus (Trucco, 1992; McDevitt, 2001). Central tolerance can be broken even in the presence of disease-resistant MHC molecules. Indeed, it has been demonstrated that disruption of thymic expression of a single tissue-specific gene self-molecule, as insulin for diabetes, is sufficient to trigger autoimmunity toward the specific tissue (Figure 2) (Fan et al., 2009).

In pre-diabetic mice, insulin specific T cells are the predominant component of islet-infiltrating T cells. Multiple CD4+ and CD8+ T cell clones, targeting different insulin epitopes, have been isolated (Wegmann et al., 1994) demonstrating that T1D development depends on both CD4+ and CD8+ T cells. Moreover, T1D can only be transferred to

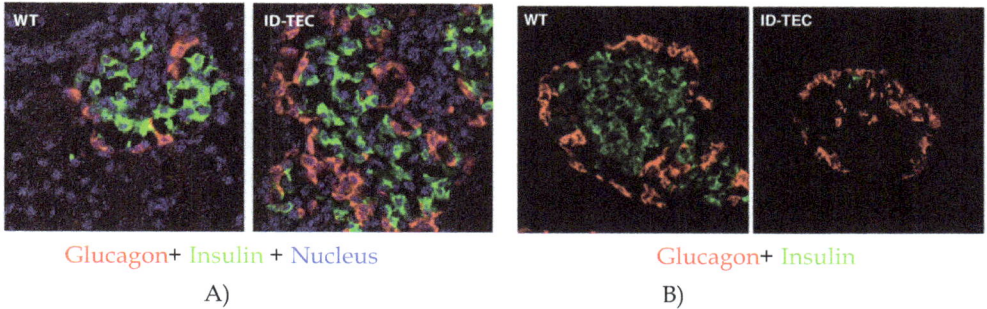

Glucagon+ Insulin + Nucleus   Glucagon+ Insulin

A)   B)

Fig. 2. Transgenic mice that do not express insulin in the thymus (ID-TEC) develop diabetes within 3 weeks. A) Normal islet development of transgenic mice at day 1 after birth; B) 4 week after birth only a small number of β-cells are still present in the islets. Pancreatic section stained using anti-insulin (green), and glucagon (red) antibodies (Fan et al., 2009).

immunocompromised syngeneic recipients by a combination of splenic CD4+ and CD8+ T cells from donor NOD mice but not by either T cell subset alone (Phillips et al., 2009).

There are several ways in which autoreactive T cells can mediate β-cell death. CD8+ T cells may kill pancreatic β-cells through MHC class I mediated cytotoxicity, and both CD4+ and CD8+ T cells produce cytokines, such as interferon-γ (IFNγ), that induce expression of the death receptor Fas (CD95) and chemokine production by β-cells. Activation of Fas by Fas ligand (FasL)-expressing activated T cells can initiate β-cell apoptosis. Chemokine production by β-cells results in further recruitment of mononuclear cells to the site, thereby enhancing inflammation (Eizirik et al., 2009). In addition, IFNγ can activate macrophages and induce increased pro-inflammatory cytokine production, including interleukin-1β (IL-1β) and tumour necrosis factor (TNF). β-cells express high levels of IL-1 receptor and seem to be more sensitive to IL-1β-induced apoptosis than other endocrine cells in the islet. This crosstalk between T cells and macrophages undoubtedly exacerbates the immune-mediated stress on β-cells and contributes to their destruction. IFNγ, IL-1β and TNF also induce the expression of reactive oxygen species (ROS) including nitric oxide by β-cells, and ROS have the potential to mediate apoptosis.

Although T cells have a pathological role in T1D onset, there is also evidence supporting a role for a subset of T cells, the T regulatory cells (Tregs), able to prevent β-cell death.

Tregs play an indispensable role in maintaining homeostatic balance within the immune system. Tregs are involved in mediating normal immune responses against pathogens and terminating such responses when they are no longer required, as well as in preventing autoimmunity. Phenotypically, most Tregs express the surface marker CD25, the high affinity interleukin 2 (IL-2) receptor ligand-binding α chain, and Foxp3, an intracellular transcription factor (Fontenot et al., 2003). Because of that they are identified as CD4+CD25+Foxp3+ cells. Both CD25 and Foxp3 coordinate Treg development and function. In the thymus, IL-2 is critical for the development of Tregs, while, in the periphery, it has been shown that interleukin 7 (IL-7) can complement potentially limiting amounts of IL-2 in promoting Treg survival and functional fitness (Di Caro et al., 2011).

Many studies in the NOD mouse strain have demonstrated the role of CD4+CD25+Foxp3+ Tregs in the maintenance of self-tolerance. Indeed, depletion of CD25-expressing T cells results in a marked acceleration of T1D and foxp3-/- NOD mice display an increased incidence and earlier onset of the disease compared to wild type mice (Brunkow et al., 2001). In humans, patients with IPEX syndrome, who have a mutation in the *FOXP3* gene, develop endocrine autoimmune disease including T1D (Bennett et al., 2001). Tregs can control or limit the activation of CD4+ and CD8+ T cells at various stages such as differentiation and/or proliferation during priming in the draining lymph node, inhibition of IL-2 production or trafficking to the pancreas.

T cells are clearly of pivotal importance for T1D development, but there are also data suggesting an involvement of B-lymphocytes in initiation and progression of the disease. Recently, it was demonstrated that B cell depletion in NOD mice, either through gene targeting or antibody treatment, impaired the development of T1D (Hu et al., 2007) .

The investigation of the roles of B cells in autoimmune inflammatory diseases has focused mainly on the ability of B cells to secrete autoantibodies. More recently, B cells have been identified as important sources of pro- and anti-inflammatory cytokines, for example IL-6 and IL-10. B cells can either provide a quantitatively or functionally dominant source of cytokines. Moreover, they can have a role as antigen-presenting cells that maintain islet antigen-specific T cell activity (Hu et al., 2007; Pescovitz et al., 2009).

4.2 Innate immune cells

As islet antigen-specific T cells can differentiate into either pathogenic effector T cells or regulatory T cells, many studies have investigated the role of innate immune cells in T1D, as these cells usually determine a specific type of immune response. Innate cells producing pro- or anti-inflammatory cytokines define the milieu in which islet antigen specific T cells are activated and whether a deleterious or protective immune response occurs in the pancreas (Figure 3).

Macrophages are one of the two major antigen-presenting cells in islet infiltrates of NOD mice. It has been shown that inhibition of the macrophage influx into the pancreas, by blocking adhesion-promoting receptors on those cells, inhibited the development of T1D (Hutchings et al., 1990). *In vitro* and *in vivo* studies in mice and rats showed that the deleterious effect of macrophages on β-cells can be mediated through the production of TNF and IL-1β (Arnush et al., 1998; Dahlen et al., 1998). Interestingly, pro-inflammatory macrophages can be detected in pancreatic islets before T cell infiltration, as well as in NOD/*scid* (severe combined immunodeficient) mice, which lack functional B and T cells. Macrophages have been shown to produce IL-12 (Alleva et al., 2000) and to promote efficient differentiation of diabetogenic CD8+ cytotoxic T lymphocytes (CTLs) leading to T1D onset (Jun et al., 1999). More recent data suggest that recruitment of macrophages to islets is mediated by the secretion of CC-chemokine ligand 1 (CCL1) and CCL2 by CD4+ T cells and pancreatic β-cells, respectively (Cantor & Haskins, 2007; Martin et al., 2008). Macrophages recruited to the pancreas produce IL-1β, TNF and ROS that can cause β-cell death, revealing an additional role for macrophages in the destructive phase of T1D. Finally, TNF and IL-1β-producing macrophages have been observed in pancreatic islet infiltrates from patients with recent-onset T1D (Ueno et al., 2007). Together, these studies support a pathogenic role for macrophages in both the initiation and destruction phases of T1D at least in the mouse.

NK cells mediate early protection against viruses and are involved in the killing of infected cells and tumours. NK cells are both cytotoxic and producers of cytokines, particularly IFNγ. Thus, NK cells could contribute directly and indirectly to the destruction of β-cells.

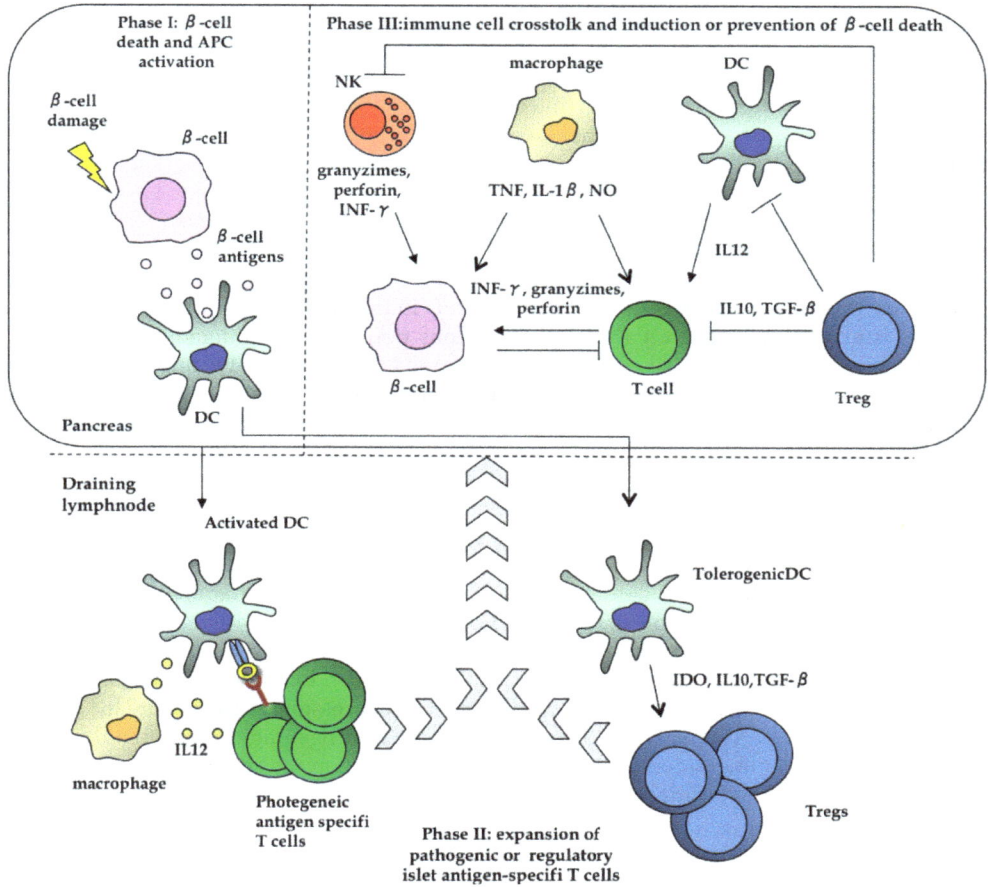

Fig. 3. Cellular and molecular mechanisms in the development or prevention of T1D. The initiation phase of T1D takes place in the pancreas, where DCs capture and process β-cell antigens. β-cell damage can occur by 'natural' apoptosis or after viral infections. Activated DCs prime pathogenic islet antigen-specific T cells after migration to the draining lymph nodes and macrophages promote this activation through IL-12 secretion. The activation of islet antigen-specific T cells can be inhibited by DCs through various mechanisms, such as expansion of Tregs through production of IDO, IL-10 and TGFβ. In the pancreas, β-cells can be killed by diabetogenic T cells and NK cells through the release of interferon-γ (IFNγ), granzymes and perforin, as well as by macrophages through the production of TNF, IL-1β and nitric oxide (NO). β-cell damage can be inhibited by Treg cells that inhibit diabetogenic T cells and innate immune cells through IL-10 and TGF-β. Tolerogenic DCs stimulated by NK cells could also control diabetogenic T cells through IDO production. Lastly, β-cells can inhibit diabetogenic T cells by expressing PDL1. This complex crosstalk between innate and adaptive immune cells results in the development or the prevention of T1D. (Figure adapted from Lehuen et al., 2010).

NK cells have been detected in the pancreas of patients with T1D and in T1D mouse models (Dotta et al., 2007; Alba et al., 2008; Brauner et al., 2010). Moreover, several reports have described a correlation between the frequency and/or activation of NK cells with the destructiveness of the pancreatic infiltrate (Poirot et al., 2004; Feuerer et al., 2009). NK cells isolated from the pancreas of diabetic mice have a more activated phenotype, proliferate more and spontaneously produce higher levels of IFNγ, which promote the effector function of diabetogenic CD4+ T cell, and express CD107a on their cell surface, a marker of granule exocytosis, reflecting their cytotoxic function (Gur et al., 2010). Interestingly, NK cells were observed in the pancreas in NOD mice before T cell infiltration and in the pancreas of NOD–Rag mice, which lack mature B and T cells, suggesting that they could have a sentinel role in the pancreas.

Besides macrophages and NK cells, an important role in the pathogenesis of an autoimmune response is played by DCs. DCs are a heterogeneous population of antigen presenting cell that check tissue homeostasis, initiate T cell mediated immunity and control the maintenance of the immune tolerant state. It is known that patients with a congenital DC deficiency develop autoimmune diseases (Ohnmacht et al., 2009). This highlights their role in mediating peripheral tolerance. DCs, depending on their subset and function, can activate Tregs. It has been shown that they mediate peripheral tolerance by inducing T cell depletion or anergy and expansion of antigen specific Tregs (Ueno et al., 2007).

Studies aimed at elucidating the role of DCs in T1D have outlined beneficial as well as detrimental roles of this cell type in the autoimmune process. In the NOD/BDC2.5 transgenic mouse model, it was demonstrated that DCs prevent the inflammation process in the pancreas by producing indole 2,3-dioxygenase (IDO), a tryptophan catabolizing enzyme that arrests T cell proliferation (Saxena et al., 2007). However, in the same model, it was shown that IFN type 1 is more intimately involved in the initiation of the destructive autoimmunity and is correlated with the increased DC expression in the pancreatic lymph nodes (Li et al., 2008). Alternatively, these two opposite findings might point to a dual role of DC in the autoimmune process most probably depending on the stage of DC maturation and capacity to activate specific immunomodulatory cell types.

5. Immunotherapy to induce immunotolerance

Individuals with T1D develop hyperglycemia due to insufficient insulin production by β-cells in the pancreas. To prevent the rise of blood glucose to pathological levels, T1D patients have to receive a life long treatment with recombinant insulin. Despite insulin supplementation, rapid excursion of glucose levels, in these patients, increases the risk for severe complications such as cardiovascular diseases, nephropathy and neuropathy. Insulin replacement therapy cannot match the precision of endogenous insulin secretion, for this reason new treatments that, ideally, can cure the disease or at least delay/prevent the onset are needed.

The new emerging therapies for T1D, aimed at regulating the autoimmune response largely involve broad based immunoregulatory strategies, including the inhibition or deletion of lymphocytes subsets and/or the use of agents that induce or re-establish immune tolerance via activation of regulatory cells (Chatenoud, 2003; Luo et al., 2010).

5.1 Immunosuppressive drugs
Several randomized clinical trials (RCT), based on preclinical study in animal models, have been performed to test the effect of different immunosuppressive drugs on diabetes

patients. Cyclosporin A (CSA) was employed in the first trials showing effects of immunosuppressive therapies on T1D. Continuous CSA treatment initiated soon after diagnosis eliminated the need for exogenous insulin (Bougneres et al., 1990; Carel et al., 1996). However, the lack of lasting effects and renal toxicity of the drug diminished enthusiasm for this approach. Indeed, in considering immunosuppressive therapies we have to remember that these drugs increase the risk of developing infections and malignancies and that some of them have been shown to inhibit β-cell regeneration (Nir et al., 2007). Within the multitude of immunosuppressive drugs, we are now focusing our overview on those drugs that are of particular interest because of their low levels of side effects and/or because they are able to induce Tregs or tolerogenic DCs.

5.1.1 Anti T-lymphocyte Globulin (ATG)

ATG is a very potent immunosuppressive drug. It depletes almost the entire T cell population in treated patients and is primarily used as inductive treatment after solid organ transplantation or in acute rejection settings in transplant patients. Since ATG is a polyclonal non-human protein mixture, common side effects include fever and serum sickness including arthralgia, rashes and lymphadenopathy. Administration over a longer period increases the risk for immunoproliferative disorders, which is why only short-term treatments are considered. A pilot trial involving new-onset T1D patients has shown a reduction of insulin requirement (Eisenbarth et al., 1985). In a more recent study, ATG (Fresenius) retarded the loss of C-peptide in new-onset patients without the need for continuous drug administration (Saudek et al., 2004) but additional studies are being performed to confirm these findings.

5.1.2 Anti-CD3

One of the most potent treatments at reversing new-onset diabetes in NOD mice is therapy with anti-CD3 mAb (Chatenoud et al., 1994). Chatenoud et al. showed that an intravenous treatment with anti-CD3 mAb resulted in a long-lasting restoration of normoglycemia in 80% of treated NOD mice. The treatment was given for only 5 days indicating that continuous administration might not be required to reach a beneficial effect through restoration of the immune balance in favor of endogens tolerance. These studies also showed that treatment was only effective if it was given shortly after the onset of hyperglycemia (Chatenoud, 2003). These results in NOD mice have led to trials in humans using humanized Fc-engineered monoclonal anti-CD3 antibodies. So far, two antibodies have been tested in diabetic patients, hOKT3 g1 Ala-Ala (Teplizumab) (Herold et al., 2005) and ChAglyCD3 (Otelixizumab) (Keymeulen et al., 2005), and both have shown positive results in patients with T1D in terms of C-peptide preservation and reduction of insulin requirements (Herold et al., 2002). Additionally, sustained C-peptide levels for approximately 2 years and in some cases up to 5 years were observed (Herold et al., 2005, Keymeulen et al., 2005). The side effects of anti-CD3 treatment were predominantly headaches, fever and arthralgia. Moreover gastrointestinal symptoms and most importantly transient EBV-viremia with symptoms of acute mononucleosis were observed. All patients however recovered spontaneously. The mechanism of action of this treatment has been extensively investigated. It can be demonstrated that anti-CD3 treatment modulates the T cell receptors in a way that renders T cells blind to antigens, induces T cell anergy, blocks the IL-2 signaling pathway, and induces apoptosis (Chatenoud & Blustone, 2007).

Interestingly, it has also been shown that Tregs are less susceptible to anti-CD3 induced apoptosis; at least when administered in low doses, thus leading to higher numbers of T regulatory cells under the generalized CD3+ T cell lymphopenia. Taken together, these data have made anti-CD3 antibody a possible candidate for future combination therapies. However, the anti CD3 based phase III clinical trial by Lilly didn't meet the target of the trial and the use of anti-CD3 is no longer being pursued by this commercial entity (http://www.fiercepharma.com/press_releases/macrogenics-and-lilly-announce-pivotal-clinical-trial-teplizumab-did-not-meet-primary).

5.1.3 Anti-CD20

B cells are implicated in the pathogenesis of diabetes. Hu et al., (2007) and Xiu et al., (2008) have shown that diabetes can be prevented in NOD mice by depleting B cells with anti-CD20 mAb before and at the time of onset of hyperglycemia (9–12-week-old mice) and can even reverse disease in about 30% of animals treated at the first appearance of hyperglycemia. Interestingly, cotransfer of B cells from the successfully treated mice diminished the rate of adoptive transfer of disease via T cells, suggesting a possible role for

Agent	Target mechanism	Phase/ ID	Details	Reference
Cyclosporin A	Immune suppression	Completed	Remission successful during treatment but severe side effects	Bougneres et al., 1990, Carel et al., 1996.
Teplizumab Anti CD3 (hOKT3) g1 Ala-Ala	T cell immunomodulation and treg generation by anti Cd3 mAb	Phase III	Primary end point not achieved	
Otelixizumab Anti CD3 (ChAgly CD3)	T cell immunomodulation and treg generation by anti Cd3 mAb	Phase II	6 day treatment: better maintenance of C-peptide levels, reduced insulin requirement out to 18 mo	Chatenoud et al., 1994; Keymeulen et al., 2005.
Rituximab (Anti-CD20 mAb)	B cell depletion	Phase II	Preservation of C-peptide levels for 3/6 months	Prescovitz et al., 2009; Hu et al., 2007.
ATG	T cell depletion generate Treg population	Phase II	Could cause cytokine release syndrome	Simon et al, 2008.

Table 1. Summary of immunotherapy approaches in T1D using antibodies.

activation of "regulatory" B cells. Others have shown that IL-10-producing B cells can be induced in mice depleted of CD20+ B cells (Yanaba et al., 2008).

In a recent phase II clinical trial, depletion of B cells using an anti-CD20 mAb (Rituximab), has shown modest (23%) but significant improvement in β-cell function 3 months after diagnosis and overall at 1 year, in antibody-treated compared to placebo-treated subjects (Pescovitz et al., 2009). There were also significant improvements in clinical parameters including glycated hemoglobin A1c, C-peptide level and insulin use. Side effects that appear frequently are mostly related to the administration itself and decrease over the course of the therapy. However the patients eventually returned to hyperglycemia as B cells reappeared to a great extent (69%) by the end of the year and the C-peptide level started to decline.

This study could ultimately prove that there is a role for B cells in disease pathogenesis, which is scientifically of great interest. However, B cell depletion in this setting does not appear to mediate a significant deceleration of disease progression.

5.2 Anti-inflammatory treatments
5.2.1 Cytokine and cytokine receptor-directed therapies

Cytokine and cytokine receptor-directed therapies are also in development for treatment of T1D. Human insulitis shows a considerably greater infiltration of innate immune cells such as macrophages and NK compared to NOD insulitis (Itoh et al., 1993; Dotta et al., 2007). Moreover, innate mediators (TNF-α, IL-1, and type 1 interferons) were among the first molecules shown to have direct cytotoxic effects on β-cells and were postulated to be the direct cause of β-cell killing (Rabinovitch et al., 1990). Possibly because of its innate role in activating adaptive immune responses, it was not surprising that IL-1 receptor-deficient NOD mice had reduced development of diabetes (Thomas et al., 2004). Treatment with the IL-1 receptor antagonist (Anakinra) was shown to improve glucose control in patients with T2D (Donath & Mandrup-Poulsen, 2008). Interestingly, the drug mechanism appeared to involve a beneficial effect on β-cells, reflected by an increase in the insulin:proinsulin ratio. β-cells may be a source of IL-1, particularly in response to glucose, suggesting a destructive cycle in which hyperglycemia induces expression of the inflammatory mediator resulting in immune activation and further β-cell destruction. Initial preclinical data do not suggest that IL-1 blockade alone will prevent or reverse T1D, but this could be an important target of a combination strategy.

TNF-α is considered to play an active role in the pathogenesis of T1D. TNF-α is directly cytotoxic to β-cells, suggesting this cytokine as an additional possible target for immune therapy. In a small pilot trial in children and adolescents early after diagnosis (< 30 days on average), the use of a TNF antagonist (Etanercept) resulted in preservation of residual insulin secretion compared with placebo (Mastrandrea et al., 2009). C-peptide loss was reduced, as well as a decrease in insulin needs. However there are contrasting data about targeting the TNF-α pathways. Indeed, it has been shown, *in vitro*, that selective CD8+ autoreactive Tcell death induction can be activated by TNF-α, suggesting the use of a TNF agonist instead of a TNF antagonist (Ban et al., 2008). The discrepancy could be due to the timing of TNF-α blockade/ TNF-α administration.

5.3 Antigen specific strategies

Establishment of a simple strategy that results in the emergence of antigen-specific regulatory T cells and the induction of tolerance to autoantigens is a desirable goal. It would ultimately stop the autoimmune process without inducing some of the major side effects that have been observed, for example, in chemical and antibody-based immunosuppressive treatments. Moreover, individuals at risk could be treated prior to significant destruction of β-cell mass and clinical onset of disease. However, the risk of boosting autoreactivity should never be underestimated. As outlined earlier, several autoantigens have been described in T1D; insulin and GAD65 are believed to be the major autoantigens that drive the autoreactivity. Consequently they have been studied most intensively in terms of inducing tolerance in humans.

5.3.1 Insulin

Several clinical trials target insulin because it is the initiating antigen in the NOD model and is also a major autoantigen in human T1D (Nakayama et al., 2005; Fan et al., 2009). There have been a number of human new-onset trials using insulin therapy. In the immunotherapy diabetes (IMDIAB) trial, a total of 82 patients with clinical T1D were randomized to receive oral insulin or placebo (Pozzilli et al., 2000). At a 1-year follow-up, there was no difference between the insulin-treated and the placebo-treated groups with respect to mean C-peptide secretion, requirement for insulin therapy, or IgG insulin antibodies. Furthermore, in patients younger than 15 years, a tendency for low C-peptide at 9 and 12 months was observed in the oral insulin group, suggesting acceleration in the decline of β-cell function. These results are consistent with those seen in murine models where oral insulin was shown not to reverse new-onset diabetes (Fousteri et al., 2007). Interestingly, if nasal insulin therapy is used in combination with anti-CD3 therapy, a significant benefit in reversing recent-onset diabetes is then achieved in two animal models of autoimmune diabetes (Bresson et al., 2006). Expansion of insulin-specific Treg cells producing IL-10, TGF-β, and IL-4, and possibly their modulation of antigen-presenting cells in local draining lymph nodes, were proposed as likely mechanisms. These findings should provide the basis for using combinatorial therapies in future trials for humans with recent-onset diabetes.

A recent phase I study using a single intramuscular injection of human insulin B chain in incomplete Freund's adjuvant in 12 subjects with recent-onset diabetes showed that this therapy led to the development of lasting (at a 2 year follow-up) insulin B chain-specific Tregs (Orban et al., 2009). This study provides the basis for testing this modality of insulin B chain therapy in a larger T1D trial to determine the effect on glycemic level. Another ongoing phase I–II clinical trial of subcutaneous BHT-3021, a plasmid encoding proinsulin, is testing the safety, dose, and preliminary efficacy of this therapeutic modality in recent-onset T1D patients

5.3.2 Glutamate decarboxylase 65

Immune therapies using GAD65 have also been tested in both animal models and human T1D. Interestingly, the initial antigenic region is confined to a few epitopes near the C terminus of the GAD protein but later spreads intramolecularly to other GAD determinants, followed by further intermolecular spreading to other β-cell antigens. Consequently, tolerance induction by intravenous or intrathymic injections of GAD in female NOD mice at 3 weeks of age eliminates the anti-GAD T cell responses, as well as subsequent spreading of the cascade of T cell responses to other β-cell antigens and the development of insulitis or clinical diabetes (Tisch et al., 1993). Intravenous injections of GAD during the later stages of disease still effectively blocked disease progression in prediabetic mice and protected syngeneic islet graft survival in diabetic NOD mice (Tian et al., 1996). The identification of Tregs in GAD-treated mice suggests a major role in the induction of tolerance by treatment with this autoantigen, which raises the question of whether GAD is targeted early in T1D (Tisch et al., 1998).

Agent	Target mechanism	Phase/ ID	Details	Reference
Anakinra (IL1 antagonist)	Anti-inflammatory and improve β-cell survival	Phase II/III	Recruiting	Pickersgill et al., 2009
Etanercept (TNF-α blockade)	Anti-inflammatory	Phase II/III	Low HbA1C and insulin need, increased C-peptide	Mastrandrea et al., 2009
Insulin in IFA	Tolerance vaccination to insulin B chain	Phase I/II	Ongoing	Orban et al., 2009.
BHT-3021	Tolerance vaccination to insulin	Phase I/II	Reduce insulin Ab titers, preserved C-peptide and reduce HbA1c	Gottlieb, 2009.
GAD-Alum	Tolerance to GAD65 skewing Th1 to Th2	Phase II / Phase III	Preservation of residual insulin secretion, GAD specific humoral and cellular response, Ongoing in Europe and USA	Agardh et al., 2009; Ludvigsson et al., 2008
Diap277	Induction of Tregs via TLRs	Phase III	Phase I: preserved C-peptide Phase II: no effect in T1D adults and children Phase III: recruiting	Raz et al., 2001; Lazar et al., 2007; Schloot et al., 2007

Table 2. Summary of immunotherapy approach in T1D using autoantigens, cytokines or cytokine-specific antibodies.

Promising preclinical data in the NOD model prompted two clinical trials using alum-formulated human recombinant GAD65. A phase II safety and dose-finding trial conducted in patients with latent autoimmune diabetes in adults (LADA) (Agardh et al., 2005) showed the approach to be safe, and administration of two subcutaneous doses led to an increase of fasting and stimulated C-peptide at 24 weeks compared to baseline, a benefit that was associated with an increase in CD4+CD25+ Treg cells. In a second trial, in recent-onset T1D children between 10 and 18 years of age, a slower decline of fasting and stimulated C-peptide in the GAD-alum group was observed compared to the placebo (Ludvigsson et al., 2008). More importantly, the protective effect of GAD-alum was preferentially seen in those who received treatment within 6 months of diagnosis, suggesting that the autoimmune process is more susceptible to GAD-based modulatory therapy if initiated at an earlier stage.

5.3.3 Heat shock protein

Early controversies existed as to whether heat shock proteins (hsp) were true autoantigens implicated in the pathogenesis of T1D (Atkinson & Eisenbarth, 2001). However, extensive preclinical studies using the hsp60 peptide p277 demonstrated efficacy of peptide vaccination in halting disease progression in NOD mice (Elias et al., 1991; Elias & Cohen, 1995). p277 treatment appeared to promote Th2-type cell responses with upregulation of IL-10 and IL-13 and downregulation of IFN-γ (Elias et al., 1997; Jin et al., 2008). p277 also has inhibitory effects on the innate immune system via signaling through TLR-2, leading to inhibition of inflammatory lymphocyte chemotaxis (Nussbaum et al., 2006). The equivalent of human hsp60 p277 is a 24 amino acid synthetic peptide derived from the C terminus of the human hsp60, termed DiaPep277. Several phase I and II clinical trials in human T1D patients have been completed in Europe, and phase III trials are underway. A phase II trial was conducted in patients with established T1D but with residual β-cell function (Huurman et al., 2007) and used a range of doses of subcutaneously administered DiaPep277. Results showed a trend of dose-dependent preservation of stimulated C-peptide secretion. Three additional trials were conducted in new-onset T1D patients (Raz et al., 2001; Lazar et al., 2007; Schloot et al., 2007). Two of these trials enrolled adult TID patients, whereas the third enrolled pediatric T1D patients. The adult trials showed significantly better preservation of insulin synthesis as measured by C-peptide production in the treated groups compared with placebo, but this effect was not seen in the pediatric trial. Similar results were observed in one other trial performed in pediatric patients (Schloot et al., 2007), although in children with less aggressive disease progression based on genetic background, there appeared to be a trend to better preserved C-peptide at the end of the study period. In summary, phase II trials with DiaPep277 have shown some promise in preserving residual β-cell function, which appears to be less effective in patients with more aggressive disease. A phase III trial is underway with results expected in later 2011.

6. Cell therapy in type 1 diabetes

Cellular adoptive-transfer-based approaches have shown significant promise preclinically in the NOD model, both in prediabetic and postdiabetic stages. The idea is to compensate a presumed deficiency in tolerogenic cells or tolerogenic cell/molecular signaling pathways by transferring cell types with immunomodulatory capacity. Specifically, both *ex vivo* expanded Tregs or induced CD4+CD25+Foxp3+ Tregs (iTreg) have been shown to control ongoing autoimmunity and either prevent progression to diabetes or protect syngeneic islet grafts and/or allow β-cell recovery, thus inducing diabetes remission in NOD mice (Tang & Bluestone, 2006; Weber et al., 2006; Luo et al., 2007; Godebu et al., 2008). It is unclear whether antigen specificity is critically important in this approach because both nonspecifically-expanded polyclonal or induced Tregs and islet antigen-specific Tregs have shown efficacy in controlling the disease. Additionally, it also appears that Tregs of one antigen specificity may be sufficient in controlling ongoing autoimmunity that is probably caused by autoaggressive T cells of multiple islet antigen specificities (Tarbell et al., 2004; Luo et al., 2007). Clearly delineating these characteristics of Treg adoptive-transfer therapy will have significant impact on the design of future clinical trials using this modality.

Another strategy for enhancing Treg numbers *in vivo* is by DC-based therapy. It has been shown that direct injection of either DC from pancreatic draining lymph nodes or β-cell antigen-pulsed immature DC protects prediabetic NOD mice from developing overt diabetes, possibly through the *in vivo* induction of Treg cells (Clare-Salzler et al., 1992; Lo et al., 2006). However, direct *ex vivo* DC therapy carries the potential risk of their acquiring an activated phenotype upon adoptive transfer, leading to immune activation to some antigen(s) rather than tolerance.

6.1 Diabetes-suppressive dendritic cells

Methods to stably maintain DC in an immature state, defined by low levels of surface costimulatory proteins that include CD80, CD86 and CD40, by downregulating these proteins or blocking their interaction with their ligands, are at the forefront of tolerogenic biologicals like the CTLA4-Ig protein. These strategies result in tolerance to allografts and prevention of autoimmune disease. We have considered two strategies to maintain DCs in a stably-immature state. The first involves *ex vivo* treatment with short double-stranded decoys of the NF-kappaB transcription factor and the second involves *ex vivo* treatment of DCs with antisense oligonucleotides (AS-ODN DC) targeting the primary transcripts of CD40, CD80 and CD86 concurrently. Both DC products are able to prevent and to reverse new onset T1D (Ma et al., 2003; Machen et al., 2004; Trucco & Giannoukakis, 2007; Giannoukakis et al., 2008). These preclinical studies have led to a recently completed phase I trial using autologous *ex vivo*-engineered DC from established diabetic patients (clinicaltrials.gov identifier NCT00445913), conducted at the University of Pittsburgh Medical Center (UPMC), to determine safety as a primary end-point (Figure 4).

Mechanistically, functionally immature DCs, with low to absent costimulatory molecule expression, mediate peripheral tolerance by inducing T cell anergy and the expansion of antigen specific Foxp3+ CD25+ CD4+ Treg (Ueno et al., 2007).

In our approach, AS-ODN DCs promote Treg cell survival through IL-7 signaling in addition to impaired provision of CD40, CD80 and CD86 costimulation (Harnaha et al., 2006). AS-ODN DCs, but not control DC, produce IL-7, in response to a secondary action of the antisense oligonucleotides on Toll Like Receptor (TLR) signaling. It is known that CpG oligonucleotides, like the AS-ODN we use to make tolerogenic DCs, can activate TLR signaling and confer an immunoregulatory phenotype to DCs (Roberts et al., 2005; Jarnicki et al., 2008) and are thus useful for treatment of autoimmune conditions (Ho et al., 2005). It is possible that the oligonucleotides act in a sequence-nonspecific manner when interacting with TLRs, TLR9 in particular, based on conformation and higher order multistrand structures (Guiducci et al., 2008; Kindrachuk et al., 2008). For example, certain multimer formations or conformations would induce non-MyD88 signaling pathways, whereas others

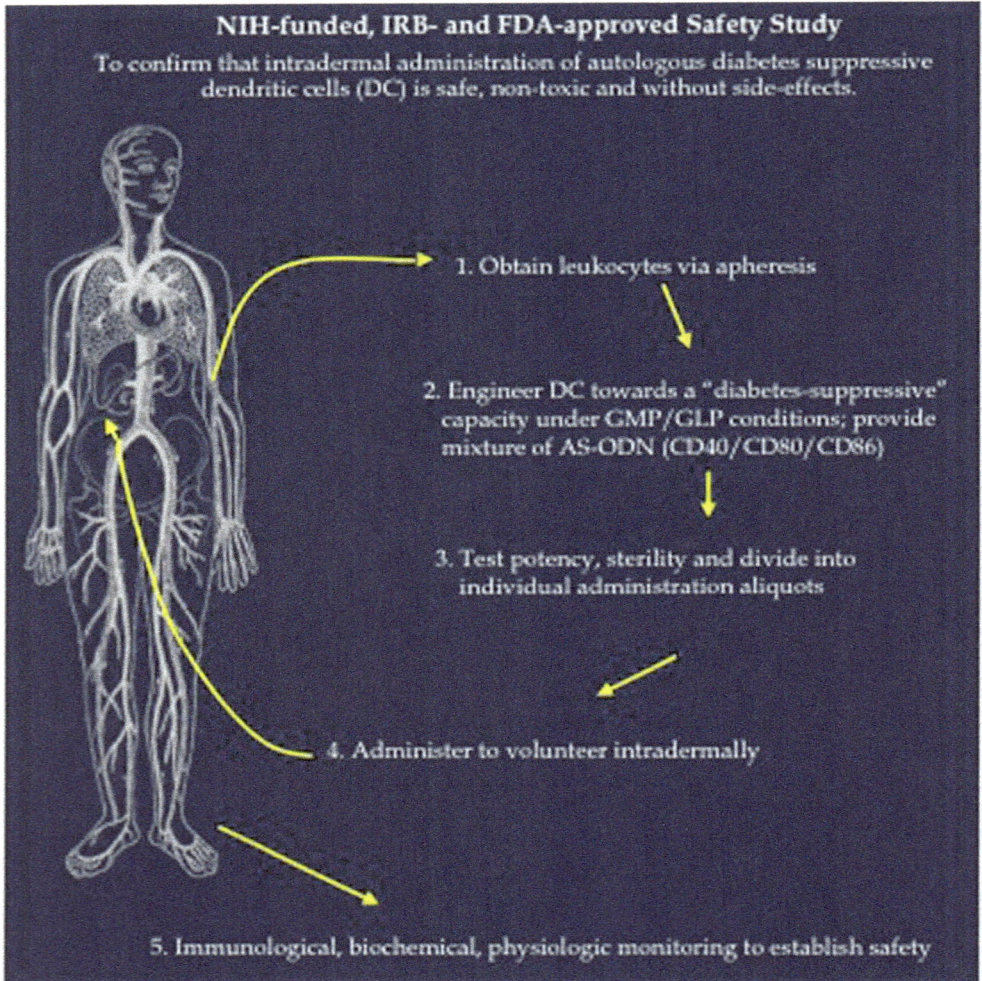

Fig. 4. DC-based clinical trial for T1D. Schematic of the procedures involved in the phase I clinical trial recently completed at the University of Pittsburgh to prove the safety of the DC-based vaccine. (Giannoukakis et al., 2008)

would recruit MyD88. We propose a model where AS-ODN treatment results in a coordinate downregulation of CD40, CD80 and CD86 and induction of IL-7 production via non-MyD88 TLR signals. At this time it is unclear which of the DNA-sensing TLRs transduces the AS-ODN effects. TLR3, TLR7, TLR8 and TLR9 are all equally possible, although the effect of chloroquine on IL- 7 production would suggest an endosomal TLR with TLR9 being the most likely candidate (Figure 5) (Di Caro & Giannoukakis, unpublished data). Indeed, the data indicating that CpG oligonucleotide-triggered TLR9 signaling confers immunosuppressive capacity to DC that can treat autoimmunity *in vivo* strengthens our hypothesis (Ho PP et al., 2005).

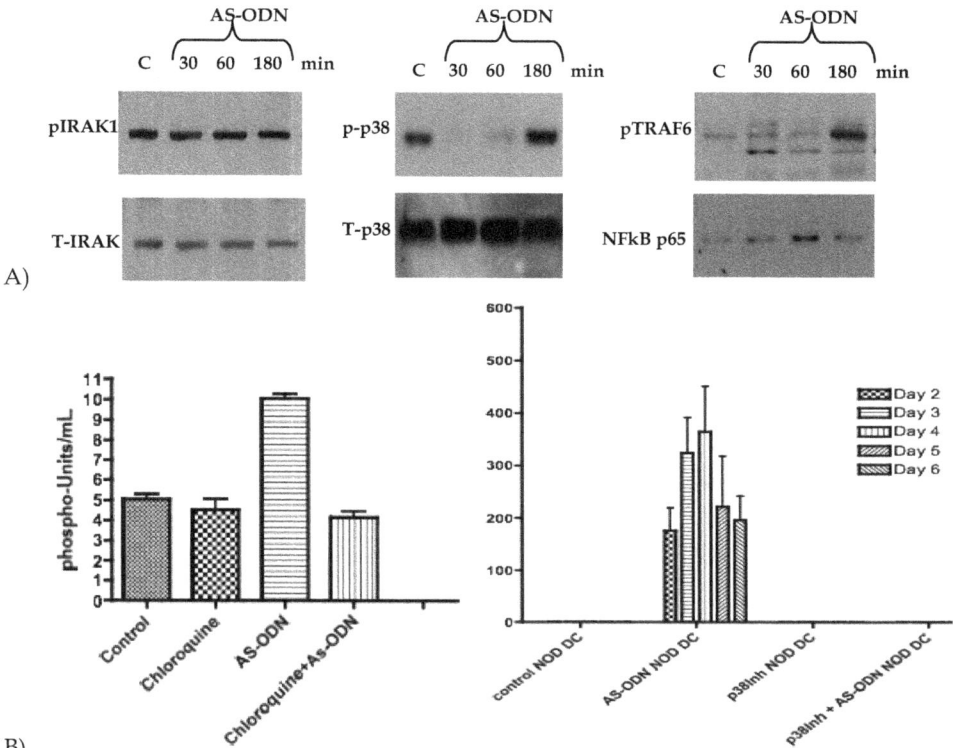

Fig. 5. AS-ODN treatment of DC *in vitro* activates TLRs signals leading to IL-7 production.
A) Western blot analysis of protein extracts from DC treated with AS-ODN for CD40, CD80
and CD86 over time, using the indicated antibodies, shows activation of NFkB after 1 hour
and activation of p38 MAP kinase and TRAF6 after 3 hours. B) p38 MAP kinase
phosphorylation in AS-ODN DC in the presence of chloroquine, a specific inhibitor of
endosomal TLR signaling (e.g. TLR9), is decreased, as demonstrated by LUMINEX-based
nuclear transcription factor analysis. C) inhibition of p38 phosphorylation, using the p38
MAP Kinase inhibitor SB203580, shows a complete abrogation of IL-7 production for each of
the 7 days of generation of the AS-ODN DC.

Recently, we identified a novel CD127+ CD25+ Foxp3+ T cell subpopulation that expresses
the IL-7 receptor (CD127) and has immunosuppressive activity (Figure 6). More
interestingly, exposure of this novel T cell subpopulation to IL-7 *in vitro* results in the
phenotypic maturation of CD127+ CD25+ Foxp3+ T cells to the classical CD25HIGH Foxp3+
Treg (Figure 7) (Di Caro et al., 2011).
IL-7 production by the AS-ODN DC could serve to mature the CD127+ Foxp3+ cells into
powerfully suppressive CD25HIGH Foxp3+ Tregs, and maintain their survival for a longer
time period, especially when the IL-2 concentration in the lymphoid environment is
expected to be limiting, given the competition among CD25+ Tregs and CD25+ effector T
cells for this critical cytokine. Furthermore, the apparent biregulation of cell surface CD25

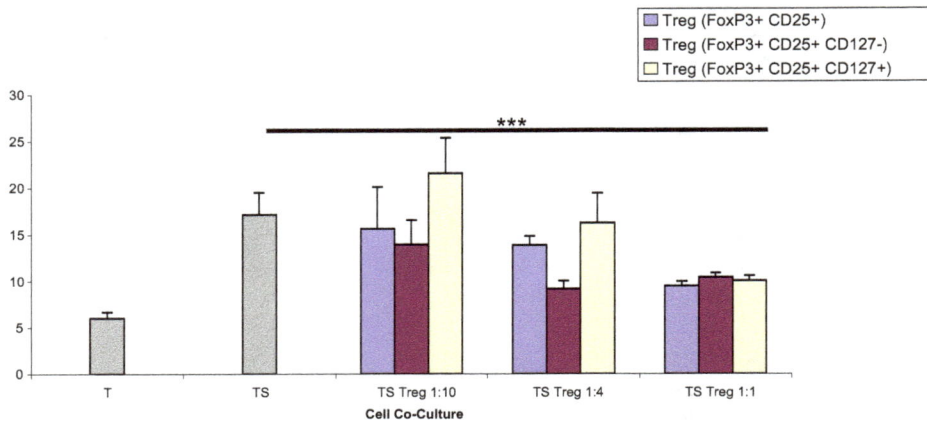

Fig. 6. CD127⁺ CD25⁺ Foxp3⁺ T cell are functionally suppressive *in vitro*. Highly enriched, flow sorted CD4⁺CD25⁺CD127⁺ splenic T cells, isolated form FoxP3 promoter-GFP transgenic mice, are suppressive when added to a co-culture of syngeneic T cells and allogeneic, irradiated, splenocytes (Di Caro et al., 2011).

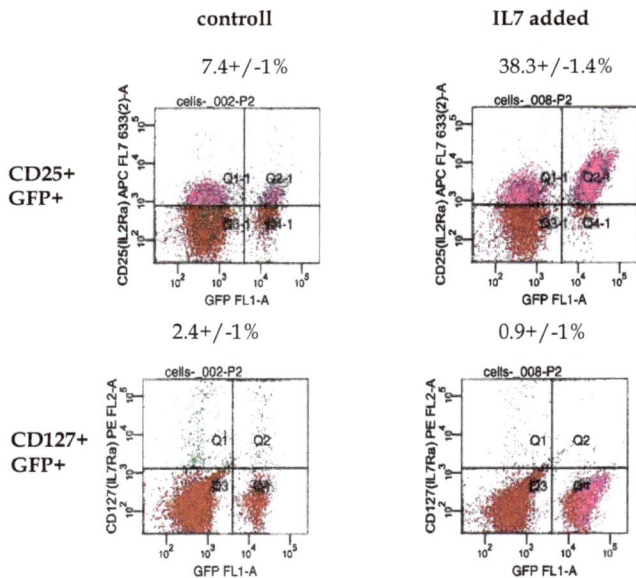

Fig. 7. IL-7 promotes an increase in prevalence of CD127⁻CD25⁺Foxp3⁺ cells. Incubation of splenic CD4⁺GFP⁺ T cells from Foxp3 promoter-GFP transgenic mice with IL-7 overnight results in an increase in CD25⁺GFP⁺ T cells, whereas IL-7 downregulates the prevalence of CD127⁺ GFP⁺ cells (Di Caro et al., 2011).

and CD127 on Tregs in response to their respective ligand availability and signaling, in peripheral lymphoid organs, could have two functions; Treg maintenance and suppressive competency. IL-7 could best serve Tregs under homeostatic conditions in the periphery where IL-2 production would be low. This would maintain a pool of CD4+ CD25[HIGH] Tregs as some type of "memory" Treg population. In contrast, in an environment where IL- 2 would be acutely produced at high levels (i.e. vigorous proliferation of autoreactive T-cells), Tregs would compete as well as the effector T cells for IL-2 and therefore, IL-7 might not be as relevant.

Through these mechanisms and others yet unknown, tolerogenic DC could modulate and restore the balance of pro and anti-inflammatory components of the immune system. Our data and the work carried out by other groups highlights the relevance of using tolerogenic DC to treat autoimmune diabetes as well as other tissue specific autoimmune disorders.

7. Conclusion

T1D most likely results from a combination of genetic susceptibility and exposure to an environmental trigger. The main effector mechanism is clearly an autoimmune reaction, which is also evident at time of clinical diagnosis. A better knowledge of the causes that lead to T1D is critical for prevention as well as for developing new therapies. Early detection is also required to maximally preserve the remaining β-cell mass, because the ability to secrete even small amounts of insulin can make disease control easier and help minimize the complications due to chronic inadequate glycemic control.

Much of our current understanding of T1D comes from the NOD mouse model, this autoimmune diabetes model, so far, has been useful to discover and develop treatments even if some of them were not as successful in humans (e.g. the anti-CD3 therapy).

Today the landscape of possible treatment has been changed by the prospect that T1D progression may be blocked by the active stimulation of tolerance induced by autoantigen-specific Tregs or tolerogenic DCs. The ultimate goal of autoimmune therapy is to silence the immune attack against self without sacrificing the patient's protective immune response to pathogens. This will most likely be achieved by a therapy that combines a nonspecific immune suppressant and the induction of Tregs/ tolerogenic DCs. Regardless of the tolerogenic method employed for therapy, we think that early intervention in T1D patients is critical to prevent ongoing islet destruction and to establish an ideal microenvironment to allow the recovery of a normal β-cell mass from endogenous progenitor cells. The chances for disease prevention will be improved by the identification of biomarkers identifying patients at risk as early in the disease process as possible.

Major efforts on several fronts are still required to fully realize the benefits of the technological and scientific advances in autoimmune diabetes research even if substantial improvements in the cure of T1D patients were indeed promoted.

8. References

Agardh, C.D.; Cilio, C.M.; Lethagen, A.; Lynch, K.; Leslie, R.D.; Palmer, M.; Harris, R.A.; Robertson, J.A. & Lernmark, A. (2005). Clinical evidence for the safety of GAD65 immunomodulation in adult-onset autoimmune diabetes. *J Diabetes Complications*, Vol.19, (4), pp.238-246, ISSN 1056-8727

Alba, A.; Planas, R.; Clemente, X.; Carrillo, J.; Ampudia, R.; Puertas, M.C.; Pastor, X.; Tolosa, E.; Pujol-Borrell, R.; Verdaguer, J.&Vives-Pi, M. (2008). Natural killer cells are required for accelerated type 1 diabetes driven by interferon-beta. *Clin Exp Immunol*, Vol.151, (3), pp.467-475, ISSN 1365-2249

Alleva, D.G.; Pavlovich, R.P.; Grant, C.; Kaser, S.B. & Beller, D.I. (2000). Aberrant macrophage cytokine production is a conserved feature among autoimmune-prone mouse strains: elevated interleukin (IL)-12 and an imbalance in tumor necrosis factor-alpha and IL-10 define a unique cytokine profile in macrophages from young nonobese diabetic mice. *Diabetes*, Vol.49, (7), pp.1106-1115, ISSN 0012-1797

Arnush, M.; Scarim, A.L.; Heitmeier, M.R.; Kelly, C.B. & Corbett, J.A. (1998). Potential role of resident islet macrophage activation in the initiation of autoimmune diabetes. *J Immunol*, Vol.160, (6), pp.2684-2691, ISSN 0022-1767

Atkinson, M.A. & Eisenbarth, G.S. (2001). Type 1 diabetes: new perspectives on disease pathogenesis and treatment. *Lancet*, Vol.358, (9277), pp.221-229, ISSN 0140-6736

Ban, L.; Zhang, J.; Wang, L.; Kuhtreiber, W.; Burger, D. & Faustman, D.L. (2008). Selective death of autoreactive T cells in human diabetes by TNF or TNF receptor 2 agonism. *Proc Natl Acad Sci U S A*, Vol.105, (36), pp.13644-13649, ISSN 1091-6490

Barinas-Mitchell, E.; Pietropaolo, S.; Zhang, Y.J.; Henderson, T.; Trucco, M.; Kuller, L.H. & Pietropaolo. M. (2004). Islet cell autoimmunity in a triethnic adult population of the Third National Health and Nutrition Examination Surveys (NHANES) III. *Diabetes*, Vol.53, pp.1293- 1302, ISSN 0012-1797

Barker, J.M. (2006). Clinical review: Type 1 diabetes-associated autoimmunity: natural history, genetic associations, and screening. *J Clin Endocrinol Metab*, Vol.91, (4), pp.1210-1217, ISSN 0021-972X

Bennett, C.L.; Christie, J.; Ramsdell, F.; Brunkow, M.E.; Ferguson, P.J.; Whitesell, L.; Kelly, T.E.; Saulsbury, F.T.; Chance, P.F. & Ochs, H.D. (2001). The immune dysregulation, polyendocrinopathy, enteropathy, X-linked syndrome (IPEX) is caused by mutations of FOXP3. *Nat Genet*, Vol.27, (1), pp.20-21, ISSN 1061-4036

Bonifacio, E.; Scirpoli, M.; Kredel, K.; Fuchtenbusch, M. & Ziegler, A.G. (1999). Early autoantibody responses in prediabetes are IgG1 dominated and suggest antigen-specific regulation. *J Immunol*, Vol.163, (1), pp.525-532, ISSN 0022-1767

Bougneres, P.F.; Landais, P.; Boisson, C.; Carel, J.C.; Frament, N.; Boitard, C.; Chaussain, J.L. & Bach, J.F. (1990). Limited duration of remission of insulin dependency in children with recent overt type I diabetes treated with low-dose cyclosporin. *Diabetes*, Vol.39, (10), pp.1264-1272, ISSN 0012-1797

Brauner, H.; Elemans, M.; Lemos, S.; Broberger, C.; Holmberg, D.; Flodstrom-Tullberg, M.; Karre, K. & Hoglund, P. (2010). Distinct phenotype and function of NK cells in the pancreas of nonobese diabetic mice. *J Immunol*, Vol.184, (5), pp.2272-2280, ISSN 1550-6606

Bresson, D.; Togher, L.; Rodrigo, E.; Chen, Y.; Bluestone, J.A.; Herold, K.C. & von Herrath, M. (2006). Anti-CD3 and nasal proinsulin combination therapy enhances remission from recent-onset autoimmune diabetes by inducing Tregs. *J Clin Invest*, Vol.116, (5), pp.1371-1381, ISSN 0021-9738

Brunkow, M.E.; Jeffery, E.W.; Hjerrild, K.A.; Paeper, B.; Clark, L.B.; Yasayko, S.A.; Wilkinson, J.E.; Galas, D.; Ziegler, S.F. & Ramsdell, F. (2001). Disruption of a new forkhead/winged-helix protein, scurfin, results in the fatal lymphoproliferative disorder of the scurfy mouse. *Nat Genet*, Vol.27, (1), pp.68-73, ISSN 1061-4036

Cantor, J.& Haskins, K. (2007). Recruitment and activation of macrophages by pathogenic CD4 T cells in type 1 diabetes: evidence for involvement of CCR8 and CCL1. *J Immunol*, Vol.179, (9), pp.5760-5767, ISSN 0022-1767

Carel, J.C.; Boitard, C.; Eisenbarth, G.; Bach, J.F. & Bougneres, P.F. (1996). Cyclosporine delays but does not prevent clinical onset in glucose intolerant pre-type 1 diabetic children. *J Autoimmun*, Vol.9, (6), pp.739-745, ISSN 0896-8411

Chatenoud, L. (2003). CD3-specific antibody-induced active tolerance: from bench to bedside. *Nat Rev Immunol*, Vol.3, (2), pp.123-132, ISSN 1474-1733

Chatenoud, L. & Bluestone, J.A. (2007). CD3-specific antibodies: a portal to the treatment of autoimmunity. *Nat Rev Immunol*, Vol.7, (8), pp.622-632, ISSN 1474-1733

Chatenoud, L.; Thervet, E.; Primo, J. & Bach, J.F. (1994). Anti-CD3 antibody induces long-term remission of overt autoimmunity in nonobese diabetic mice. *Proc Natl Acad Sci U S A*, Vol.91, (1), pp.123-127, ISSN 0027-8424

Clare-Salzler, M.J.; Brooks, J.; Chai, A.; Van Herle, K. & Anderson, C. (1992). Prevention of diabetes in nonobese diabetic mice by dendritic cell transfer. *J Clin Invest*, Vol.90, (3), pp.741-748, ISSN 0021-9738

Dahlen, E.; Dawe, K.; Ohlsson, L. & Hedlund, G. (1998). Dendritic cells and macrophages are the first and major producers of TNF-alpha in pancreatic islets in the nonobese diabetic mouse. *J Immunol*, Vol.160, (7), pp.3585-3593, ISSN 0022-1767

Di Caro, V.; D'Anneo, A.; Phillips, B.; Engman, C.; Harnaha, J.; Lakomy, R.; Styche, A.; Trucco, M. & Giannoukakis, N. (2011). Interleukin-7 matures suppressive CD127(+) forkhead box P3 (FoxP3)(+) T cells into CD127(-) CD25(high) FoxP3(+) regulatory T cells. *Clin Exp Immunol*, ISSN 1365-2249

Donath, M.Y. & Mandrup-Poulsen, T. (2008). The use of interleukin-1-receptor antagonists in the treatment of diabetes mellitus. *Nat Clin Pract Endocrinol Metab*, Vol.4, (5), pp.240-241, ISSN 1745-8374

Dotta, F.; Censini, S.; van Halteren, A.G.; Marselli, L.; Masini, M.; Dionisi, S.; Mosca, F.; Boggi, U.; Muda, A.O.; Prato, S.D.; Elliott, J.F.; Covacci, A.; Rappuoli, R.; Roep, B.O. & Marchetti, P. (2007). Coxsackie B4 virus infection of beta cells and natural killer cell insulitis in recent-onset type 1 diabetic patients. *Proc Natl Acad Sci U S A*, Vol.104, (12), pp.5115-5120, ISSN 0027-8424

Eisenbarth, G.S. (1986). Type I diabetes mellitus. A chronic autoimmune disease. *N Engl J Med*, Vol.314, (21), pp.1360-1368, ISSN 0028-4793

Eisenbarth, G.S.; Srikanta, S.; Jackson, R.; Rabinowe, S.; Dolinar, R.; Aoki, T. & Morris, M.A. (1985). Anti-thymocyte globulin and prednisone immunotherapy of recent onset type 1 diabetes mellitus. *Diabetes Res*, Vol.2, (6), pp.271-276, ISSN 0265-5985

Eizirik, D.L.; Colli, M.L. & Ortis, F. (2009). The role of inflammation in insulitis and beta-cell loss in type 1 diabetes. *Nat Rev Endocrinol*, Vol.5, (4), pp.219-226, ISSN 1759-5037

Elias, D. & Cohen, I.R. (1995). Treatment of autoimmune diabetes and insulitis in NOD mice with heat shock protein 60 peptide p277. *Diabetes*, Vol.44, (9), pp.1132-1138, ISSN 0012-1797

Elias, D.; Meilin, A.; Ablamunits, V.; Birk, O.S.; Carmi, P.; Konen-Waisman, S. & Cohen, I.R. (1997). Hsp60 peptide therapy of NOD mouse diabetes induces a Th2 cytokine burst and downregulates autoimmunity to various beta-cell antigens. *Diabetes*, Vol.46, (5), pp.758-764, ISSN 0012-1797

Elias, D.; Reshef, T.; Birk, O.S.; van der Zee, R.; Walker, M.D. & Cohen, I.R. (1991). Vaccination against autoimmune mouse diabetes with a T-cell epitope of the human 65-kDa heat shock protein. *Proc Natl Acad Sci U S A*, Vol.88, (8), pp.3088-3091, ISSN 0027-8424

Fan, Y.; Rudert, W.A.; Grupillo, M.; He, J.; Sisino, G.&Trucco, M. (2009). Thymus-specific deletion of insulin induces autoimmune diabetes. *EMBO J*, Vol.28, (18), pp.2812-2824, ISSN 1460-2075

Feuerer, M.; Shen, Y.; Littman, D.R.; Benoist, C. & Mathis, D. (2009). How punctual ablation of regulatory T cells unleashes an autoimmune lesion within the pancreatic islets. *Immunity*, Vol.31, (4), pp.654-664, ISSN 1097-4180

Fontenot, A.P.; Gharavi, L.; Bennett, S.R.; Canavera, S.J.; Newman, L.S. & Kotzin, B.L. (2003). CD28 costimulation independence of target organ versus circulating memory antigen-specific CD4+ T cells. *J Clin Invest*, Vol.112, (5), pp.776-784, ISSN 0021-9738

Fousteri, G.; von Herrath, M. & Bresson, D. (2007). Mucosal exposure to antigen: cause or cure of type 1 diabetes? *Curr Diab Rep*, Vol.7, (2), pp.91-98, ISSN 1534-4827

Giannoukakis, N.; Phillips, B. & Trucco, M. (2008). Toward a cure for type 1 diabetes mellitus: diabetes-suppressive dendritic cells and beyond. *Pediatr Diabetes*, Vol.9, (3 Pt 2), pp.4-13, ISSN 1399-5448

Godebu, E.; Summers-Torres, D.; Lin, M.M.; Baaten, B.J. & Bradley, L.M. (2008). Polyclonal adaptive regulatory CD4 cells that can reverse type I diabetes become oligoclonal long-term protective memory cells. *J Immunol*, Vol.181, (3), pp.1798-1805, ISSN 1550-6606

Gottlieb, P.A. BHT-3021 DNA vaccine trial type 1 diabetes. *ADA conference*, June 2009, new Orlens LA.

Guiducci, C.; Ghirelli, C.; Marloie-Provost, M.A.; Matray, T.; Coffman, R.L.; Liu, Y.J.; Barrat, F.J. & Soumelis, V. (2008). PI3K is critical for the nuclear translocation of IRF-7 and type I IFN production by human plasmacytoid predendritic cells in response to TLR activation. *J Exp Med*, Vol.205, (2), pp.315-322, ISSN 1540-9538

Gur, C.; Porgador, A.; Elboim, M.; Gazit, R.; Mizrahi, S.; Stern-Ginossar, N.; Achdout, H.; Ghadially, H.; Dor, Y.; Nir, T.; Doviner, V.; Hershkovitz, O.; Mendelson, M.; Naparstek, Y. & Mandelboim, O. (2010). The activating receptor NKp46 is essential for the development of type 1 diabetes. *Nat Immunol*, Vol.11, (2), pp.121-128, ISSN 1529-2916

Harnaha, J.; Machen, J.; Wright, M.; Lakomy, R.; Styche, A.; Trucco, M.; Makaroun, S. & Giannoukakis, N. (2006). Interleukin-7 is a survival factor for CD4+ CD25+ T-cells and is expressed by diabetes-suppressive dendritic cells. *Diabetes*, Vol.55, (1), pp.158-170, ISSN 0012-1797

Herold, K.C.; Gitelman, S.E.; Masharani, U.; Hagopian, W.; Bisikirska, B.; Donaldson, D.; Rother, K.; Diamond, B.; Harlan, D.M. & Bluestone, J.A. (2005). A single course of anti-CD3 monoclonal antibody hOKT3gamma1(Ala-Ala) results in improvement in C-peptide responses and clinical parameters for at least 2 years after onset of type 1 diabetes. *Diabetes*, Vol.54, (6), pp.1763-1769, ISSN 0012-1797

Herold, K.C.; Hagopian, W.; Auger, J.A.; Poumian-Ruiz, E.; Taylor, L.; Donaldson, D.; Gitelman, S.E.; Harlan, D.M.; Xu, D.; Zivin, R.A. & Bluestone, J.A. (2002). Anti-CD3 monoclonal antibody in new-onset type 1 diabetes mellitus. *N Engl J Med*, Vol.346, (22), pp.1692-1698, ISSN 1533-4406

Ho, P.P.; Fontoura, P.; Platten, M.; Sobel, R.A.; DeVoss, J.J.; Lee, L.Y.; Kidd, B.A.; Tomooka, B.H.; Capers, J.; Agrawal, A.; Gupta, R.; Zernik, J.; Yee, M.K.; Lee, B.J.; Garren, H.; Robinson, W.H. & Steinman, L. (2005). A suppressive oligodeoxynucleotide enhances the efficacy of myelin cocktail/IL-4-tolerizing DNA vaccination and treats autoimmune disease. *J Immunol*, Vol.175, (9), pp.6226-6234, ISSN 0022-1767

Hu, C.Y.; Rodriguez-Pinto, D.; Du, W.; Ahuja, A.; Henegariu, O.; Wong, F.S.; Shlomchik, M.J. & Wen, L. (2007). Treatment with CD20-specific antibody prevents and reverses autoimmune diabetes in mice. *J Clin Invest*, Vol.117, (12), pp.3857-3867, ISSN 0021-9738

Hutchings, P.; Rosen, H.; O'Reilly, L.; Simpson, E.; Gordon, S. & Cooke, A. (1990). Transfer of diabetes in mice prevented by blockade of adhesion-promoting receptor on macrophages. *Nature*, Vol.348, (6302), pp.639-642, ISSN 0028-0836

Huurman, V.A.; Decochez, K.; Mathieu, C.; Cohen, I.R.&Roep, B.O. (2007). Therapy with the hsp60 peptide DiaPep277 in C-peptide positive type 1 diabetes patients. *Diabetes Metab Res Rev*, Vol.23, (4), pp.269-275, ISSN 1520-7552

Itoh, N.; Hanafusa, T.; Miyazaki, A.; Miyagawa, J.; Yamagata, K.; Yamamoto, K.; Waguri, M.; Imagawa, A.; Tamura, S.; Inada, M. & et al. (1993). Mononuclear cell infiltration and its relation to the expression of major histocompatibility complex antigens and adhesion molecules in pancreas biopsy specimens from newly diagnosed insulin-dependent diabetes mellitus patients. *J Clin Invest*, Vol.92, (5), pp.2313-2322, ISSN 0021-9738

Jarnicki, A.G.; Conroy, H.; Brereton, C.; Donnelly, G.; Toomey, D.; Walsh, K.; Sweeney, C.; Leavy, O.; Fletcher, J.; Lavelle, E.C.; Dunne, P. & Mills, K.H. (2008). Attenuating regulatory T cell induction by TLR agonists through inhibition of p38 MAPK signaling in dendritic cells enhances their efficacy as vaccine adjuvants and cancer immunotherapeutics. *J Immunol*, Vol.180, (6), pp.3797-3806, ISSN 0022-1767

Jin, L.; Zhu, A.; Wang, Y.; Chen, Q.; Xiong, Q.; Li, J.; Sun, Y.; Li, T.; Cao, R.; Wu, J. & Liu, J. (2008). A Th1-recognized peptide P277, when tandemly repeated, enhances a Th2 immune response toward effective vaccines against autoimmune diabetes in nonobese diabetic mice. *J Immunol*, Vol.180, (1), pp.58-63, ISSN 0022-1767

Jun, H.S.; Yoon, C.S.; Zbytnuik, L.; van Rooijen, N. & Yoon, J.W. (1999). The role of macrophages in T cell-mediated autoimmune diabetes in nonobese diabetic mice. *J Exp Med*, Vol.189, (2), pp.347-358, ISSN 0022-1007

Keymeulen, B.; Vandemeulebroucke, E.; Ziegler, A.G.; Mathieu, C.; Kaufman, L.; Hale, G.; Gorus, F.; Goldman, M.; Walter, M.; Candon, S.; Schandene, L.; Crenier, L.; De Block, C.; Seigneurin, J.M.; De Pauw, P.; Pierard, D.; Weets, I.; Rebello, P.; Bird, P.; Berrie, E.; Frewin, M.; Waldmann, H.; Bach, J.F.; Pipeleers, D. & Chatenoud, L. (2005). Insulin needs after CD3-antibody therapy in new-onset type 1 diabetes. *N Engl J Med*, Vol.352, (25), pp.2598-2608, ISSN 1533-4406

Kindrachuk, J.; Potter, J.; Wilson, H.L.; Griebel, P.; Babiuk, L.A. & Napper, S. (2008). Activation and regulation of toll-like receptor 9: CpGs and beyond. *Mini Rev Med Chem*, Vol.8, (6), pp.590-600, ISSN 1389-5575

Knip, M.; Kukko, M.; Kulmala, P.; Veijola, R.; Simell, O.; Akerblom, H.K. & Ilonen, J. (2002). Humoral beta-cell autoimmunity in relation to HLA-defined disease susceptibility in preclinical and clinical type 1 diabetes. *Am J Med Genet*, Vol.115, (1), pp.48-54, ISSN 0148-7299

Lazar, L.; Ofan, R.; Weintrob, N.; Avron, A.; Tamir, M.; Elias, D.; Phillip, M. & Josefsberg, Z. (2007). Heat-shock protein peptide DiaPep277 treatment in children with newly diagnosed type 1 diabetes: a randomised, double-blind phase II study. *Diabetes Metab Res Rev*, Vol.23, (4), pp.286-291, ISSN 1520-7552

Lehuen, A.; Diana, J.; Zaccone, P. & Cooke, A. (2010). Immune cell crosstalk in type 1 diabetes. *Nat Rev Immunol*, Vol.10, (7), pp.501-513, ISSN 1474-1741

Li, Q.; Xu, B.; Michie, S.A.; Rubins, K.H.; Schreriber, R.D. & McDevitt, H.O. (2008). Interferon-alpha initiates type 1 diabetes in nonobese diabetic mice. *Proc Natl Acad Sci U S A*, Vol.105, (34), pp.12439-12444, ISSN 1091-6490

Lo, J.; Peng, R.H.; Barker, T.; Xia, C.Q. & Clare-Salzler, M.J. (2006). Peptide-pulsed immature dendritic cells reduce response to beta cell target antigens and protect NOD recipients from type I diabetes. *Ann N Y Acad Sci*, Vol.1079, pp.153-156, ISSN 0077-8923

Ludvigsson, J.; Faresjo, M.; Hjorth, M.; Axelsson, S.; Cheramy, M.; Pihl, M.; Vaarala, O.; Forsander, G.; Ivarsson, S.; Johansson, C.; Lindh, A.; Nilsson, N.O.; Aman, J.; Ortqvist, E.; Zerhouni, P. & Casas, R. (2008). GAD treatment and insulin secretion in recent-onset type 1 diabetes. *N Engl J Med*, Vol.359, (18), pp.1909-1920, ISSN 1533-4406

Luo, X.; Herold, K.C. & Miller, S.D. (2010). Immunotherapy of type 1 diabetes: where are we and where should we be going? *Immunity*, Vol.32, (4), pp.488-499, ISSN 1097-4180

Luo, X.; Tarbell, K.V.; Yang, H.; Pothoven, K.; Bailey, S.L.; Ding, R.; Steinman, R.M. & Suthanthiran, M. (2007). Dendritic cells with TGF-beta1 differentiate naive CD4+CD25- T cells into islet-protective Foxp3+ regulatory T cells. *Proc Natl Acad Sci U S A*, Vol.104, (8), pp.2821-2826, ISSN 0027-8424

Ma, L.; Qian, S.; Liang, X.; Wang, L.; Woodward, J.E.; Giannoukakis, N.; Robbins, P.D.; Bertera, S.; Trucco, M.; Fung, J.J. & Lu, L. (2003). Prevention of diabetes in NOD mice by administration of dendritic cells deficient in nuclear transcription factor-kappaB activity. *Diabetes*, Vol.52, (8), pp.1976-1985, ISSN 0012-1797

Machen, J.; Bertera, S.; Chang, Y.; Bottino, R.; Balamurugan, A.N.; Robbins, P.D.; Trucco, M. & Giannoukakis, N. (2004). Prolongation of islet allograft survival following ex vivo transduction with adenovirus encoding a soluble type 1 TNF receptor-Ig fusion decoy. *Gene Ther*, Vol.11, (20), pp.1506-1514, ISSN 0969-7128

Martin, A.P.; Rankin, S.; Pitchford, S.; Charo, I.F.; Furtado, G.C. & Lira, S.A. (2008). Increased expression of CCL2 in insulin-producing cells of transgenic mice promotes mobilization of myeloid cells from the bone marrow, marked insulitis, and diabetes. *Diabetes*, Vol.57, (11), pp.3025-3033, ISSN 1939-327X

Mastrandrea, L.; Yu, J.; Behrens, T.; Buchlis, J.; Albini, C.; Fourtner, S. & Quattrin, T. (2009). Etanercept treatment in children with new-onset type 1 diabetes: pilot randomized, placebo-controlled, double-blind study. *Diabetes Care*, Vol.32, (7), pp.1244-1249, ISSN 1935-5548

McDevitt, H. (2001). Closing in on type 1 diabetes. *N Engl J Med*, Vol.345, (14), pp.1060-1061, ISSN 0028-4793

Morel, P.A.; Dorman, J.S.; Todd, J.A.; McDevitt, H.O. & Trucco, M. (1988). Aspartic acid at position 57 of the HLA-DQ beta chain protects against type I diabetes: a family study. *Proc Natl Acad Sci U S A*, Vol.85, (21), pp.8111-8115, ISSN 0027-8424

Morran, M.P.; Casu, A.; Arena, V.C.; Pietropaolo, S.; Zhang, Y.J.; Satin, L.S.; Trucco, M.; Becker, D.J. & Pietropaolo, M. (2010). Humoral autoimmunity against theextracellular domain of the neuroendocrine autoantigen IA-2 heightens the risk of type 1 diabetes. *Endocrinology*, Vol.151, pp.2528-2537, ISSN 1945-7170

Nakayama, M.; Abiru, N.; Moriyama, H.; Babaya, N.; Liu, E.; Miao, D.; Yu, L.; Wegmann, D.R.; Hutton, J.C.; Elliott, J.F. & Eisenbarth, G.S. (2005). Prime role for an insulin epitope in the development of type 1 diabetes in NOD mice. *Nature*, Vol.435, (7039), pp.220-223, ISSN 1476-4687

Nir, T.; Melton, D.A. & Dor, Y. (2007). Recovery from diabetes in mice by beta cell regeneration. *J Clin Invest*, Vol.117, (9), pp.2553-2561, ISSN 0021-9738

Nussbaum, G.; Zanin-Zhorov, A.; Quintana, F.; Lider, O. & Cohen, I.R. (2006). Peptide p277 of HSP60 signals T cells: inhibition of inflammatory chemotaxis. *Int Immunol*, Vol.18, (10), pp.1413-1419, ISSN 0953-8178

Ohnmacht, C.; Pullner, A.; King, S.B.; Drexler, I.; Meier, S.; Brocker, T. & Voehringer, D. (2009). Constitutive ablation of dendritic cells breaks self-tolerance of CD4 T cells and results in spontaneous fatal autoimmunity. *J Exp Med*, Vol.206, (3), pp.549-559, ISSN 1540-9538

Orban, T.; Sosenko, J.M.; Cuthbertson, D.; Krischer, J.P.; Skyler, J.S.; Jackson, R.; Yu, L.; Palmer, J.P.; Schatz, D. & Eisenbarth, G. (2009). Pancreatic islet autoantibodies as predictors of type 1 diabetes in the Diabetes Prevention Trial-Type 1. *Diabetes Care*, Vol.32, (12), pp.2269-2274, ISSN 1935-5548

Patterson, C.C.; Dahlquist, G.G.; Gyurus, E.; Green, A. & Soltesz, G. (2009). Incidence trends for childhood type 1 diabetes in Europe during 1989-2003 and predicted new cases 2005-20: a multicentre prospective registration study. *Lancet*, Vol.373, (9680), pp.2027-2033, ISSN 1474-547X

Pescovitz, M.D.; Greenbaum, C.J.; Krause-Steinrauf, H.; Becker, D.J.; Gitelman, S.E.; Goland, R.; Gottlieb, P.A.; Marks, J.B.; McGee, P.F.; Moran, A.M.; Raskin, P.; Rodriguez, H.; Schatz, D.A.; Wherrett, D.; Wilson, D.M.; Lachin, J.M. & Skyler, J.S. (2009). Rituximab, B-lymphocyte depletion, and preservation of beta-cell function. *N Engl J Med*, Vol.361, (22), pp.2143-2152, ISSN 1533-4406

Phillips, J.M.; Parish, N.M.; Bland, C.; Sawyer, Y.; De La Pena, H. & Cooke, A. (2009). Type 1 Diabetes Development Requires Both CD4+ and CD8+ T cells and Can Be Reversed by Non-Depleting Antibodies Targeting Both T Cell Populations. *Rev Diabet Stud*, Vol.6, (2), pp.97-103, ISSN 1614-0575

Pickersgill, L.M. & Mandrup-Poulsen, T.R. (2009). The anti-interleukin-1 in type 1 diabetes action trial–background and rationale. *Diabetes Metab Res Rev*, Vol.25, pp. 321–324, ISSN1520-7560

Pietropaolo, M.; Yu, S.; Libman, I.M.; Pietropaolo, S.L.; Riley, K.; LaPorte, R.E.; Drash, A.L.; Mazumdar, S.; Trucco, M. & Becker, D.J. (2005). Cytoplasmic islet cell antibodies remain valuable in defining risk of progression to Type 1 diabetes in subjects with other islet autoantibodies. *Pediatric Diabetes,* Vol.6, pp.184-192, ISSN 1399-543X

Poirot, L.; Benoist, C. & Mathis, D. (2004). Natural killer cells distinguish innocuous and destructive forms of pancreatic islet autoimmunity. *Proc Natl Acad Sci U S A*, Vol.101, (21), pp.8102-8107, ISSN 0027-8424

Pozzilli, P.; Pitocco, D.; Visalli, N.; Cavallo, M.G.; Buzzetti, R.; Crino, A.; Spera, S.; Suraci, C.; Multari, G.; Cervoni, M.; Manca Bitti, M.L.; Matteoli, M.C.; Marietti, G.; Ferrazzoli, F.; Cassone Faldetta, M.R.; Giordano, C.; Sbriglia, M.; Sarugeri, E. & Ghirlanda, G. (2000). No effect of oral insulin on residual beta-cell function in recent-onset type I diabetes (the IMDIAB VII). IMDIAB Group. *Diabetologia*, Vol.43, (8), pp.1000-1004, ISSN 0012-186X

Rabinovitch, A.; Sumoski, W.; Rajotte, R.V. & Warnock, G.L. (1990). Cytotoxic effects of cytokines on human pancreatic islet cells in monolayer culture. *J Clin Endocrinol Metab*, Vol.71, (1), pp.152-156, ISSN 0021-972X

Raz, I.; Elias, D.; Avron, A.; Tamir, M.; Metzger, M. & Cohen, I.R. (2001). Beta-cell function in new-onset type 1 diabetes and immunomodulation with a heat-shock protein peptide (DiaPep277): a randomised, double-blind, phase II trial. *Lancet*, Vol.358, (9295), pp.1749-1753, ISSN 0140-6736

Roberts, T.L.; Sweet, M.J.; Hume, D.A. & Stacey, K.J. (2005). Cutting edge: species-specific TLR9-mediated recognition of CpG and non-CpG phosphorothioate-modified oligonucleotides. *J Immunol*, Vol.174, (2), pp.605-608, ISSN 0022-1767

Roep, B.O. (2003). The role of T-cells in the pathogenesis of Type 1 diabetes: from cause to cure. *Diabetologia*, Vol.46, (3), pp.305-321, ISSN 0012-186X

Saudek, F.; Havrdova, T.; Boucek, P.; Karasova, L.; Novota, P.&Skibova, J. (2004). Polyclonal anti-T-cell therapy for type 1 diabetes mellitus of recent onset. *Rev Diabet Stud*, Vol.1, (2), pp.80-88, ISSN 1614-0575

Saxena, V.; Ondr, J.K.; Magnusen, A.F.; Munn, D.H. & Katz, J.D. (2007). The countervailing actions of myeloid and plasmacytoid dendritic cells control autoimmune diabetes in the nonobese diabetic mouse. *J Immunol*, Vol.179, (8), pp.5041-5053, ISSN 0022-1767

Schloot, N.C.; Meierhoff, G.; Lengyel, C.; Vandorfi, G.; Takacs, J.; Panczel, P.; Barkai, L.; Madacsy, L.; Oroszlan, T.; Kovacs, P.; Suto, G.; Battelino, T.; Hosszufalusi, N. & Jermendy, G. (2007). Effect of heat shock protein peptide DiaPep277 on beta-cell function in paediatric and adult patients with recent-onset diabetes mellitus type 1: two prospective, randomized, double-blind phase II trials. *Diabetes Metab Res Rev*, Vol.23, (4), pp.276-285, ISSN 1520-7552

Simon, G.; Parker, M.; Ramiya, V.; Wasserfall, C. & Huang, Y. (2008). Murine antithymocyte globulin therapy alters disease progression in NOD mice by a time-dependent induction of immunoregulation. *Diabetes* Vol.57, pp.405–414, ISSN1939-327X

Tang, Q. & Bluestone, J.A. (2006). Regulatory T-cell physiology and application to treat autoimmunity. *Immunol Rev*, Vol.212, pp.217-237, ISSN 0105-2896

Tarbell, K.V.; Yamazaki, S.; Olson, K.; Toy, P. & Steinman, R.M. (2004). CD25+ CD4+ T cells, expanded with dendritic cells presenting a single autoantigenic peptide, suppress autoimmune diabetes. *J Exp Med*, Vol.199, (11), pp.1467-1477, ISSN 0022-1007

Thomas, H.E.; Irawaty, W.; Darwiche, R.; Brodnicki, T.C.; Santamaria, P.; Allison, J. & Kay, T.W. (2004). IL-1 receptor deficiency slows progression to diabetes in the NOD mouse. *Diabetes*, Vol.53, (1), pp.113-121, ISSN 0012-1797

Tian, J.; Clare-Salzler, M.; Herschenfeld, A.; Middleton, B.; Newman, D.; Mueller, R.; Arita, S.; Evans, C.; Atkinson, M.A.; Mullen, Y.; Sarvetnick, N.; Tobin, A.J.; Lehmann, P.V. & Kaufman, D.L. (1996). Modulating autoimmune responses to GAD inhibits disease progression and prolongs islet graft survival in diabetes-prone mice. *Nat Med*, Vol.2, (12), pp.1348-1353, ISSN 1078-8956

Tisch, R.; Liblau, R.S.; Yang, X.D.; Liblau, P. & McDevitt, H.O. (1998). Induction of GAD65-specific regulatory T-cells inhibits ongoing autoimmune diabetes in nonobese diabetic mice. *Diabetes*, Vol.47, (6), pp.894-899, ISSN 0012-1797

Tisch, R.; Yang, X.D.; Singer, S.M.; Liblau, R.S.; Fugger, L. & McDevitt, H.O. (1993). Immune response to glutamic acid decarboxylase correlates with insulitis in non-obese diabetic mice. *Nature*, Vol.366, (6450), pp.72-75, ISSN 0028-0836

Todd, J.A.; Walker, N.M.; Cooper, J.D.; Smyth, D.J.; Downes, K.; Plagnol, V.; Bailey, R.; Nejentsev, S.; Field, S.F.; Payne, F.; Lowe, C.E.; Szeszko, J.S.; Hafler, J.P.; Zeitels, L.; Yang, J.H.; Vella, A.; Nutland, S.; Stevens, H.E.; Schuilenburg, H.; Coleman, G.; Maisuria, M.; Meadows, W.; Smink, L.J.; Healy, B.; Burren, O.S.; Lam, A.A.; Ovington, N.R.; Allen, J.; Adlem, E.; Leung, H.T.; Wallace, C.; Howson, J.M.; Guja, C.; Ionescu-Tirgoviste, C.; Simmonds, M.J.; Heward, J.M.; Gough, S.C.; Dunger, D.B.; Wicker, L.S. & Clayton, D.G. (2007). Robust associations of four new chromosome regions from genome-wide analyses of type 1 diabetes. *Nat Genet*, Vol.39, (7), pp.857-864, ISSN 1061-4036

Trucco, M. (1992). To be or not to be Asp 57, that is the question. *Diabetes Care*, Vol.15, (5), pp.705-715, ISSN 0149-5992

Trucco, M. & Giannoukakis, N. (2007). Immunoregulatory dendritic cells to prevent and reverse new-onset Type 1 diabetes mellitus. *Expert Opin Biol Ther*, Vol.7, (7), pp.951-963, ISSN 1744-7682

Turley, S.; Poirot, L.; Hattori, M.; Benoist, C. & Mathis, D. (2003). Physiological beta cell death triggers priming of self-reactive T cells by dendritic cells in a type-1 diabetes model. *J Exp Med*, Vol.198, (10), pp.1527-1537, ISSN 0022-1007

Ueno, H.; Klechevsky, E.; Morita, R.; Aspord, C.; Cao, T.; Matsui, T.; Di Pucchio, T.; Connolly, J.; Fay, J.W.; Pascual, V.; Palucka, A.K. & Banchereau, J. (2007). Dendritic cell subsets in health and disease. *Immunol Rev*, Vol.219, pp.118-142, ISSN 0105-2896

van Belle, T.L.; Coppieters, K.T. & von Herrath, M.G. (2011). Type 1 diabetes: etiology, immunology, and therapeutic strategies. *Physiol Rev*, Vol.91, (1), pp.79-118, ISSN 1522-1210

von Herrath, M.; Sanda, S. & Herold, K. (2007). Type 1 diabetes as a relapsing-remitting disease? *Nat Rev Immunol*, Vol.7, (12), pp.988-994, ISSN 1474-1741

von Herrath, M.G.; Fujinami, R.S. & Whitton, J.L. (2003). Microorganisms and autoimmunity: making the barren field fertile? *Nat Rev Microbiol*, Vol.1, (2), pp.151-157, ISSN 1740-1526

Weber, S.E.; Harbertson, J.; Godebu, E.; Mros, G.A.; Padrick, R.C.; Carson, B.D.; Ziegler, S.F. & Bradley, L.M. (2006). Adaptive islet-specific regulatory CD4 T cells control autoimmune diabetes and mediate the disappearance of pathogenic Th1 cells in vivo. *J Immunol*, Vol.176, (8), pp.4730-4739, ISSN 0022-1767

Wegmann, D.R.; Gill, R.G.; Norbury-Glaser, M.; Schloot, N. & Daniel, D. (1994). Analysis of the spontaneous T cell response to insulin in NOD mice. *J Autoimmun*, Vol.7, (6), pp.833-843, ISSN 0896-8411

Wenzlau, J.M.; Juhl, K.; Yu, L.; Moua, O.; Sarkar, S.A.; Gottlieb, P.; Rewers, M.; Eisenbarth, G.S.; Jensen, J.; Davidson, H.W. & Hutton, J.C. (2007). The cation efflux transporter ZnT8 (Slc30A8) is a major autoantigen in human type 1 diabetes. *Proc Natl Acad Sci U S A*, Vol.104, (43), pp.17040-17045, ISSN 0027-8424

Xiu, Y.; Wong, C.P.; Bouaziz, J.D.; Hamaguchi, Y.; Wang, Y.; Pop, S.M.; Tisch, R.M. & Tedder, T.F. (2008). B lymphocyte depletion by CD20 monoclonal antibody prevents diabetes in nonobese diabetic mice despite isotype-specific differences in Fc gamma R effector functions. *J Immunol*, Vol.180, (5), pp.2863-2875, ISSN 0022-1767

Yanaba, K.; Bouaziz, J.D.; Haas, K.M.; Poe, J.C.; Fujimoto, M. & Tedder, T.F. (2008). A regulatory B cell subset with a unique CD1dhiCD5+ phenotype controls T cell-dependent inflammatory responses. *Immunity*, Vol.28, (5), pp.639-650, ISSN 1097-4180

12

Autoimmunity in Vitiligo

E. Helen Kemp[1], Sherif Emhemad[1],
David J. Gawkrodger[2] and Anthony P. Weetman[1]
[1]Department of Human Metabolism, The Medical School, University of Sheffield, Sheffield,
[2]Department of Dermatology, Royal Hallamshire Hospital, Sheffield,
United Kingdom

1. Introduction

Vitiligo is an idiopathic disorder of pigmentation characterised by the presence of depigmented skin macules due to the chronic and progressive loss of melanocytes from the cutaneous epidermis. Large population surveys have shown a worldwide incidence of 1-2% (Boisseau-Garsaud et al., 2000; Howitz et al., 1977; Majumder et al. 1993; Mehta et al., 1973), although a prevalence of 8.8% has been reported in India (Sehgal & Srivastava, 2007). The disease occurs independently of age and race, and both sexes are equally affected (Behl et al., 2003; Cho et al., 2000; Handa & Dogra, 2003; Hann & Lee, 1996; LePoole & Boissy, 1997; Zaima & Koga, 2002). In approximately half of all cases, vitiligo appears before the age of 20 years, and 70-80% of patients develop the disease by the age of 30 years (Behl et al., 2003; Herane, 2003). Frequently, patients with vitiligo also suffer from other autoimmune conditions (Alkhateeb et al., 2003; Laberge et al., 2005).

Usually, vitiligo is viewed as a minor disease, but the impact on patients' psychological well-being and social interactions is often underestimated (Kent & Al' Abadie, 1996; Ongenae et al., 2006; Porter et al., 1986). The treatment of choice in vitiligo is dependent upon factors which include vitiligo type (non-segmental, segmental), patient age, and location and stability of depigmented lesions (Taieb & Picardo, 2010). However, despite the many available therapeutic modalities (Abu Tahir et al., 2010; Olsson, 2010), repigmentation in the majority of vitiligo patients is rarely complete or long-lasting, so a better understanding of the precise aetiology and pathogenesis of the disease is crucial to improving the efficacy of treatment regimens.

Currently, the exact aetiology of vitiligo remains obscure, but many factors have been implicated in the development of the disease including infections (Grimes et al., 1996; Shegan, 1971), stress (Al'Abadie et al., 1994a), neural abnormalities (Al'Abadie et al., 1994b), defective melanocyte adhesion (Gauthier et al., 2003), and genetic susceptibility (Spritz, 2010). The biochemical hypothesis argues that melanocyte destruction is due to the accumulation of toxic metabolites from melanogenesis, the break-down of free-radical defence and an excess of hydrogen peroxide (Dell'Anna & Picardo, 2006; Schallreuter et al., 1991; Schallreuter et al., 2001; Schallreuter et al., 2005). In addition, many studies have indicated a role for both cellular (Ogg et al., 1998; Van den Boorn et al., 2009; Wankowicz-Kalinska et al., 2003) and humoral (Gilhar et al., 1995; Naughton et al., 1983a; Norris et al., 1988a) immunity in the pathogenesis of vitiligo. Ultimately, these different factors may act independently or together to yield the same effect, namely the disappearance of melanocytes from the skin and this is proposed in the convergence theory (Le Poole et al., 1993a). For example, autoimmunity might arise as a secondary phenomenon following the self-destruction of pigment cells and this might then amplify the damage to melanocytes. In addition, different pathogenic mechanisms could account for the various clinical types of vitiligo: the possible neural mechanisms are usually related to segmental vitiligo, whereas autoimmunity is most often associated with the non-segmental (generalised) form (Taieb, 2000).

2. Immunological factors in vitiligo aetiology and pathogenesis

The evidence for the role of autoimmunity in the aetiology and pathogenesis of vitiligo will be discussed in the next sections.

2.1 Immuno-genetic factors

The majority of cases of vitiligo are sporadic without a family history of the disease. Nevertheless, 15-20% of patients report at least one affected first-degree relative (Alkhateeb et al., 2003), lending evidence for a genetic role in the aetiology of vitiligo. Furthermore, among Caucasians, the risk of vitiligo developing in a patient's sibling is approximately 6.1% (Alkhateeb et al., 2003), an increase of 16-fold compared to the general Caucasian population where the prevalence of the disease is 0.38% (Howitz et al., 1977). Similarly, an increased risk among first-degree relatives is found in Indian-Pakistanis at 6.1% (Alkhateeb et al., 2003), in American Hispanic-Latinos at 4.8% (Alkhateeb et al., 2003) and in Han Chinese at 2.6% (Sun et al., 2006). A simple Mendelian inheritance pattern is not displayed in these familial aggregations of vitiligo cases (Alkhateeb et al., 2003; Bhatia et al., 1992; Carnevale et al., 1980; Das et al., 1985; Hafez et al., 1983; Laberge et al., 2005; Majumder et al., 1988; Majumder et al., 1993; Mehta et al., 1973; Nath et al., 1994; Sun et al., 2006), suggesting that the disease is probably transmitted as a polygenic trait. Indeed, earlier disease onset in familial cases (Alkhateeb et al., 2003; Laberge et al., 2005) and reduced risk of vitiligo with increasing genetic distance from the patient (Alkhateeb et al. 2003) are indicative of a polygenic disorder. Formal genetic segregation analyses of vitiligo have also suggested that multiple loci contribute to vitiligo susceptibility (Majumder et al., 1993; Nath et al., 1994; Sun et al., 2006). Seldomly have large multi-generation families been reported where vitiligo segregates in an autosomal dominant pattern (Alkhateeb et al., 2005). Twin studies have also provided evidence of a genetic component to vitiligo aetiology. For vitiligo in monozygotic twins, the concordance is 23% (Alkhateeb et al. 2003), a disease risk that is 60-fold greater than that in the general population (Howitz et al., 1977) and 4-fold higher than that for a patient's sibling (Alkhateeb et al., 2003).

The genetic epidemiological evidence has prompted the search for genes which predispose an individual to vitiligo. Investigations have included families with vitiligo as well as cohorts of patients without a familial history of the disease (Cantón et al., 2005; Fain et al., 2003). In addition, different approaches have been employed to identify genes which confer susceptibility to vitiligo including candidate gene association studies (Blomhoff et al., 2005; Cantón et al., 2005), genome-wide linkage studies (Chen et al., 2005; Fain et al., 2003; Liang et al., 2007; Spritz et al., 2004), and genome-wide association studies (Birlea et al., 2010; Jin et al., 2010a; Quan et al., 2010). The majority of genes and genetic loci so far identified have a role in the function of the immune system (Spritz, 2010), and these are summarised in the following sections.

2.1.1 Human leukocyte antigen alleles of the major histocompatibility complex

Initial case-control analyses demonstrated an association between predisposition to vitiligo and several different human leukocyte antigen (HLA) alleles of the major histocompatibility complex (MHC), and these are summarised in Table 1. Although these studies showed weak and variable associations, a significant association of HLA-DR4 and vitiligo was demonstrated in several populations (Dunston et al. 1990; Foley et al. 1983; Venneker et al. 1992) and a subsequent meta-analysis of a series of case-control studies reported association of vitiligo with HLA-A2 (Liu et al., 2007).

Population	Associated HLA Allele	Reference
American (Caucasian)	DR4	Foley et al., 1983
American (African)	DR4, DQw3	Dunston et al., 1990
American and British (European-derived, Caucasian)	DRB1A*04-DQB1*0301	Fain et al., 2006
American and British (European-derived, Caucasian)	Class I (specifically A*0201) and II antigens	Jin et al., 2010a
Chinese (Han)	DQA1*0302, DQB1*0303, DQB1*0503	Yang et al., 2005
Chinese (Han)	A25-Cw*0602-DQA1*0302	Xia et al., 2006
Chinese (Han and Uygar)	Class I and II antigens	Quan et al., 2010
Dutch	DR4, DR6, Cw6	Venneker et al., 1993; Venneker et al., 1992
Dutch	DRB4*0101, DQB1*0303	Zamani et al., 2001
German (Northern)	A2	Schallreuter et al., 1993
Hungarian	DR1, DR3	Poloy et al., 1991
Italian	A30, B27, Cw6, DQw3	Finco et al., 1991
Italian (Northern)	A3	Lorini et al., 1992
Italian (Northern)	A30, Cw6, DQw3	Orecchia et al., 1992
Japanese	A31, Bw46, Cw4	Ando et al., 1993
Kuwaiti	B21, Cw6	Al-Fouzan et al., 1995
Moroccan (Jewish)	B13	Metzker et al., 1980
Omani	Bw6, DR7	Venkataram et al., 1995
Slovak	A2, Dw7	Buc et al., 1996
Turkish	DRB1*03, DRB1*04, DRB1*07	Tastan et al., 2004
Yemeni	Bw35	Metzker et al., 1980

Table 1. Association of human leukocyte antigen (HLA) alleles with vitiligo susceptibility

More recently, the use of better analytical and statistical methods has revealed associations of vitiligo with HLA-DRB1*04, HLA-DRB1*03 and HLA-DRB1*07 alleles in Turkish patients (Tastan et al., 2004), with HLA-DRB4*0101 and HLA-DQB1*0303 in Dutch patients (Zamani et al., 2001), and HLA-A25-Cw*0602-DQA1*0302, HLA-DQA1*0302, HLA-DQB1*0303 and HLA-DQB1*0503 in Han Chinese patients (Xia et al., 2006; Yang et al., 2005). Furthermore, a study of 76 Caucasian multiplex vitiligo families found the HLA-DRB1A*04-DQB1*0301 haplotype to be associated with a higher risk of developing vitiligo and with an earlier onset of the disease (Fain et al., 2006). Finally, two genome-wide association studies undertaken on populations of vitiligo patients have reported that predisposition of vitiligo is associated with HLA class I and II antigens (Jin et al., 2010a; Quan et al., 2010).

2.1.2 Immune-response genes and loci

Variations in several immune-response genes, including CCR6, FOXP1, FOXP3, TSLP and XBP1, have a confirmed association with predisposition to vitiligo and these are summarised in Table 2 (Birlea et al., 2011; Cheong et al., 2009; Jin et al., 2010a; Jin et al., 2010b; Quan et al., 2010; Ren et al., 2009). Of particular note, the allelic variation R620W of the PTPN22 gene, which encodes lymphoid protein tyrosine phosphatase, a molecule involved in T cell signalling, has been shown to confer vitiligo susceptibility in several independent reports (Cantón et al., 2005; Jin et al., 2010a; Laberge et al., 2008a; Laberge et al., 2008b). In addition, allelic variants in the NLRP1 gene (previously NALP1 or SLEV1), which encodes a key regulator of the innate immune system, have been reproducibly associated with an increased risk of vitiligo in different populations (Jin et al., 2007a; Jin et al., 2007b; Nath et al., 2001; Spritz et al., 2004).

The study of variations in the cytotoxic T lymphocyte antigen 4 (CTLA4) gene has yielded conflicting results with respect to vitiligo susceptibility (Birlea et al., 2011; Birlea et al., 2009; Blomhoff et al., 2005; Deeba et al., 2010; Itirli et al., 2005; Kemp et al., 1999; Laberge et al., 2008a; Pehlivan et al., 2009). Presently, allelic differences in CTLA4 appear to be predominantly associated with vitiligo occurring together with other autoimmune diseases (Blomhoff et al., 2005), and it has been suggested, therefore, that the association of CTLA4 with vitiligo is probably secondary to its primary association with disorders such as autoimmune thyroid disease (Spritz, 2010).

2.2 Associated autoimmune disease

Vitiligo is frequently associated with other autoimmune disorders, particularly autoimmune thyroid disease (Boelaert et al., 2010; Ochi & DeGroot, 1969), autoimmune polyendocrine syndromes (Ahonen et al., 1990; Neufeld et al., 1990), pernicious anaemia (Dawber, 1970), Addison's disease (Zelissen et al., 1995), and alopecia areata (Ahmed et al., 2007). Furthermore, patients with vitiligo are more likely to suffer from autoimmune conditions than those in the general population (Birlea et al., 2008; Cunliffe et al., 1968; Liu et al., 2005; Turnbridge et al., 1977). In a survey of more than 2,600 unselected Caucasian vitiligo patients, elevated frequencies of autoimmune thyroid disease, Addison's disease, systemic lupus erythematosus and pernicious anaemia were found, with approximately 30% of patients being affected with at least one additional autoimmune disorder (Alkhateeb et al., 2003). Moreover, these same autoimmune diseases occurred at an increased frequency in the first-degree relatives of the patients studied (Alkhateeb et al., 2003). Similarly, in multiplex generalised vitiligo families, higher frequencies of psoriasis, rheumatoid arthritis and type 1 diabetes mellitus were noted in addition to autoimmune thyroid disease, Addison's disease, systemic lupus erythematosus and pernicious anaemia (Laberge et al., 2005). Such data indicate that individuals can be genetically predisposed to a specific group of autoimmune diseases that includes vitiligo, and are also evidence for an autoimmune aetiology for this depigmenting disorder.

Gene or Locus	Function/Comment	Reference
AIS2	Autoimmune susceptibility locus 2. Function undefined. Associated with autoimmune disease.	Spritz et al., 2004
CCR6	Cytokine-chemokine receptor for CCL20. Recruits immune cells on binding of ligand. Associated with inflammatory bowel disease.	Jin et al., 2010a; Jin et al., 2010b; Quan et al., 2010
C1QTNF6	C1q and tumour necrosis factor-related protein- 6. Associated with rheumatoid arthritis and type 1 diabetes mellitus.	Jin et al., 2010a
FOXP1	Forkhead box P1. Transcription factor which regulates development of immune cells.	Jin et al., 2010a; Jin et al., 2010b
FOXP3	Forkhead box P3. Transcription factor which regulates regulatory T cell development. Causes autoimmune IPEX syndrome.	Birlea et al., 2011
GZMB	Granzyme B. Regulates cell-mediated immune responses.	Jin et al., 2010a
IL2RA	Interleukin (IL)-2 receptor alpha chain. Receptor for cytokine IL2 which induces T and B cell proliferation. Associated with many autoimmune diseases.	Jin et al., 2010a
LPP	LIM domain-containing preferred translocation partner in lipoma. Function unknown. Associated with celiac disease and rheumatoid arthritis.	Jin et al., 2010a
NLRP1 (NALP1; SLEV1)	NACHT leucine-rich-repeat protein 1. Functions in the innate immune response. Associated with many autoimmune diseases.	Jin et al., 2007a; Jin et al., 2007b; Nath et al., 2001; Spritz et al., 2004
PTPN22	Lymphoid protein tyrosine phosphatase. Negatively regulates T cell activation. Associated with many autoimmune diseases.	Cantón et al., 2005; Jin et al., 2010a; Laberge et al., 2008a; Laberge et al., 2008b
TSLP	Thymic stromal lymphopoietin. Cytokine which induces naïve CD4+ T cells to produce T helper cell 2 cytokines.	Birlea et al., 2011; Cheong et al., 2009
UBASH3A	Ubiquitin-associated and SH3 domain-containing A gene. Regulates T cell receptor signalling. Associated with type 1 diabetes mellitus.	Jin et al., 2010a
XBP1	X-box binding protein 1. Transcription factor which regulates MHC class II gene expression. Associated with inflammatory bowel disease.	Birlea et al., 2011; Ren et al., 2009

Table 2. Confirmed associations of immune-response gene variants with vitiligo susceptibility

2.3 Animal models

The study of animal models has added credence to the theory that immune mechanisms play a part in the development of vitiligo. Several spontaneous animal models of vitiligo exist, although the exact relevance of such models to the equivalent human disorder remains to be established (Boissy & Lamoreux, 1988). The well-documented Smyth chickens express a genetically inherited form of vitiligo-like depigmentation resulting from the loss of melanocytes in feather and ocular tissues (Smyth, 1989). In this avian model, vitiligo begins with an inherent melanocyte defect that is followed by an autoimmune response involving both humoral and cellular reactions that eliminate abnormal pigment cells (Boissy et al., 1984; Boyle et al., 1987; Lamont & Smyth, 1981; Pardue et al., 1988). An increase in T cells in the feather pulp and circulating inflammatory leukocytes has been shown in Smyth chickens prior to the onset, and during the development of, vitiligo (Erf & Smyth, 1996; Erf et al., 1995). Antibodies to chicken melanocytes have also been detected in the sera of 100% of Smyth chicks but not in the sera of normally pigmented birds (Austin et al., 1992). These antibodies were found to be present both before and during the presentation of vitiligo (Searle et al., 1991), and the primary target antigen was identified as the melanogenic enzyme tyrosinase-related protein-1 (Austin & Boissy, 1995). In other animals with vitiligo including horses, cats and dogs, antibody reactivity occurs against a similar pattern of melanocyte antigens to that found in patients with the disease (Naughton et al., 1983b; Naughton et al., 1986a), suggesting that similar immunological responses occur in both animals and humans.

2.4 Vitiligo melanocytes

Several studies have shown abnormal expression of MHC class II antigen HLA-DR and increased expression of intercellular adhesion molecule-1 by perilesional melanocytes in vitiligo compared with melanocytes from normal skin (Al Badri et al., 1993a; Hedley et al., 1998; Van den Wijngaard et al., 2000). Since these molecules have important roles in antigen presentation and in the activation of helper T cells, their expression by melanocytes could contribute to the anti-melanocyte cellular immune responses that are seen in vitiligo (Ogg et al., 1998; Van den Boorne et al., 2009). Both vitiligo and normal melanocytes are also capable of expressing MHC class I molecules (Hedley et al., 1998), which could allow interaction with destructive cytotoxic T cells. Furthermore, melanocytes have an antigen processing and presenting capability which can make them target cells for T cell-mediated cytotoxicity (Le Poole et al., 1993b). In perilesional vitiligo biopsies, melanocytes express macrophage markers CD68 and CD36 (Van den Wijngaard et al., 2000) and reduced levels of membrane regulators of complement activation, including decay acceleration factor and membrane cofactor protein (Van den Wijngaard et al., 2002), which suggests a vulnerability of these cells to attack by macrophages and the complement system, respectively.

2.5 Vitiligo treatments

Repigmentation in vitiligo patients receiving treatment with immunosuppressive agents indirectly supports the theory that immune-mediated processes are involved in vitiligo pathogenesis. Topically applied tacrolimus (FK506), a therapeutic agent which exerts a potent immunosuppressive effect on T cells by blocking the action of the cytokine gene-activating cofactor calcineurin (Homey et al., 1998), has resulted in successful repigmentation responses in vitiligo patients (Boone et al., 2007; Hartmann et al., 2008).

Topical corticosteroids, which have anti-inflammatory and immunosuppressive actions, are considered to be an effective first-line treatment in children and adults with segmental or non-segmental vitiligo of recent onset (Abu Tahir et al., 2010; Gawkrodger et al., 2010), and, indeed, following treatment of vitiligo patients with systemic steroids, a reduction in anti-melanocyte antibody levels and in antibody-mediated anti-melanocyte cytotoxicity has been demonstrated (Hann et al., 1993; Takei et al., 1984).

Psoralen with ultraviolet radiation (PUVA) is used as a second-line therapy for vitiligo (Alomar, 2010; Gawkrodger et al., 2010). Following PUVA treatment, a reduction in the number of Langerhans cells and a decrease in the expression of vitiligo-associated melanocyte antigens, which could lead to a blocking of antibody-dependent cell-mediated cytotoxicity against melanocytes, have been noted in vitiligo patients (Kao & Yu, 1992; Viac et al., 1997). In addition, ultraviolet radiation can induce the expression of anti-inflammatory cytokines, modulate the expression of intercellular adhesion molecule-1, and induce apoptosis of skin-infiltrating T lymphocytes (Duthie et al., 1999; Krutmann & Morita, 1999).

2.6 Humoral immune responses
2.6.1 Melanocyte antibodies

Antibodies to melanocytes occur at a significantly increased frequency in the sera of vitiligo patients compared with healthy individuals (Cui et al., 1992; Cui et al., 1995; Farrokhi et al., 2005; Hann et al., 1996a; Hann et al., 1996b; Naughton et al., 1983a; Naughton et al., 1983b; Rocha et al., 2002). As well as circulating antibodies, antibody deposits have been noted in the basement membrane zones of depigmented areas in patients with vitiligo (Uda et al., 1984). However, no B cells or antibody has yet been isolated from vitiligo lesions. Interestingly, correlations can also exist between the incidence and level of melanocyte antibodies and both the activity and extent of vitiligo (Aronson & Hashimoto, 1987; Harning et al., 1991; Kemp et al., 2011; Naughton et al., 1986b; Yu et al., 1993), indicating that melanocyte antibodies are possible markers of disease progression.

Predominantly, melanocyte antibodies have been characterised as IgG (Cui et al., 1992; Cui et al., 1995; Farrokhi et al., 2005; Hann et al., 1996a; Hann et al., 1996b; Naughton et al., 1983a; Naughton et al., 1983b; Rocha et al., 2002; Uda et al., 1984) and as belonging to subclasses IgG1, IgG2 and IgG3 (Xie et al., 1991), although anti-melanocyte IgA antibodies have also been reported (Aronson & Hashimoto, 1987). Initial immunoprecipitation studies using melanoma cell extracts revealed that antibodies in vitiligo patients were most commonly directed against antigens with molecular weights of 35, 40-45, 75, 90 and 150 kDa (Cui et al., 1992). Several of the proteins (40-45, 75 and 150 kDa) appeared to be common tissue antigens, while others (35 and 90 kDa) were preferentially expressed on melanocytes (Cui et al., 1992). In immunoblotting studies with melanocyte extracts, antigens of 45, 65, and 110 kDa have been identified (Hann et al., 1996b; Park et al., 1996), while vitiligo-associated antibodies have been demonstrated to recognise melanoma cell proteins of 68, 70, 88, 90, 110 and 165 kDa (Hann et al., 1996a; Rocha et al., 2002).

The identity of several vitiligo-associated antibody targets has been reported and these are summarised in Table 3. Included are the melanogenic enzymes tyrosinase (Baharav et al., 1996; Kemp et al., 1997a; Song et al., 1994) and tyrosinase-related protein-2 (Kemp et al., 1997b; Okamoto et al., 1998), and the melanosomal matrix protein gp100 (Pmel17) (Kemp et al., 1998a). The technique of peptide phage-display has identified the melanin-concentrating hormone receptor 1 (MCHR1) and tyrosine hydroxylase as targets of vitiligo patient antibodies (Kemp et al., 2002). Recent proteomic analysis has also revealed lamin A is a vitiligo-associated antigen (Li et al., 2010).

Antigen	Number of Patients with Antibodies (%)	Number of Controls with Antibodies (%)	Reference
Lamin A	24/84 (28.6)	2/64 (3.1)	Li et al., 2010
MCHR1	9/55 (16.4)	0/28 (0)	Kemp et al., 2002
MCHR1	12/84 (14.3)	Not reported	Li et al., 2010
Pmel17	3/53 (5.9)	0/20 (0)	Kemp et al., 1998a
SOX10	3/93 (3.2)	0/65 (0)	Hedstrand et al., 2001
SOX9	1/93 (1.1)	0/65 (0)	Hedstrand et al., 2001
Tyrosinase	16/26 (61)	0/31 (0)	Song et al., 1994
Tyrosinase	7/18 (39)	0/12 (0)	Baharav et al., 1996
Tyrosinase	5/46 (10.9)	0/20 (0)	Kemp et al., 1997a
TRP-1	3/53 (5.9)	0/20 (0)	Kemp et al., 1998b
TRP-1	8/84 (9.5)	Not reported	Li et al., 2010
TRP-2	3/53 (5.9)	0/20 (0)	Kemp et al., 1997b
TRP-2	10/15 (67)	0/21 (0)	Okamoto et al., 1998
TRP-2	20/30 (67)	1/35 (2)	Okamoto et al., 1998
Tyrosine hydroxylase	18/79 (23)	0/28 (0)	Kemp et al., 2011

Table 3. Defined antibody targets in patients with vitiligo

2.6.2 Pathogenic mechanisms

With respect to pathogenic effects, vitiligo-associated antibodies are able to destroy melanocytes and melanoma cells *in vitro* and *in vivo* by complement-mediated damage and antibody-dependent cellular cytotoxicity (Fishman et al., 1993; Gottumukkala et al., 2006; Norris et al., 1998a). Complement-mediated cytolysis of melanocytes by vitiligo patient antibodies appears to be cell selective and more common in individuals with active disease (Cui et al., 1993). Passive immunisation of nude mice grafted with human skin has also indicated that IgG from vitiligo patients can induce melanocyte destruction (Gilhar et al., 1995). Furthermore, IgG melanocyte antibodies from individuals with vitiligo can induce HLA-DR and intercellular adhesion molecule-1 expression on and release of interleukin-8 from melanocytes (Yi et al., 2000). Such changes that may enhance the antigen-presenting activity of melanocytes allowing antigen-specific immune effector cell attack resulting in melanocyte destruction.

Antibodies against MCHR1 have been shown to block the function of the receptor in a heterologous cell line (Gottumukkala et al., 2006). Stimulation of MCHR1 in cultured melanocytes with melanin-concentrating hormone (MCH) can down regulate the actions of α-melanocyte-stimulating hormone, including the production of melanin, suggesting that the MCH/MCHR1 signalling pathway has a role with the melanocortins in regulating melanocyte function (Hoogduijn et al., 2002). Any adverse effects of MCHR1 antibodies upon the functioning of the receptor in melanocytes could potentially disrupt normal melanocyte behaviour, a feature that could precede the clinical manifestation of vitiligo. However, this has not yet been reported and is still the object of study. More recent work has found that 69% (9/13) of vitiligo patient sera tested induced melanocyte detachment in a reconstructed epidermis model, although this was unrelated to either the extent or the activity of the disease (Cario-Andre et al., 2007). Further studies are needed to confirm that this serum effect is antibody mediated and, if so, that the antibody activity is specific to vitiligo patient sera.

2.6.3 Other antibodies

Circulating organ-specific autoantibodies, particularly to the thyroid, adrenal glands, gastric parietal cells, and pancreatic islet cells are commonly detected in the sera of vitiligo patients (Brostoff, 1969; Betterle et al., 1976; Mandry et al., 1996; Zauli et al., 1986). Moreover, antinuclear antibody and IgM-rheumatoid factor have been detected at a significant frequency in vitiligo patients (Farrokhi et al., 2005). Anti-keratinocyte intracellular antibodies that correlate with disease extent and activity have also been detected in vitiligo patients (Yu et al., 1993).

2.7 Cellular immune responses
2.7.1 Cytokines

An imbalance of cytokines, which can affect melanocyte activity and survival, has been shown in vitiligo lesional skin (Moretti et al., 2002). The level of granulocyte-macrophage colony-stimulating factor is reduced in patients with active vitiligo compared with healthy controls (Yu et al., 1997; Moretti et al., 2002). This cytokine has been found to act as a growth factor for melanocytes and a decrease in its production slows down the proliferation of surviving melanocytes in vitiligo lesions (Imokawa et al., 1996). Other melanogenic cytokines, including stem cell factor and endothelin-1, are also lowered in depigmented lesions (Moretti et al., 2002).

Serum levels of soluble interleukin-2 receptor can be used to monitor *in vivo* immune activation, and its elevation has been correlated with T cell-mediated immune disease. Indeed, the level of the soluble interleukin-2 receptor level in vitiligo patients is significantly increased compared with that of controls, indicating that the activation of T cells is a component in the pathogenesis of vitiligo (Tu et al., 1999; Yeo et al., 1999). The production of interleukin-6 by mononuclear cells is also elevated in vitiligo patients (Yu et al., 1997). This cytokine can induce the expression of intercellular adhesion molecule-1 on melanocytes thereby facilitating leukocyte-melanocyte interactions and consequently cause immunological damage (Kirnbauer et al., 1992). Increased production of interleukin-8, which can attract neutrophils to vitiligo lesions amplifying destructive inflammatory reactions, has also been reported in the mononuclear cells of vitiligo patients (Yu et al., 1997). Furthermore, the expression of tumour necrosis factor-alpha, an inflammatory mediator involved in the pathogenesis of autoimmune disease, is significantly elevated in vitiligo skin (Moretti et al., 2002). However, the exact roles in vitiligo pathogenesis of these inflammatory cytokines, which can also act as paracrine inhibitors of melanocyte proliferation and of melanogenesis, remain to be determined.

2.7.2 Macrophages

Macrophage infiltration has been demonstrated in vitiligo lesions, with increased numbers present in perilesional skin (Le Poole et al., 1996; Van den Wijngaard et al., 2000). It is possible that macrophages are involved in clearing melanocytes that have been induced to apoptose by cytotoxic T lymphocytes. Additional evidence for the active involvement of macrophages in vitiligo pathogenesis is demonstrated by their expression of immunoglobulin receptors: in a mouse model, it has been shown that macrophages, expressing the common gamma chain of the activating Fc gamma receptors, can mediate vitiligo in the presence and absence of complement C3 fraction (Trcka et al., 2002)

2.7.3 Dendritic cells

The density of Langerhans cells in vitiliginous skin has been variously reported as normal, increased and decreased compared with pigmented skin from the same patients and from control subjects (Claudy & Rouchouse, 1984; Hatchcome et al., 1987; Riley, 1967; Searle et al., 1991). The differences in the documented Langerhans cells densities may be due to the type of vitiligo, the sampling techniques used or the site of skin biopsies. An increase in the number of Langerhans cells could contribute to the immunological processes that damage melanocytes. However, although degenerative changes in Langerhans cells have been observed in vitiligo skin lesions, their role in vitiligo still remains unclear. More recently, dendritic cell-mediated destruction of melanocytes has been demonstrated *in vivo* and *in vitro* (Kroll et al., 2005). This process is related to the release of heat-shock protein 70 by stressed melanocytes, which induces an immune response against the cells from which it is produced, and to the increased expression of tumour-necrosis factor-related apoptosis inducing ligand receptors on stressed melanocytes making them more prone to killing by dendritic cells (Denman et al., 2008; Kroll et al., 2005).

2.7.4 T cells

Autoimmune disorders are often associated with an expansion of peripheral helper T cells. However, with respect to vitiligo, inconsistent data regarding abnormalities in circulating helper T cells have been reported. An increase in the number of activated helper T cells was detected in patients with stable vitiligo as well as in their first-degree relatives when compared with healthy individuals (Abdel-Naser et al., 1992; D'Amelio et al., 1990; Soubiran et al., 1985). In contrast, a decrease in the helper T cell population has also been observed in individuals with vitiligo (Grimes et al., 1986; Halder et al., 1986). No simple explanation exists for these differences but they could be attributable to the factors such as the population of patients under study, disease characteristics and received treatments.

Circulating melanocyte-specific cytotoxic T lymphocytes that target melanocyte-specific antigens, including Melan-A (MART-1), gp100 (Pmel17) and tyrosinase, have been detected in vitiligo patients (Lang et al., 2001; Ogg et al., 1998; Palermo et al., 2001). They express high levels of the skin-homing receptor cutaneous lymphocyte-associated antigen and their frequency correlates with both the extent and activity of the disease (Lang et al., 2001). In addition, melanocyte-specific T cells have cytotoxic reactivity towards melanocytes (Ogg et al., 1998). Such findings are consistent with a role for skin-homing, autoreactive, melanocyte-specific T cells in causing the destruction of melanocytes in vitiligo.

Histological studies of skin biopsies from vitiligo patients have demonstrated that infiltrating cytotoxic and helper T cells are most prominent at the periphery of vitiligo lesions (Al Badri et al., 1993b; Van den Wijngaard et al., 2000). Many of the inflammatory cells are activated, as indicated by the expression of the MHC class II antigen HLA-DR, and a significant number also exhibit high levels of the receptor cutaneous lymphocyte-associated antigen, typical of skin-homing T cells (Al Badri et al., 1993b; Van den Wijngaard et al., 2000). Local activation of cytotoxic T cells at the perilesional epidermal/dermal junction of vitiliginous skin is also suggested by the presence of granzyme B+ and perforin+ cells (Van den Wijngaard, et al., 2000). There is evidence for interleukin-2 receptor and interferon-gamma receptor expression by the lymphocytic infiltrate (Abdel-Naser et al., 1994), and also for down-regulation of the helper T cell 2-dependent CDw60 molecule in the vitiliginous epidermis suggesting that infiltrating T cells may exhibit a helper T cell 1-type cytokine production pattern which is consistent with cell-mediated organ-specific autoimmunity (Le Poole et al., 2003). In addition, perilesional T cell clones exhibit a predominant type-1-like cytokine secretion profile (Wankowicz-Kalinska et al., 2003). More recently it has been demonstrated that T lymphocytes obtained from perilesional skin biopsies are enriched for cytotoxic T cells that recognise melanocyte antigens tyrosinase, gp100 and MelanA (Van den Boorn et al., 2009). Moreover, upon infiltration of autologous pigmented skin, isolated perilesional T lymphocytes efficiently kill melanocytes, providing direct evidence that cytotoxic T cells can cause the depigmentation seen in vitiligo (Van den Boorn et al., 2009). Additional to this, are findings that regulatory T cells occur at a reduced level in the skin of vitiligo patients (Klarquist et al., 2010). This may allow the unchecked destruction of melanocytes by cytotoxic T cells in vitiligo lesions (Klarquist et al., 2010).

3. Conclusion

Autoimmunity is one hypothesis forwarded to explain the development of vitiligo due to the evidence presented in this review. However, it is most likely that interacting mechanisms, of which immune responses are a part, are responsible for the clinical manifestations of the disease (Le Poole et al., 1993a). In addition, although the evidence for the role of immune-related genes in the aetiology of vitiligo is clear, the limited concordance in identical twins (Alkhateeb et al., 2003) indicates that other factors, probably environmental, are also involved in its development, making the disease   complex, polygenic, and multi-factorial. Notably, *in vitro* studies have provided a link and a temporal sequence connecting cellular oxidative stress (Dell'Anna & Picardo, 2006; Schallreuter et al., 1991; Schallreuter et al., 2001; Schallreuter et al., 2005) and the immune response in vitiligo: stressed melanocytes were found to mediate dendritic cell-activation with the consequent dendritic cell effector functions playing a role in the destruction of melanocytes (Kroll et al., 2005). This work suggests that intrinsic damage to melanocytes could be the initiating event in vitiligo development followed by a secondary immune response by cytotoxic T cells which exacerbates the destruction of melanocytes and progresses the disease (Hariharan et al., 2010; Le Poole & Luiten, 2008; Van den Boorn et al., 2011). Indeed, 50% of vitiligo patients experience a Koebner phenomenon, whereby depigmented lesions develop at a site previously exposed to a physical stress (Le Poole & Luiten, 2008).

As indicated, it is most likely that immune responses in vitiligo are of a secondary nature following melanocyte damage. Indeed, several vitiligo-associated autoantigens such as tyrosinase and gp100 are located intracellularly, and it has been suggested that either the formation of neo-antigens due to haptenation, the exposure of cryptic epitopes or the modification of proteins during apoptosis could account for immune responses to these molecules (Namazi, 2007; Westerhof & d'Ischia, 2007). Following processing by mature Langerhans cells, antigenic peptides could be presented to T cells which have escaped clonal deletion or to naïve T lymphocytes which have not been tolerised against cryptic epitopes (Namazi, 2007; Westerhof & d'Ischia, 2007). Antibodies could then be produced following the stimulation of B lymphocytes by activated helper T cells (Namazi, 2007), and activated cytotoxic T cells could directly attack melanocytes expressing antigenic peptides on their surface in the context MHC class I molecules (Hedley et al., 1998; Le Poole et al., 1993b). In the case of immune reactivities against common cellular antigens, the selective destruction of melanocytes in vitiligo might occur because they are intrinsically more sensitive to immune-mediated injury than other skin cells (Norris et al., 1988b).

4. References

Abdel-Naser, M.B., Ludwig, W.D., Gollnick, H. & Orfanos, C.E. (1992). Non-segmental vitiligo: decrease of the CD45R+ T cell subset and evidence for T cell activation. *Int J Dermatol*, Vol.31, pp. 321-326

Abdel-Naser, M.B., Kruger-Krasagakes, S., Krasagakis, K., Gollnick, H., Abdel-Fattah, A. & Orfanos, C.E. (1994). Further evidence for involvement of both cell mediated and humoral immunity in generalized vitiligo. *Pigment Cell Res*, Vol.7, pp. 1-8

Abu Tahir, M., Pramod, K., Ansari, S.H. & Ali, J. (2010). Current remedies for vitiligo. *Autoimmun Rev*, Vol.9, pp. 516-520

Ahmed, I., Nasreen, S. & Bhatti, R. (2007). Alopecia areata in children. *J Coll Physicians Surg Pak*, Vol.17, pp. 587-590

Ahonen, P., Myallarniemi, S., Sipila, I. & Perheentupa, J. (1990). Clinical variation of autoimmune endocrinopathy-candidiasis-ectodermal dystrophy (APECED) in a series of 68 patients. *N Eng J Med*, Vol.322, pp. 1829-1836

Al'Abadie, M.S., Kent, G.G. & Gawkrodger, D.J. (1994a). The relationship between stress and the onset and exacerbation of psoriasis and other skin conditions. *Br J Dermatol*, Vol.130, pp. 199-203

Al'Abadie, M.S., Senior, H.J., Bleehen, S.S. & Gawkrodger, D.J. (1994b). Neuropeptide and neuronal marker studies in vitiligo. *Br J Dermatol*, Vol.131, pp. 160-165

Al Badri, A.M., Fouli, A.K., Todd, P.M., Gariouch, J.J., Gudgeon, J.E., Stewart, D.G., Gracie, J.A. & Goudie, R.B. (1993a). Abnormal expression of MHC class II and ICAM-1 by melanocytes in vitiligo. *J Pathol*, Vol.169, pp. 203-206

Al Badri, A.M.T., Todd, P.M., Garioch, J.J., Gudgeon, J.E., Stewart, D.G. & Goudie, R.B. (1993b). An immunohistological study of cutaneous lymphocytes in vitiligo. *J Pathol*, Vol.170, pp. 149-155

Al-Fouzan, A., Al-Arbash, M., Fouad, F., Kaaba, S.A., Mousa, M.A. & Al-Harbi, S.A. (1995). Study of HLA class I/IL and T lymphocyte subsets in Kuwaiti vitiligo patients. *Eur J Immunogenet*, Vol.22, pp. 209-213

Alomar, A. (2010). PUVA and related treatment. In: *Vitiligo*, M. Picardo & A. Taïeb (Eds.), pp. 345-350, Springer–Verlag, Berlin, Germany

Alkhateeb, A., Fain, P.R., Thody, A., Bennett, D.C. & Spritz, R.A. (2003). Epidemiology of vitiligo and associated autoimmune diseases in Caucasian probands and their relatives. *Pigment Cell Res*, Vol.16, pp. 208-214

Alkhateeb, A., Fain, P.R. & Spritz, R.A. (2005). Candidate functional promoter variant in the FOXD3 melanoblast developmental regulator gene in autosomal dominant vitiligo. *J Invest Dermatol*, Vol.125, pp. 388-391

Ando, I., Chi, H.I., Nakagawa, H. & Otsuka, F. (1993). Difference in clinical features and HLA antigens between familial and non-familial vitiligo of non-segmental type. *Br J Dermatol*, Vol.129, pp. 408-410

Aronson, P.J. & Hashimoto, K. (1987). Association of IgA anti-melanoma antibodies in the sera of vitiligo patients with active disease. *J Invest Dermatol*, Vol.88, 475

Austin, L.M., Boissy, R.E., Jacobsen, B.S. & Smyth, J.R. (1992). The detection of melanocyte autoantibodies in the Smyth chicken model for vitiligo. *Clin Immunol Immunopathol*, Vol.64, pp. 112-120

Austin, L.M. & Boissy, R.E. (1995). Mammalian tyrosinase-related protein-1 is recognised by autoantibodies from vitiliginous Smyth chickens. *Am J Pathol*, Vol.146, 1529-1541

Baharav, E., Merimski, O., Shoenfeld, Y., Zigelman, R., Gilbrud, B., Yecheskel, G., Youinou, P. & Fishman, P. (1996). Tyrosinase as an autoantigen in patients with vitiligo. *Clin Exp Immunol*, Vol.105, pp. 84–88

Behl, P.N., Aggarwal, A. & Srivastava, G, (2003). Vitiligo, In: *Practice of Dermatology*, P.N. Behl & G. Srivastava (Eds.), pp. 238-241, CBS Publishers, New Delhi, India

Betterle, C., Del Prete, G.F., Peserico, A., Bersani, G., Caracciolo, F., Trisotto, A. & Poggi, F. (1976). Autoantibodies in vitiligo. *Arch Dermatol*, Vol.112, pp. 1328

Bhatia, P.S., Mohan, L., Pandey, O.N., Singh, K.K., Arora, S. K. & Mukhija, R.D. (1992). Genetic nature of vitiligo. *J Dermatol Sci*, Vol.4, pp. 180-184

Birlea, S.A., Fain, P.R. & Spritz, R.A. (2008). A Romanian population isolate with high frequency of vitiligo and associated autoimmune diseases. *Arch Dermatol*, Vol.144, pp. 310-316

Birlea, S.A., Labergem G.S., Procopciucm, L.M., Fain, P.R. & Spritz, R.A. (2009). CTLA4 and generalized vitiligo: two genetic association studies and a meta-analysis of published data. *Pigment Cell Melanoma Res*, Vol.22, pp. 230-234

Birlea, S.A., Gowan K., Fain, P.R. & Spritz, R.A. (2010). Genome-wide association study of generalized vitiligo in an isolated European founder population identifies SMOC2, in close proximity to IDDM8. *J Invest Dermatol*, Vol.130, pp. 798-803

Birlea, S.A., Jin, Y., Bennett, D.C., Herbstman, D.M., Wallace, M.R., McCormack, W.T., Kemp, E.H., Gawkrodger, D.J., Weetman, A.P., Picardo, M., Leone, G., Taïeb, A., Jouary, T., Ezzedine, K., Van Geel, N., Lambert, J., Overbeck, A., Fain, P.R. & Spritz, R.A. (2011). Comprehensive association analysis of candidate genes for generalized vitiligo supports XBP1, FOXP1, and TSLP. *J Invest Dermatol*, Vol.131, pp. 371-381

Blomhoff, A., Kemp, E.H., Gawkrodger, D.J., Weetman, A.P, Husebye, E.S., Akselsen, H.E., Lie, B.A. & Undlien, D.E. (2005). CTLA4 polymorphisms are associated with vitiligo, in patients with concomitant autoimmune diseases. *Pigment Cell Res*, Vol.18, pp. 55-58

Boelaert, K., Newby, P.R., Simmonds, M.J., Holder, R.L., Carr-Smith, J.D., Heward, J.M., Manji, N., Allahabadia, A., Armitage, M., Chatterjee, K.V., Lazarus, J.H., Pearce, S.H., Vaidya, B., Gough, S.C. & Franklyn, J.A. (2010). Prevalence and relative risk of other autoimmune diseases in subjects with autoimmune thyroid disease. *Am J Med*, Vol.123, pp. 183.e1-183.e9

Boisseau-Garsaud, A.M., Garsaud, P., Cales-Quist, D., Helenon, R., Queneherve, C. & Claire, R.C. (2000). Epidemiology of vitiligo in the French West Indies (Isle of Martinique). *Int J Dermatol*, Vol.39, pp. 18-20

Boissy, R.E., Lamont, S.J. & Smyth, J.R. (1984). Persistence of abnormal melanocytes in immunosuppressed chickens of the autoimmune "DAM" line. *Cell Tissue Res*, Vol.235, pp. 663-668

Boissy, R.E. & Lamoreux, M.L. (1988). Animal models of an acquired pigmentary disorder: vitiligo. In: *Advances in Pigment Cell Research,* J. Bagnara J, (Ed.), pp. 207-218, Alan R. Liss Inc., New York, USA

Boone, B., Ongenae, K., Van Geel, N., Vernijns, S., De Keyser, S. & Naeyaert, J.M. (2007). Topical pimecrolimus in the treatment of vitiligo. *Eur J Dermatol,* Vol.17, pp. 55-61

Boyle, M.L., Pardue, S.L., Smyth, J.R. Effect of corticosterone on the incidence of amelanosis in Smyth delayed amelanotic line chickens. (1987). *Poultry Sci,* Vol.66, pp. 363-367

Brostoff, J. (1969). Autoantibodies in patients with vitiligo. *Lancet,* Vol.2 pp. 177-178

Buc, M., Busová, B., Hegyi, E. and Kolibásová, K. (1996). Vitiligo is associated with HLA-A2 and HLA-Dw7 in the Slovak populations. *Folia Biol (Praha),* Vol.42, pp. 23-25

Cario-Andre, M., Pain, C., Gauthier, Y. & Taieb A. (2007). The melanocytorrhagic hypothesis of vitiligo tested on pigmented, stressed, reconstructed epidermis. *Pigment Cell Res,* Vol.20, pp. 385-393

Cantón, I., Akhtar. S., Gavalas, N.G., Gawkrodger, D.J., Blomhoff, A., Watson, P.F., Weetman, A.P. & Kemp, E.H. (2005). A single nucleotide polymorphism in the gene encoding lymphoid protein tyrosine phosphatase (PTPN22) confers susceptibility to generalised vitiligo. *Genes Immunol,* Vol.6, pp. 584-587

Chen, J.J., Huang, W., Gui, J.P., Yang, S., Zhou, F.S., Xiong, Q.G., Wu, H.B., Cui,Y., Gao, M., Li, W., Li, J. X., Yan, K.L., Yuan, W.T., Xu, S.J., Liu, J.J. & Zhang, X.J. (2005). A novel linkage to generalized vitiligo on 4q13-q21 identified in a genomewide linkage analysis of Chinese families. *Am J Hum Genet,* Vol.76, pp. 1057-1065

Cheong, K.A., Chae, S.C., Kim, Y.S., Kwon, H.B., Chung, H.T. & Lee, A.Y. (2009). Association of thymic stromal lymphopoietin gene -847C>T polymorphism in generalized vitiligo. *Exp Dermatol,* Vol.18, pp. 1073-1075

Cho, S., Kang, H.C. & Hahm, J.H. (2000). Characteristics of vitiligo in Korean children. *Pediatr Dermatol,* Vol.17, pp. 189-193

Claudy, A. & Rouchouse, B. (1984). Langerhans cells and vitiligo: quantitative study of T6 and HLA-DR-antigen expressing cells. *Acta Dermatol Venereol,* Vol.64, pp. 334-336

Cui, J., Harning, R., Henn, M. & Bystryn, J.-C. (1992). Identification of pigment cell antigens defined by vitiligo antibodies. *J Invest Dermatol,* Vol.98, pp. 162-165

Cui, J., Arita, Y. & Bystryn, J.-C. (1993). Cytolytic antibodies to melanocytes in vitiligo. *J Invest Dermatol,* Vol.100, pp. 812-815

Cui, J., Arita, Y. & Bystryn, J.-C. (1995). Characterisation of vitiligo antigens. *Pigment Cell Res,* Vol.8, pp.53-59

Cunliffe, W.J., Hall, R., Newell, D.J. & Stevenson, C.J. (1968). Vitiligo, thyroid disease and autoimmunity. *Br J Dermatol,* Vol.80, pp. 135-139

D'Amelio, R., Frati, C., Fattorossi, A. & Aiuti, F. (1990). Peripheral T cell subset imbalance in patients with vitiligo and their apparently healthy first-degree relatives. *Ann Allergy,* Vol.65, pp. 143-145

Das, S.K., Majumder, P.P., Majumdar, T.K. & Haldar, B. (1985). Studies on vitiligo. II. Familial aggregation and genetics. *Genet Epidemiol,* Vol.2, pp. 255-262

Dawber, R.P. (1970). Integumentary association of pernicious anaemia. *Br J Dermatol,* Vol.82, pp. 221-222

Deeba, F., Syed, R., Quareen, J., Waheed, M.A., Jamil, K. & Rao, H. (2010). CTLA-4 A49G gene polymorphism is not associated with vitiligo in South Indian population. *Indian J Dermatol,* Vol.55, 29-32

Dell'Anna, M.L. & Picardo, M. (2006). A review and a new hypothesis for non-immunological pathogenetic mechanisms in vitiligo. *Pigment Cell Res*, Vol.19, pp. 406-411

Denman, C.J., McCracken, J., Hariharan, V., Klarquist, J., Oyarbide-Valencia, K., Guevara-Patiño, J.A. & Le Poole, I.C. (2008). HSP70i accelerates depigmentation in a mouse model of autoimmune vitiligo. *J Invest Dermatol*, Vol.128, pp. 2041-2048

Dunston, G.M & Halder, R.M. (1990). Vitiligo is associated with HLA-DR4 in black patients. A preliminary report. *Arch Dermatol*, Vol.126, pp. 56-60

Duthie, M.S., Kimber, I., Norval, M. (1999). The effects of ultraviolet radiation on the immune system. *Br J Dermatol*, Vol.140, pp. 995-1009

Erf, G.F., Trejo-Skalli, A.V. & Smyth, J.R. (1995). T cells in regenerating feathers of Smyth line chickens in vitiligo. *Clin Immunol Immunopathol*, Vol.76, pp. 120-126

Erf, G.F. & Smyth, J.R. (1996). Alterations in blood leukocyte populations in Smyth line chickens with autoimmune vitiligo. *Poultry Sci*, Vol.75, pp. 351-356

Fain, P.R., Gowan, K., LaBerge, G.S., Alkhateeb, A., Stetler, G.L., Talbert, J., Bennett, D.C. & Spritz, R.A. (2003). A genome-wide screen for generalized vitiligo: confirmation of AIS1 on chromosome 1p31 and evidence for additional susceptibility loci. *Am J Hum Genet*, Vol.72, pp. 1560–1564

Fain, P.R., Babu, S.R., Bennett, D.C. & Spritz, R.A. (2006). HLA class II Haplotype DRB1*04-DQB1*0301 contributes to risk of familial generalized vitiligo and early disease onset. *Pigment Cell Res*, Vol.19, pp. 51-57

Farrokhi, S., Farsangi-Hojjat, M., Noohpisheh. M.K., Tahmasbi, R. & Rezaei, N. (2005). Assessment of the immune system in 55 Iranian patients with vitiligo. *J Eur Acad Dermatol Venereol*, Vol.19, pp. 706-711

Finco, O., Cuccia, M., Martinetti, M., Ruberto, G., Orecchia, G. & Rabbiosi, G. (1991). Age of onset in vitiligo: relationship with HLA supratypes. *Clin Genet*, Vol.39, pp. 448-454

Fishman, P., Azizi, E., Shoenfeld, Y., Sredni, B., Yecheskel, G., Ferrone, S., Zigelman, R., Chaitchik, S., Floro, S. & Djaldetti, M. (1993). Vitiligo autoantibodies are effective against melanoma. *Cancer*, Vol.72, pp. 2365-2369

Foley, L.M, Lowe, N.J., Misheloff, E. & Tiwari, J.L. (1983). Association of HLA-DR4 with vitiligo. *J Am Acad Dermatol*, Vol.8, pp. 39-40

Gauthier, Y., Cario-Andre, M. & Taieb, A. (2003). A critical appraisal of vitiligo etiologic theories. Is melanocyte loss a melanocytorrhagy? *Pigment Cell Res*, Vol.16, pp. 322-332

Gawkrodger, D. J., Ormerod, A. D., Shaw, L., Mauri-Sole, I., Whitton, M. E., Watts, M. J., Anstey, A. V., Ingham, J. & Young, K. (2010). Vitiligo: concise evidence based guidelines on diagnosis and management. *Postgrad Med J*, Vol.86, pp. 466-471

Gilhar, A., Zelickson, B., Ulman, Y. & Etzioni, A. (1995). In vivo destruction of melanocytes by the IgG fraction of serum from patients with vitiligo. *J Invest Dermatol*, Vol.105, pp. 683-686

Gottumukkala, R.V.S.R.K., Gavalas, N.G., Akhtar, S., Metcalfe, R.A., Gawkrodger, D. J., Haycock, J.W., Waston, P.F., Weetman, A.P. & Kemp, E. H. (2006). Function blocking autoantibodies to the melanin-concentrating hormone receptor in vitiligo patients. *Lab Invest*, Vol.86, pp. 781-789

Grimes, P.E., Ghoneum, M., Stockton, T., Payne, C., Kelly, A.P. & Alfred, L. (1986). T cell profiles in vitiligo. *J Am Acad Dermatol*, Vol.14, pp. 196-201

Grimes, P.E., Sevall, J.S. & Vojdani, A. (1996). Cytomegalovirus DNA identified in skin biopsy specimens of patients with vitiligo. *J Am Acad Dermatol*, Vol.35, pp. 21-26

Halder, R.M., Walters, C.S., Johnson, B.A., Chakarabarti, S.G. & Kenney, J.A. (1986). Aberrations in T lymphocytes and natural killer cells in vitiligo: a flow cytometric study. *J Am Acad Dermatol*, Vol.14, pp. 733-737

Handa, S. & Dogra, S. (2003). Epidemiology of childhood vitiligo: a study of 625 patients from north India. *Pediatr Dermatol*, Vol.20, pp. 207-210

Hann, S.K., Kim, H.I., Im, S., Park, Y.K., Cui, J. & Bystryn, J.-C. (1993). The change of melanocyte cytotoxicity after systemic steroid treatment in vitiligo patients. *J Dermatol Sci*, Vol.6, pp. 201-205

Hann, S.K. & Lee, H.J. (1996). Segmental vitiligo: clinical findings in 208 patients. *J Am Acad Dermatol*, Vol.35, pp. 671-674

Hann, S.K., Koo, S.W., Kim, J.B. & Park, Y.K. (1996a). Detection of antibodies to human melanoma cells in vitiligo and alopecia areata by Western blot analysis. *J Dermatol*, Vol.23, pp. 100-103

Hann, S.K., Shin, H.K., Park, S.H., Reynolds, S.R. & Bystryn, J.-C. (1996b). Detection of antibodies to melanocytes in vitiligo by western blotting. *Yonsei Med J*, Vol.37, pp. 365-370

Hariharan, V., Klarquist, J., Reust, M.J., Koshoffer, A., McKee, M.D., Boissy, R.E. & Le Poole, I.C. (2010). Monobenzyl ether of hydroquinone and 4-tertiary butyl phenol activate markedly different physiological responses in melanocytes: relevance to skin depigmentation. *J Invest Dermatol*, Vol.130, pp. 211-220

Harning, R., Cui, J. & Bystryn, J.-C. (1991). Relation between the incidence and level of pigment cell antibodies and disease activity in vitiligo. *J Invest Dermatol*, Vol.97, 1078-1080

Hartmann, A., Brocker, E.B. & Hamm, H. (2008). Occlusive treatment enhances efficacy of tacrolimus 0.1% ointment in adult patients with vitiligo: results of a placebo-controlled 12-month prospective study. *Acta Derm Venereol*, Vol.88, pp. 474-479

Hatchome, N., Aiba, S., Kato, T., Torinuki, W. & Tagami, H. (1987). Possible functional impairment of Langerhans' cells in vitiliginous skin. Reduced ability to elicit dinitrochlorobenzene contact sensitivity reaction and decreased stimulatory effect in the allogeneic mixed skin cell lymphocyte culture reaction. *Arch Dermatol*, Vol.123, pp. 51-54

Hedley, S.J., Metcalfe, R., Gawkrodger, D.J., Weetman A.P. & MacNeil, S. (1998). Vitiligo melanocytes in long-term culture show normal constitutive and cytokine-induced expression of intercellular adhesion molecule-1 and major histocompatibility complex class I and class II molecules. *Br J Dermatol*, Vol.139, pp. 965-973

Hedstrand, H., Ekwall, O., Olsson, M.J., Landgren, E., Kemp, E.H., Weetman, A.P., Perheentupa, J., Husebye, E., Gustafsson, J., Betterle, C., Kämpe, O. & Rorsman, F. (2001). The transcription factors SOX9 and SOX10 are vitiligo autoantigens in autoimmune polyendocrine syndrome type I. *J Biol Chem*, Vol.276, pp. 35390-35395

Herane, M.I. (2003). Vitiligo and leukoderma in children. *Clin Dermatol*, Vol.21, pp. 283-295

Homey, B., Assmann, T., Vohr, H.W., Ulrich, P., Lauerma, A.I., Ruzicka, T., Lehmann, P. & Schuppe, H.C. (1998). Topical FK506 suppresses cytokine and costimulatory molecule expression in epidermal and local draining lymph node cells during primary skin immune responses. *J Immunol*, Vol.160, pp. 5331-5340

Hoogduijn, M.J., Ancans, J., Suzuki, I., Estdale, S. & Thody, A.J. (2002). Melanin-concentrating hormone and its receptor are expressed and functional in human skin. *Biochem Biophys Res Commun*, Vol.296, pp. 698-701

Howitz, J., Brodthagen, H., Schwartz, M. & Tomsen, K. (1977). Prevalence of vitiligo: Epidemiological survey on the Isle of Bornholm, Denmark. *Arch Dermatol*, Vol.113, pp. 47-52

Imokawa, G., Yada, Y., Kimura, M. & Morisaki, N. (1996). Granulocyte/macrophage colony-stimulating factor is an intrinsic keratinocyte-derived growth factor for human melanocytes in UVA-induced melanosis. *Biochem J*, Vol.313, pp. 625-631

Itirli, G., Pehlivan, M., Alper, S., Yuksel, S.E., Onay, H., Ozkinay, F. & Pehlivan, S. (2005). Exon-3 polymorphism of CTLA-4 gene in Turkish patients with vitiligo. *J Dermatol Sci*, Vol.38, pp. 225-227

Jin, Y., Birlea, S.A., Fain, P.R. & Spritz, R.A. (2007a). Genetic variations in NALP1 are associated with generalized vitiligo in a Romanian population. *J Invest Dermatol*, Vol.127, pp. 2558-2562

Jin, Y., Mailloux, C.M., Gowan, K., Riccardi, S.L., LaBerge, G., Bennett, D.C., Fain, P.R. & Spritz, R.A. (2007b). NALP1 in vitiligo-associated multiple autoimmune disease. *N Engl J Med*, Vol.356, pp. 1216-1225

Jin, Y., Birlea, S.A., Fain, P.R., Gowan, K., Riccardi, S.L., Holland, P.J., Mailloux C.M., Sufit, A.J., Hutton, S.M., Amadi-Myers, A., Bennett, D.C., Wallace, M.R., McCormack, W.T., Kemp, E.H., Gawkrodger, D.J., Weetman, A.P., Picardo, M., Leone, G., Taieb, A., Jouary, T., Ezzedine, K., van Geel, N., Lambert, J., Overbeck, A. & Spritz, R.A. (2010a). Variant of TYR and autoimmunity susceptibility loci in generalized vitiligo. *N Engl J Med*, Vol.362, pp. 1686-1697

Jin, Y., Birlea, S.A., Fain, P.R., Mailloux, C.M., Riccardi, S.L., Gowan, K., Holland, P.J., Bennett, D.C., Wallace, M.R., McCormack, W.T., Kemp, E.H., Gawkrodger, D.J., Weetman, A.P., Picardo, M., Leone, G., Taieb, A., Jouary, T., Ezzedine, K., van Geel, N., Lambert, J., Overbeck, A. & Spritz, R.A. (2010b). Common variants in FOXP1 are associated with generalized vitiligo. *Nat Genet*, Vol.42, pp. 576-578

Kao, C.H. & Yu, H.S. (1992). Comparison of the effect of 8-Methoxypsoralen (8-MOP) plus UVA (PUVA) on human melanocytes in vitiligo vulgaris and *in vitro*. *J Invest Dermatol*, Vol.98, pp. 734-740

Kemp, E.H., Gawkrodger, D.J., MacNeil, S., Watson, P.F. & Weetman, A.P. (1997a). Detection of tyrosinase autoantibodies in patients with vitiligo using ^{35}S-labeled recombinant human tyrosinase in a radioimmunoassay. *J Invest Dermatol*, Vol.109, pp. 69-73.

Kemp, E.H., Gawkrodger, D.J., Watson, P.F. & Weetman, A.P. (1997b). Immunoprecipitation of melanogenic enzyme autoantigens with vitiligo sera: evidence for cross-reactive autoantibodies to tyrosinase and tyrosinase-related protein-2 (TRP-2). *Clin Exp Immunol*, Vol.109, pp. 495–500

Kemp, E.H., Gawkrodger, D.J., Watson, P.F. & Weeman, A.P. (1998a). Autoantibodies to human melanocyte-specific protein Pmel17 in the sera of vitiligo patients: a sensitive and quantitative radioimmunoassay (RIA). *Clin Exp Immunol*, Vol.114, pp. 333-338

Kemp, E.H., Waterman, E.A., Gawkrodger, D.J., Watson, P.F. & Weetman, A.P. (1998b). Autoantibodies to tyrosinase-related protein-1 detected in the sera of vitiligo patients using a quantitative radiobinding assay. *Br J Dermatol*, Vol.139, pp. 798-805

Kemp, E.H., Ajjan, R.A., Waterman, E.A., Gawkrodger, D.J., Cork, M.J., Watson, P.F. & Weetman, A.P. (1999). Analysis of a microsatellite polymorphism of the cytotoxic T-lymphocyte antigen-4 gene in patients with vitiligo. *Br J Dermatol*, Vol.140, pp. 73-78

Kemp, E.H., Waterman, E.A., Hawes, B.E., O'Neill, K., Gottumukkala, R.V., Gawkrodger, D.J., Weetman, A.P. & Watson, P.F. (2002). The melanin-concentrating hormone receptor 1, a novel target of autoantibody responses in vitiligo. *J Clin Invest*, Vol.109, pp. 923-930

Kemp, E.H., Emhemad, S., Akhtar, S., Watson, P.F., Gawkrodger, D.J. & Weetman, A.P. (2011). Autoantibodies against tyrosine hydroxylase in patients with non-segmental (generalised) vitiligo. *Exp Dermatol*, Vol.20, pp. 35-40

Kent, G. & Al' Abadie, M.S.K. (1996). Psychologic effects of vitiligo: a critical incident analysis. *J Am Acad Dermatol*, Vol.35, pp. 895-898

Kirnbauer, R., Charvat, B., Schauer, E., Kock, A., Urbanshi, A., Forster, E., Neuner, P., Assmann, I., Luger, T.A. & Schwarz, T. (1992). Modulation of intercellular adhesion molecule-1 expression on human melanocytes and melanoma cells: evidence for a regulatory role of IL-6, IL-7, TNF beta, and UVB light. *J Invest Dermatol*, Vol.98, pp. 320-326

Klarquist, J., Denman, C.J., Hernandez, C., Wainwright, D.A., Strickland, F.M., Overbeck, A. Mehrotra, S., Nishimura, M.I. & Le Poole, I.C. (2010). Reduced skin homing by functional Treg in vitiligo. *Pigment Cell Melanoma Res*, Vol.23, pp. 276-286

Kroll, T.M., Bommiasamy, H., Boissy, R.E., Hernandez, C., Nickoloff, B.J., Mestril, R. & Le Poole, I.C. (2005). 4-tertiary butyl phenol exposure sensitizes human melanocytes to dendritic cell-mediated killing: relevance to vitiligo. *J Invest Dermatol*, Vol.124, pp. 798-806

Krutmann, J. & Morita, A. (1999). Mechanisms of ultraviolet (UV) B and phototherapy. *J Invest Dermatol Symp Proc*, Vol.4, pp. 70-72

Laberge, G., Mailloux, C.M., Gowan, K., Holland, P., Bennett, D.C., Fain, P.R. & Spritz, R.A. (2005). Early onset and increased risk of other autoimmune diseases in familial generalized vitiligo. *Pigment Cell Res*, Vol.18, pp. 300-305

Laberge, G.S., Bennett, D.C., Fain, P.R. & Spritz, R.A. (2008a). PTPN22 is genetically associated with risk of generalized vitiligo, but CTLA4 is not. *J Invest Dermatol*, Vol.128, pp. 1757-1762

Laberge, G. S., Birlea, S.A., Fain, P.R. & Spritz, R.A. (2008b). The PTPN22-1858C>T (R620W) functional polymorphism is associated with generalized vitiligo in the Romanian population. *Pigment Cell Melanoma Res*, Vol.21, pp. 206-208

Lamont, S.J. & Smyth, J.R. (1981). Effect of bursectomy on development of a spontaneous postnatal amelanosis. *Clin Immunol Immunopathol*, Vol.21, pp. 407-411

Lang, K.S., Caroli, C.C., Muhm, D., Wernet, D., Moris, A., Schittek, B., Knauss-Scherwitz, E., Stevanovic, S., Rammensee, H.-G. & Garbe, C. (2001). HLA-A2 restricted, melanocyte-specific CD8+ T lymphocytes detected in vitiligo patients are related to disease activity and are predominantly directed against MelanA/MART1. *J Invest Dermatol*, Vol.116, pp.891-897

Le Poole, I.C. & Boissy, R.E. (1997). Vitiligo. *Semin Cutan Med Surg*, Vol.16, pp. 3-14

Le Poole, I.C. & Luiten, R.M. (2008). Autoimmune etiology of generalized vitiligo. *Curr Dir Autoimmun*, Vol.10, pp. 227-243

Le Poole, I.C., Das, P.K., van den Wijngaard, R.M., Bos, J.D. & Westerhof, W. (1993a). Review of the etiopathomechanism of vitiligo: a convergence theory. *Exp Dermatol*, Vol.2, pp. 145-153

Le Poole, I.C., Mutis, T., van den Wijngaard, R.M., Westerhof, W., Ottenhoff, T., de Vries, R.R. & Das, P.K. (1993b). A novel, antigen-presenting function of melanocytes and its possible relationship to hypopigmentary disorders. *J Immunol*, Vol.151, pp. 7284-7292

Le Poole, I.C., van den Wijngaard, R.M.J.G.J., Westerhof, W. & Das, P.K. (1996). Presence of T cells and macrophages in inflammatory vitiligo skin parallels melanocyte disappearance. *Am J Pathol*, Vol.148, 1219-1228

Le Poole, I.C., Stennett. L.S., Bonish, B.K., Dee L., Robinson, J.K., Hernandez, C., Hann, S.K., & Nickoloff, B.J. (2003). Expansion of vitiligo lesions is associated with reduced epidermal CDw60 expression and increased expression of HLA-DR in perilesional skin. *Br J Dermatol*, Vol.149, pp. 739-748

Li, Q., Lv, Y., Li, C., Yi, X., Long, H.A., Qiao, H., Lu, T., Luan, Q., Li, K., Wang, X., Wang, G. & Gao, T. (2010). Vitiligo autoantigen VIT75 is identified as lamin A in vitiligo by serological proteome analysis based on mass spectrometry. *J Invest Dermatol*, Vol.131, pp. 727-734

Liang, Y., Yang S., Zhou, Y., Gui, J., Ren, Y., Chen, J., Fan, X., Sun, L., Xiao, F., Gao, M., Du, W., Fang, Q., Xu, S., Huang, W. & Zhang, X. (2007). Evidence for two susceptibility loci on chromosomes 22q12 and 6p21-p22 in Chinese generalized vitiligo families. *J Invest Dermatol*, Vol.127, pp. 2552-2557

Liu, J. B., Li, M., Yang, S., Gui, J. P., Wang, H. Y., Du, W. H., Zhao, X. Y., Ren, Y. Q., Zhu, Y. G. & Zhang, X. J. (2005). Clinical profiles of vitiligo in China: an analysis of 3742 patients. *Clin Exp Dermatol*, Vol.30, pp. 327-331

Liu, J.B., Li, M., Chen, H., Zhong, S. Q., Yang, S., Du, W.D., Hao, J. H., Zhang, T.S., Zhang, X.J. & Zeegers, M.P. (2007). Association of vitiligo with HLA-A2: a meta-analysis. *J Eur Acad Dermatol Venereol*, Vol.21, pp. 205-213

Lorini, R., Orecchia, G., Martinetti, M., Dugoujon, J.M. & Cuccia, M. (1992). Autoimmunity in vitiligo: relationship with HLA, Gm and Km polymorphisms. *Autoimmunity*, Vol.11, 255-260

Majumder, P.P., Das, S.K. & Li, C.C. (1988). A genetical model for vitiligo. *Am J Hum Genet*, Vol.43, pp. 119-125

Majumder, P.P., Nordlund, J.J. & Nath, S.K. (1993). Pattern of familial aggregation of vitiligo. *Arch Dermatol*, Vol.129, pp. 994-998

Mandry, R.C., Ortiz, L.J., Lugo-Somolinos, A. & Sanchez J.L. (1996). Organ-specific autoantibodies in vitiligo patients and their relatives. *Int J Dermatol*, Vol.35 pp. 18-21

Mehta, N.R., Shah, K.C., Theodore, C., Vyas, V.P . & Patel, A.B. (1973). Epidemiological study of vitiligo in Surat area, South Gujarat. *Indian J Med Res*, Vol.61, pp. 145-154

Metzker, A., Zamir, R., Gazit, E., David, M. & Feuerman, E.J. (1980). Vitiligo and the HLA system. *Dermatologica*, Vol.160, pp. 100-105

Moretti, S., Spallanzani, A., Amato, L., Hautmann, G., Gallerani, I., Fabiani, M. & Fabbri, P. (2002). New insights into the pathogenesis of vitiligo: imbalance of epidermal cytokines at sites of lesions. *Pigment Cell Res,* Vol.15, pp. 87-92

Namazi, M.R. (2007). Neurogenic dysregulation, oxidative stress, and melanocytorrhagy in vitiligo: can they be interconnected? *Pigment Cell Res,* Vol.20, pp. 360-363

Nath, S.K., Majumder, P.P. & Nordlund, J.J. (1994). Genetic epidemiology of vitiligo: multilocus recessivity cross-validated. *Am J Hum Genet,* Vol.55 pp. 981-990

Nath, S.K., Kelly, J.A., Namjou, B., Lam, T., Bruner, G.R., Scofield, R.H., Aston, C.E. & Harley, J.B. (2001). Evidence for a susceptibility gene, SLEV1, on chromosome 17p13 in families with vitiligo-related systemic lupus erythematosus. *Am J Hum Genet,* Vol.69, pp. 1401-1406

Naughton, G.K., Eisinger, M. & Bystryn, J.C. (1983a). Detection of antibodies to melanocytes in vitiligo by specific immunoprecipitation. *J Invest Dermatol,* Vol.81, pp. 540-542

Naughton G.K., Eisinger, M. & Bystryn, J.-C. (1983b). Antibodies to normal human melanocytes in vitiligo. *J Exp Med,* Vol.158, pp. 246-251

Naughton, G.K., Mahaffey, M. & Bystryn, J.-C. (1986a). Antibodies to surface antigens of pigmented cells in animals with vitiligo. *Proc Soc Exp Biol Med,* Vol.181, pp. 423-426

Naughton, G.K., Reggiardo, M.D. & Bystryn, J.-C. (1986b). Correlation between vitiligo antibodies and extent of depigmentation in vitiligo. *J Am Acad Dermatol,* Vol.15, pp. 978-981

Neufeld, M., Maclaren, N.K. & Blizard, R.M. (1981). Two types of autoimmune Addison's disease associated with different polyglandular autoimmune (PGA) syndrome. *Medicine,* Vol.60, pp. 355-362

Norris, D.A., Kissinger, R.M., Naughton, G.M. & Bystryn, J.-C. (1988a). Evidence for immunologic mechanisms in human vitiligo: patients' sera induce damage to human melanocytes in vitro by complement-mediated damage and antibody-dependent cellular cytotoxicity. *J Invest Dermatol,* Vol.90, pp.783-789

Norris, D.A., Capin, L., Muglia, J.J., Osborn, R.L., Zerbe, G.O., Bystryn J.-C. & Tonnesen, M.G. (1988b) Enhanced susceptibility of melanocytes to different immunologic effector mechanisms in vitro: potential mechanisms for post-inflammatory hypopigmentation and vitiligo. *Pigment Cell Res,* Vol.1 (Supplement), pp. 113-123

Ochi, Y. & DeGroot, L.J. (1969). Vitiligo in Graves' disease. *Ann Intern Med,* Vol.71, pp. 935-940

Ogg, G.S., Dunbar P.R., Romero P., Chen, J.L. & Cerundolo, V. (1998). High frequency of skin-homing melanocyte-specific cytotoxic T lymphocytes in autoimmune vitiligo. *J Exp Med,* Vol.188, pp. 1203–1208

Okamoto, T., Irie, R.F., Fujii, S., Huang, S., Nizze, A.J., Morton, D.L. & Hoon, D.S. (1998). Anti-tyrosinase-related protein-2 immune response in vitiligo and melanoma patients receiving active-specific immunotherapy. *J Invest Dermatol,* Vol.111, pp. 1034-1039

Olsson, M.J. (2010). Surgical therapies. In: *Vitiligo,* M. Picardo & A. Taïeb (Eds.), pp. 394-406, Springer-Verlag, Berlin, Germany

Ongenae, K., Beelaert, L., van Geel, N. & Naeyaert, J.M. (2006). Psychosocial effects of vitiligo. *J Eur Acad Dermatol Venereol,* Vol.20, pp. 1-8

Orecchia, G., Perfetti, L., Malagoli, P., Borghini, F. & Kipervarg, Y. (1992). Vitiligo is associated with a significant increase in HLA-A30, Cw6 and Dqw3 and a decrease in C4AQ0 in northern Italian patients. *Dermatology*, Vol.185, pp. 123-127

Palermo, B., Campanelli, R., Garbelli, S., Mantovani, S., Lantelme, E., Brazzelli, V., Ardigo, M., Borroni, G., Martinetti, M., Badulli, C., Necker, A. & Giachino, C. (2001). Specific cytotoxic T lymphocyte responses against Melan-A/MART1, tyrosinase and gp100 in vitiligo by the use of major histocompatibility complex/peptide tetramers: the role of cellular immunity in the etiopathogenesis of vitiligo. *J Invest Dermatol*, Vol.117, pp. 326-332

Pardue, S.L., Fite, K.V., Bengston, L., Lamont, S.J., Boyle, M.L. & Smyth J.R. (1988). Enhanced integumental and ocular amelanosis following the termination of cyclosporin administration. *J Invest Dermatol*, Vol.88, pp. 758-761

Park, Y.K., Kim, N.S., Hann, S.K. & Im, S. (1996). Identification of autoantibody to melanocytes and characterisation of vitiligo antigen in vitiligo patients. *J Dermatol Sci*, Vol.11, pp. 111-120

Pehlivan, S., Ozkinay, F., Alper, S., Onay, H., Yuksel, E., Pehlivan, M. & Ozkinay, C. (2009). Association between IL4 (-590), ACE (I)/(D), CCR5 (Delta32), CTLA4 (+49) and IL1-RN (VNTR in intron 2) gene polymorphisms and vitiligo. *Eur J Dermatol*, Vol.19, pp. 126-128

Poloy, A., Tibor, L., Kramer, J., Anh-Tuan, N., Kraszits, E., Medgyessy, I., Füst, G., Stenszky, V. & Farid, N.R. (1991). HLA-DR1 is associated with vitiligo. *Immunol Lett*, Vol.27, pp. 59-62

Porter, J.R., Beuf, A.H., Lerner, A. & Nordlund, J. (1986). Psychosocial effect of vitiligo: a comparison of vitiligo patients with "normal" control subjects, with psoriasis patients, and with patients with other pigmentary disorders. *J Am Acad Dermatol*, Vol.15, pp. 220-224

Quan, C., Ren, Y.Q., Xiang, L.H., Sun, L.D., Xu, A.E., Gao, X.H., Chen, H.D., Pu, X.M., Wu, R.N., Liang, C.Z., Li, J.B., Gao, T.W., Zhang, J.Z., Wang, X.L., Wang, J., Yang, R.Y., Liang, L., Yu, J.B., Zuo, X.B., Zhang, S.Q., Zhang, S.M., Chen, G., Zheng, X.D., Li, P., Zhu, J., Li, Y.W., Wei, X.D., Hong. W.S., Ye, Y., Zhang, Y., Wu, W.S., Cheng, H., Dong, P.L., Hu, D. Y., Li, Y., Li, M., Zhang, X., Tang, H.Y., Tang, X.F., Xu, S.X., He, S. M., Lv, Y. M., Shen, M., Jiang, H.Q., Wang, Y., Li, K., Kang, X.J., Liu, Y. Q., Sun, L., Liu, Z.F., Xie, S.Q., Zhu, C.Y., Xu, Q., Gao, J.P., Hu, W.L., Ni, C., Pan, T.M., Yao, S., He, C.F., Liu, Y.S., Yu, Z.Y., Yin, X.Y., Zhang, F.Y., Yang, S., Zhou, Y. & Zhang, X.J. (2010). Genome-wide association study for vitiligo identifies susceptibility loci at 6q27 and the MHC. *Nat Genet*, Vol.42, pp. 614-618

Ren, Y., Yang, S., Xu, S., Gao, M., Huang, W., Gao, T., Fang, Q., Quan, C., Zhang, C., Sun, L., Liang, Y., Han, J., Wang, Z., Zhang, F., Zhou, Y., Liu, J. & Zhang, X. (2009). Genetic variation of promoter sequence modulates XBP1 expression and genetic risk for vitiligo. *PLoS Genet*, Vol.5, e1000523

Riley, P. (1967). A study of the distribution of epidermal dendritic cells in pigmented and unpigmented skin. *J Invest Dermatol*, Vol.48, pp. 28-38

Rocha, I.M., Oliveira, L.J., De Castro, L.C., ., De Araujo Pereira, L.I., Chaul, A., Guerra, J.G., Silvestre, M.C., Batista, K.M., Pereira, F.A., Gomide, M.A. & Guillo, L.A. (2002). Recognition of melanoma cell antigens with antibodies present from patients with vitiligo. *Int J Dermatol*, Vol.39, pp. 840-843

Schallreuter, K.U., Wood, J.M. & Berger, J. (1991). Low catalase levels in the epidermis of patients with vitiligo. *J Invest Dermatol*, Vol.97, pp. 1081-1085

Schallreuter, K.U, Levenig, C., Kühnl, P., Löliger, C., Hohl-Tehari, M. & Berger, J. (1993). Histocompatibility antigens in vitiligo: Hamburg study on 102 patients from northern Germany. *Dermatology*, Vol.187, pp. 186-192

Schallreuter, K.U., Moore, J., Wood, J.M., Beazley, W.D., Peters, E.M.J., Marles, L.K., Behrens-Williams, S.C., Dummer, R., Blau, N. & Thony, B. (2001). Epidermal H2O2 accumulation alters tetrahydrobiopterin (6BH4) recycling in vitiligo: identification of a general mechanism in regulation of all 6BH4-dependent processes? *J Invest Dermatol*, Vol.116, pp. 167–174

Schallreuter, K.U., Chavan, B., Rokos, H., Hibberts, N., Panske, A. & Wood, J.M. (2005). Decreased phenylalanine uptake and turnover in patients with vitiligo. *Mol Genet Metabol*, Vol.86, pp. S27-S33

Searle, E.A., Boissy, R.E., Austin, L.M. & Nordlund, J.J. (1991). Smyth chicken melanocyte autoantibodies: cross-reactivity, in vivo binding, and plasma membrane location of the antigen(s). *J Invest Dermatol*, Vol.96, pp. 631

Sehgal, V.N. & Srivastava, G. (2007). Vitiligo: compendium of clinico-epidemiological features. *Indian J Dermatol Venereol Leprol*, Vol.73, pp. 149-156

Shegan, V.N. (1971). Hypopigmented lesions in leprosy. *Br J Dermatol*, Vol.4, pp. 91-93

Smyth, J.R. The Smyth chicken: a model for autoimmune amelanosis. (1989). *CRC Crit Rev Poultry Biol*, Vol.2, pp. 1-19

Song, Y.H., Connor, E., Li, Y., Zorovich, B., Balducci, P. & Maclaren, N. (1994). The role of tyrosinase in autoimmune vitiligo. *Lancet*, Vol.344, pp. 1049-1052

Soubiran, P., Bezaken, S., Bellet, C., Lacour, J.P. & Ortonne, J.-P. (1985). Vitiligo: peripheral T cell subset imbalance as defined by monoclonal antibodies. *Br J Dermatol*, Vol.113, pp. 124-127

Spritz, R.A. (2010). Shared genetic relationships underlying generalized vitiligo and autoimmune thyroid disease. *Thyroid*, Vol.20, pp. 745-754

Spritz, R.A., Gowan, K., Bennett, D.C. & Fain, P.R. (2004). Novel vitiligo susceptibility loci on chromosomes 7 (AIS2) and 8 (AIS3), confirmation of SLEV1 on chromosome 17, and their roles in an autoimmune diathesis. *Am J Hum Genet*, Vol.74, pp. 188-191

Sun, X., Xu, A., Wei, X., Ouyang, J., Lu, L., Chen, M. & Zhang, D. (2006). Genetic epidemiology of vitiligo: a study of 815 probands and their families from south China. *Int J Dermatol*, Vol.45, 1176-1181

Taïeb, A. (2000). Intrinsic and extrinsic pathomechanisms in vitiligo. *Pigment Cell Res*, Vol.13, pp. 41-47

Taïeb, A. & Picardo, M. (2010). Epidemiology, definitions and classification. In: *Vitiligo*, M. Picardo & A. Taïeb (Eds.), pp. 13-24, Springer–Verlag, Berlin, Germany

Takei, M., Mishima, Y. & Uda, H. (1984). Immunopathology of vitiligo vulgaris, Sutton's leukoderma and melanoma-associated vitiligo in relation to steroid effects. I. Circulating antibodies for cultured melanoma cells. *J Cutan Pathol*, Vol.11, pp. 107-113.

Tastan, H.B., Akar, A., Orkunoglu, F.E., Arca, E. & Inal, A. (2004). Association of class I HLA antigens and class II HLA alleles with vitiligo in a Turkish population. *Pigment Cell Res*, Vol.17, pp. 181-184

Trcka J., Moroi, Y., Clynes, R.A., Goldberg, S.M., Bergtold, A., Perales, M.A., Ma, M., Ferrone, C.R., Carroll, M.C., Ravetch, J.V. & Houghton, A.N. (2002). Redundant and alternative roles for activating Fc receptors and complement in an antibody-dependent model of autoimmune vitiligo. *Immunity*, Vol.16, pp. 861-868

Tu, C.X., Fu, H.W. & Lin, X.R. (1999). Levels of soluble interleukin-2 receptor in the sera and skin tissue fluids of patients with vitiligo. *J Dermatol Sci*, Vol.21, pp. 59-62

Turnbridge, W.M., Evered, D.C., Hall, R., Appleton, D., Brewis, M., Clark, F., Evans, J.J., Young, E., Bird, T. & Smith, P.A. (1977). The spectrum of thyroid disease in a community: the Whickham survey. *Clin Endocrinol*, Vol.7, pp. 481-492

Uda, H., Takei, M. & Mishima, Y. (1984). Immunopathology of vitiligo vulgaris, Sutton's leukoderma and melanoma-associated vitiligo in relation to steroid effects. II. The IgG and C3 deposits in the skin. *J Cut Pathol*, Vol.11, pp. 114-124

Van den Boorn, J.G., Konijnenberg, D., Dellemijn, T.A., van der Veen, J.P., Bos, J.D., Melief, C. J., Vyth-Dreese, F.A. & Luiten, R.M. (2009). Autoimmune destruction of skin melanocytes by perilesional T cells from vitiligo patients. *J Invest Dermatol*, Vol.129, pp. 2220-2232

Van den Boorn, J.G., Picavet, D.I., van Swieten, P.F., van Veen, H.A., Konijnenberg, D., van Veelen, P.A., van Capel, T., Jong, E.C., Reits, E.A., Drijfhout, J.W., Bos, J.D., Melief, C.J. & Luiten, R.M. (2011). Skin-depigmenting agent monobenzone induces potent T-cell autoimmunity toward pigmented cells by tyrosinase haptenation and melanosome autophagy. *J Invest Dermatol*, in press

Van den Wijngaard, R., Wankowicz-Kalinska, A., Le Poole, C., Tigges, A.J., Westerhof, W. & Das, P. (2000). Local immune response in skin of generalised vitiligo patients. Destruction of melanocytes is associated with the prominent presence of CLA+ T cells at the perilesional site. *Lab Invest*, Vol.80, pp. 1299-1309

Van den Wijngaard, R.M., Asghar, S.S., Pijnenborg, AC., Tigges, A.J., Westerhof, W. & Das, P. (2002). Aberrant expression of complement regulatory proteins, membrane cofactor protein and decay accelerating factor, in the involved epidermis of patients with vitiligo. *Br J Dermatol*, Vol.146, pp. 80-87

Venkataram, M.N., White, A.G., Leeny, W.A., al Suwaid, A.R. & Daar, A.S. (1995). HLA antigens in Omani patients with vitiligo. *Clin Exp Dermatol*, Vol.20, pp. 35-37.

Venneker, G.T., Westerhof, W., de Vries, I.J., Drayer, N.M., Wolthers, B.G., de Waal, L.P., Bos, J.D. & Asghar, S.S. (1992). Molecular heterogeneity of the fourth component of complement (C4) and its genes in vitiligo. *J Invest Dermatol*, Vol.99, pp. 853-858.

Venneker, G.T., de Waal, L.P., Westerhof, W., D'Amaro, J., Schreuder, G.M. & Asghar, S.S. (1993). HLA associations in vitiligo patients in the Dutch population. *Dis Markers*, Vol.11, pp. 187-190

Viac, J., Groujon, C., Misery, L., Staniek, V., Faure, M., Schmitt, D. & Claudy, A. (1997). Effect of UVB 311 mm irradiation on normal human skin. *Photodermatol Photoimmunol Photomed*, Vol.13, pp. 103-108

Wankowicz-Kalinska, A., Van Den Wijngaard, R.M., Tigges, B.J., Westerhof, W., Ogg, G.S., Cerundolo, V., Storkus, W.J. & Das, P.K. (2003). Immunopolarization of CD4+ and CD8+ T cell to type-1-like is associated with melanocyte loss in human vitiligo. *Lab Invest*, Vol.83, pp. 683–695

Westerhof, W. & d'Ischia, M. (2007). Vitiligo puzzle: the pieces fall in place. *Pigment Cell Res*, Vol.20, pp. 345-359

Xia, Q., Zhou, W.M,, Liang, Y.H., Ge, H.S., Liu, H.S., Wang, J.Y., Gao, M., Yang, S. & Zhang, X.J. (2006). MHC haplotypic association in Chinese Han patients with vitiligo. *J Eur Acad Dermatol Venereol*, Vol.20, pp. 941-946

Xie, P., Geohegan, W.D. & Jordan, R.E. (1991). Vitiligo autoantibodies. Studies of subclass distribution and complement activation. *J Invest Dermatol*, Vol.96, pp. 627

Yang, S., Wang, J.Y., Gao, M., Liu, H.S., Sun, L.D., He, P.P., Liu, J.B., Zhang, A.P., Cui, Y., Liang, Y.H., Wang, Z.X. & Zhang, X.J. (2005). Association of HLA-DQA1 and DQB1 genes with vitiligo in Chinese Hans. *Int J Dermatol*, Vol.44, pp. 1022-1027

Yeo, U.C., Yang, Y.S., Park, K.B., Sung, H.T., Jung, S.Y., Lee, E.S. & Shin, M.H. (1999). Serum concentration of the soluble interleukin-2 receptor in vitiligo patients. *J Dermatol Sci*, Vol.19, pp. 182-188

Yi, Y.L., Yu, C.H. & Yu, H.S. (2000). IgG anti-melanocyte antibodies purified from patients with active vitiligo induce HLA-DR and intercellular adhesion molecule-1 expression and an increase in interleukin-8 release by melanocytes. *J Invest Dermatol*, Vol.115, 969-973

Yu, H.S., Kao, C.H. & Yu, C.L. (1993). Coexistence and relationship of antikeratinocyte and antimelanocyte antibodies in patients with non-segmental-type vitiligo. *J Invest Dermatol*, Vol.100, pp. 823-828

Yu, H.S., Chang, K.L., Yu, C.L., Li, H.F., Wu, M.T., Wu, C.S. & Wu, C.S. (1997). Alterations in IL-6, IL-8, GM-CSF, TNF-alpha, and IFN-gamma release by peripheral mononuclear cells in patients with active vitiligo *J Invest Dermatol*, Vol.108, pp. 527-529

Zaima, H. & Koga, M. (2002). Clinical course of 44 cases of localized type vitiligo. *J Dermatol*, Vol.29, pp. 15-19

Zamani, M., Spaepen, M., Sghar, S.S., Huang, C., Westerhof, W., Nieuweboer-Krobotova, L. & Cassiman, J.J. (2001). Linkage and association of HLA class II genes with vitiligo in a Dutch population. *Br J Dermatol*, Vol.145, pp. 90-94

Zauli, D., Tosti, A., Biasco, G., Miserocchi, F., Patrizi, A., Azzaroni, D., Andiani, G., Di Febo, G. & Callegari, C. (1986). Prevalence of autoimmune atrophic gastritis in vitiligo. *Digestion*, Vol.34, pp. 169-172

Zelissen, P.M., Bast, E.J. & Croughs, R.J. (1995). Associated autoimmunity in Addison's disease. *J Autoimmun*, Vol.8, pp. 121-130

13

Graves' Disease - The Interaction of Lymphocytes and Thyroid Cells

Ben-Skowronek Iwona
Medical University in Lublin,
Poland

1. Introduction

Human autoimmune thyroid disorders (AITD), Graves' disease (GD) and Hashimoto's thyroiditis, are characterized by reactivity to self-thyroid antigens. Graves' disease is the archetype for organ-specific autoimmune disorders, very important to our understanding the mechanisms responsible for progression of autoimmunity.
It has been known for years that hyperthyroidism in Graves'disease is induced by immunological reaction, in which TSH receptor antibodies bind to the receptors on the surface of thyrocytes, activate them and initiate thyroid hormone production independent of the hypothalamic-hypophyseal control. It is known nowadays that, probably for environmental or endogenous reasons, Graves'disease may develop in genetically predisposed individuals [Weetman, 2004].

2. Antigen presentation

A small number of antigen presenting cells (APCs) as CD1a+ presenting dendritic cells (DC) were observed in the thyroids without AITD, but their number was significantly higher in the thyroids from Graves' disease patients [Ben-Skowronek et al., 2007, 2008]. There are indications that such DCs are able to proliferate, which indicates that not all of the thyroid DCs need to have recently immigrated with the blood stream [Quadbeck et al. 2002]. CD1a antigen has the structure of an α-chain connected with β-microglobulins and is characteristic for immature APCs [Brigl & Brenner, 2004]. Thyroidal DCs are often in close contact with thyrocytes; they are clearly in an immature state and often show monocyte marker characteristics. The presence of positive reaction to CD1a protein in the granules of the apical part of some thyrocytes suggested that the thyrocytes may probably be antigen presenting cells in the thyroid autoimmune reactivity [Ben-Skowronek et al., 2007,2008]. The investigations of transgenic mice by Kimura et al. [Kimura et al., 2004] indicated that expression of class II MHC molecules on epithelial thyroid cells is not required for the initiation of an autoimmune attack to the thyroid. The initiation, then, seems to be mainly mediated by the professional antigen presenting cells in the lymphoid tissue. The antigen can be presented to CD4+ cells by conventional antigen presenting cells, particularly dendritic cells and also by B-cells and activated T-cells, and less effectively by thyrocytes. The antigen presentation by thyroid epithelial cells sustains the autoimmune reaction.

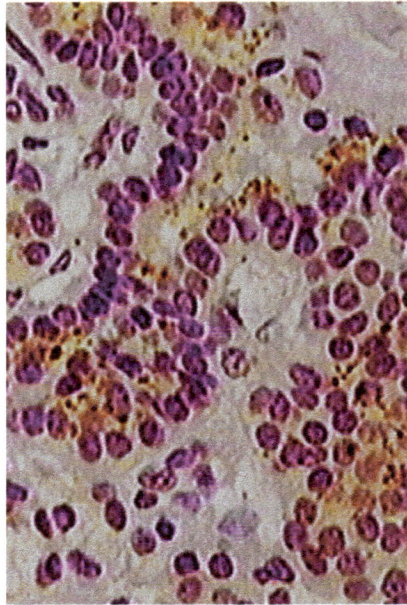

Fig. 1. The thyrocytes are antigen presenting cells and show reaction with the CD1a
monoclonal antibody. Magn. 400x

While analyzing the process of antigen presentation in thyroids sampled from patients, the
treatment process should be taken into account. Metimazole and carbimazole change the
presentation of antigens by thyrocytes. Thionamides have been reported to influence the
expression the antigens of the major histocompatibility complex class I, IL-1 (interleukin-1),
IL-6 (interleukin- 6), prostaglandins E2 produced by thyrocytes [Zantut-Wittmann et al.,
2001]. The expression of major histocompatibility complex class II is unchanged by
thionamides [Dedecjus et al. 2010].

Numerous investigations indicate that adhesion molecules are engaged in the process of
migration of lymphocytes to the thyroid and lymphocyte adhesion [Arao et al., 2000].
Adhesion molecule ICAM-1 (Inter-Cellular Adhesion Molecule 1) belonging to the
superfamily IgG is a natural ligand of antigen located on lymphocytes LFA-1 (Lymphocytic
function-associated antigen - 1). This antigen belongs to the integrin-β2 superfamily
[Springer, 1990]. ICAM-1 is located on different cells: fibroblasts, endotheliocytes, and
thymocytes. It was identified on thyrocytes as well [Weetman et al., 1989, Martin et al., 1990,
Springer,1990].The expression of ICAM-1 is regulated by proinflammatory cytokines:
interferon γ, interleukin 1β (IL 1β) and TNF-α (Tumor Necrosis Factor -1) [Dustin et al.,
1986, Martin et al., 1990, Springer 1990, Bagnasco et al., 1991]. In Graves' disease, the ICAM-
1/LFA-1 pathway plays a key role in migration and settlement of lymphocytes in the
thyroid, and particularly in the process of adhesion of lymphocytes to thyrocytes [Arao et
al.,2000]. In vitro experiments have shown that thyrocytes behave like antigen presenting
cells and can induce lymphocyte migration [Estienne et al., 2002].

Expression of HLA DR II and the immunoglobulin Fc receptor (FcγRIIB2) has been found on
the basal and apical surfaces of thyrocytes [Botazzo et al., 1983, Wu et al., 1999]. The

presentation of the latter antigen is dependent on the low level of androgens, which is probably connected with higher prevalence of AITD in women [Estienne et al., 2002]. Presentation of antigens by thyrocytes without the costimulatory molecule B7 does not lead to activation of T-cells [Marelli-Berg et al., 1997]. The expression APC characteristic antigens are dependent on TSH [Todd et al., 1987, Estienne et al., 2004]. Thyrocytes may produce HLA I under the influence of cytokines of lymphocytes present in the thyroid. In this way, the autoimmunologic reaction is sustained [Catalfamo et al., 1999].

3. The development of autoimmune reaction

When immune tolerance to thyroid antigens is broken, the endothelial cells of regional postcapillary venules are activated, allowing extravasation of blood leukocytes. In Graves' disease, the lymphatic tissue arranged in lymphoid follicles containing T- cells may be formed in the thyroid. T-cells form infiltrations and lymphatic follicles but do not damage thyrocytes [Kuby et al., 2007].

Graves' disease patients seem to have mixed Th1/Th2 profiles. The lymphocyte subsets produce signal interleukin: Th1 – IL2 and Th2- IL4.The immunological response proceeds via T-cell receptor (TCR) antigen recognition, followed by activation of the T- cell through a combined effect of antigen recognition and co-stimulatory signals, including interleukin -1 (IL-1) action leading to T- cell IL 2 secretion and IL-2 receptor expression and, subsequently, to proliferation of the T- cell into an active clone. [Janeway et al., 2001 Janeway & Medzhitov 2002]

In Graves' disease, the increased percentage of CD4+ T helper cells, in comparison to non-AITD, leads to development of humoral autoimmune response. Antigens of self-thyrocytes are presented in such a way that they are recognized by self – T-helper CD4+ lymphocytes. T-helper cells CD4+ sporadic occurred in thyroids of children from the control group, seldom in the simple goiter and slightly more often in the nontoxic nodular goiter. The number of T-helper cells in Graves' disease was the largest [Ben-Skowronek et al., 2007, 2008].

The subset of CD4+cells includes the regulatory lymphocytes - Tregs, which play a fundamental role in modulation of immunological response through their inhibitive effect on autoreactive T-cells [Piccirillo & Shevach,2004, Piccirillo & Thornton, 2004, Shewach, 2006]. The mechanism of this suppression is unknown, but many investigators consider it to be dependent on the contact between lymphocytes and independent of secretion of IL-10 and TGFβ [Piccirillo et.al. 2002,2003]. In the remission phase during thyrotoxic treatment, the subsets of lymphocytes were not different from the control group and from children with the simple goiter and nontoxic goiter [Bossowski et al. 2003]. The cells were characterized by expression of CD25 (the α-chain of IL2) and intracellular expression of FoxP3 (Forkhead winged helix box3). Only the subset of CD4+cells with maximal expression of CD25 (CD4+CD25+high) is responsible for the suppressor – regulatory effect of these lymphocytes [Cao et al., 2003, Baecher-Allan et al., 2001, 2003, Bossowski 2010]. The CD4+CD25+ cells can occur natural or can be induced – they are generated in the lymphatic tissue from CD4+CD25+ cells by different stimulant agents: by immature dendritic cells, IL-10, TGFβ, supply of vitamin D3 or dexamethasone, anti-lymphatic treatment or small doses of antigens. The Treg cells not need costimulation of CD28-B7 for their development or activity. They play a pivotal role in sustenance of immunologic tolerance [Piccirillo & Shewach, 2004, Piccirillo & Thornton, 2004]. TGF-β is assumed to be necessary for the regulatory function of Treg cells; it also prevents activation of lymphocytes and autoimmune reactions [Bommireddy et al., 2008]. The quantity of lymphocytes in this subset is decreased in Graves' disease [Deshun et al., 2009].

An increase in T-helper lymphocytes, especially in Th1 lymphocytes, results in activation of B lymphocytes and their transformation into plasma cells which produce thyroid antibodies, predominantly TRAB (TSH receptor antibody), TSI (TSH stimulated immunoglobulin), and also TPO Ab (Antithyroperoxidase antibody) and TG Ab (Antithyroglobulin antibody).

T cells CD8+ are observed in the thyroid more often in Graves' disease than in non-AITD; they have a regulatory T-cell function. Electron microscopy examinations did not demonstrate any damage to thyrocytes, but CD8+ lymphocytes frequently entered the thyroid follicles through the basal membrane [Ben-Skowronek et al., 2009].

The T-suppressor-cytotoxic CD8+ cells were observed in thyroid follicles between thyrocytes, in mononuclear infiltrations and in lymphatic follicles in the mantle zone. In light microscopy, CD8+ T-cells and adherent normal thyrocytes were visible in high magnifications. Bossowski et al. have found a correlation between expression of costimulatory molecules CTLA-4 and CD28 on T-cells and the level of antibodies against the TSH receptor [Bossowski et al., 2005]. The investigations of Negrini et al. [Negrini et al., 2006] indicate a possibility of presentation of GITR receptors on the surface T-cells CD8+ characteristic for Treg cells. Own observations have confirmed this character of CD8+ T-cells, because they are located between thyrocytes and do not cause apoptosis.

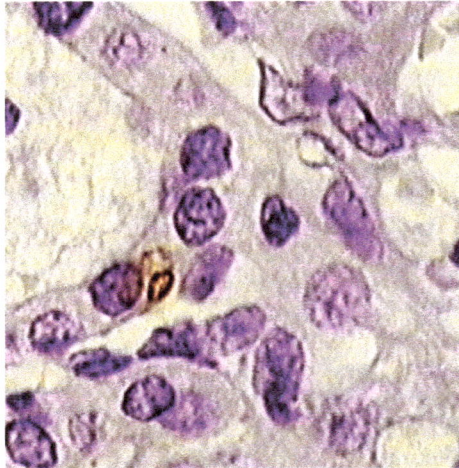

Fig. 2. The CD8+ T-cell between thyrocytes in thyroid follicle wall. The thyrocytes are active and present no signs of apoptosis or cell damage. Magn. 400x.

In vitro investigations and observations of the thyroid tissue in electron microscopy indicate the possibility of formation of the so-called immunological synapse of a character of a tight junction between lymphocytes and thyrocytes with participation of adhesive proteins. This physical contact may result in establishment of an immunological synapse able to stimulate intra thyroid T lymphocyte proliferation and differentiation.

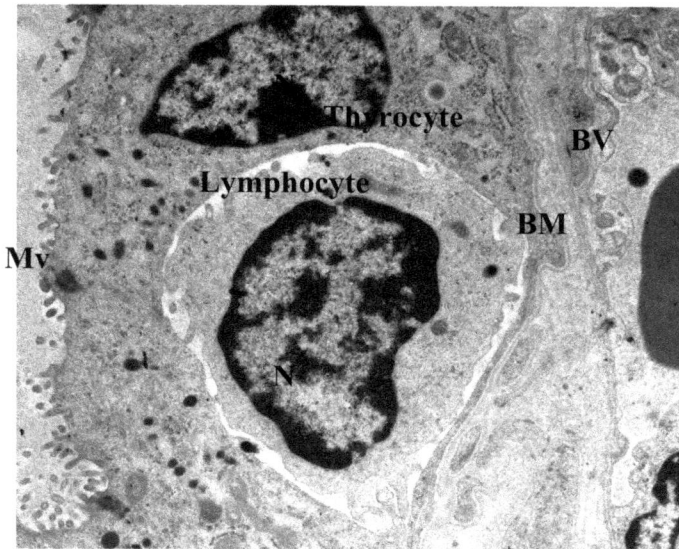

Fig. 3. T cells among thyrocytes in the thyroid epithelium. The thyrocytes are active without destruction signs. N- nucleus, Mv – microvilli, BM – basal membrane, BV – blood vessel. Transmission Electron Microscopy Magn. 15 000x.

Recent investigations have suggested that a crucial role in peripheral tolerance or autoreactive T- cells is played by T regulatory subsets (Tregs) divided into two populations: naturally occurring and inducible [Wieczorek *et al.*, 2009]. Tregs so far identified as participating in the pathogenesis of Graves' disease include naturally occurring CD4+,CD25+T cells , C8+CD122+T cells and natural killer cells [Bossowski et al., 2010]. Comparison of immunohistochemical localization of CD4+ T cells in ultrastructural investigations has shown that lymphocytes CD4+T were small cells with large nuclei and a small amount of cytoplasm in contact with thyrocytes and other lymphocytes [Ben-Skowronek et al., 2009].

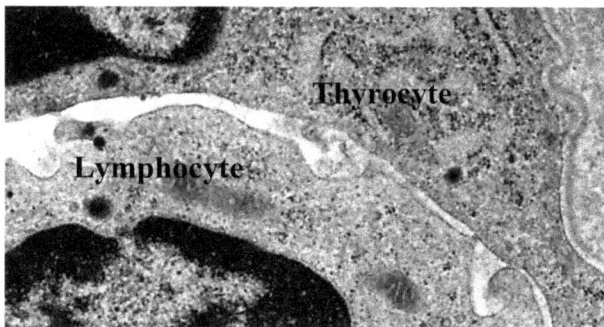

Fig. 4. The immunological synapse between T-cells and thytrocytes in Graves' disease. Transmission Electron Microscopy Magn. 20 000x

Rifa'i et al. [Rifa'i et al., 2004] have described subsets of naturally occurring Tregs CD8+CD25+. It is possible that CD8+T cells in contact with thyrocytes play the role of Tregs in the pathogenesis of Graves' disease. The investigations of Negrini et al. [Negrini et al. 2006] have characterized a subpopulation of CD8 T suppressor lymphocytes able to inhibit both cell proliferation and cytotoxicity; they have observed that glucocorticoid–induced TNF-like receptor (GITR) is expressed on such CD8 T suppressor cells. The papers of Nakano et al. [Nakano et al., 2006] and Nagayama [Nagayama et al., 2007] suggest a preventive role of Tregs in autoimmune reaction in the thyroid with AITD.

Patients with Graves' disease have an increased number of circulating B-cells but plasma cells predominate in the thyroid. The close contact with T-cells (probably Th2 cells) and plasma cells has been frequently observed only in Graves' disease and sporadically in the non-AITD and suggested the regulation function of the T-cells stimulating plasma cells to produce autoantibodies [Ben-Skowronek et al., 2008].

The plasma cells in Graves' disease penetrate between thyreocytes; nevertheless, they caused no destruction of thyroid follicles and epithelial cells. Ultrastructural changes in plasma cells were observed in patients with Graves' disease: a large, active nucleus with a nucleolus, a well-developed rough endoplasmic reticulum in which antibodies were

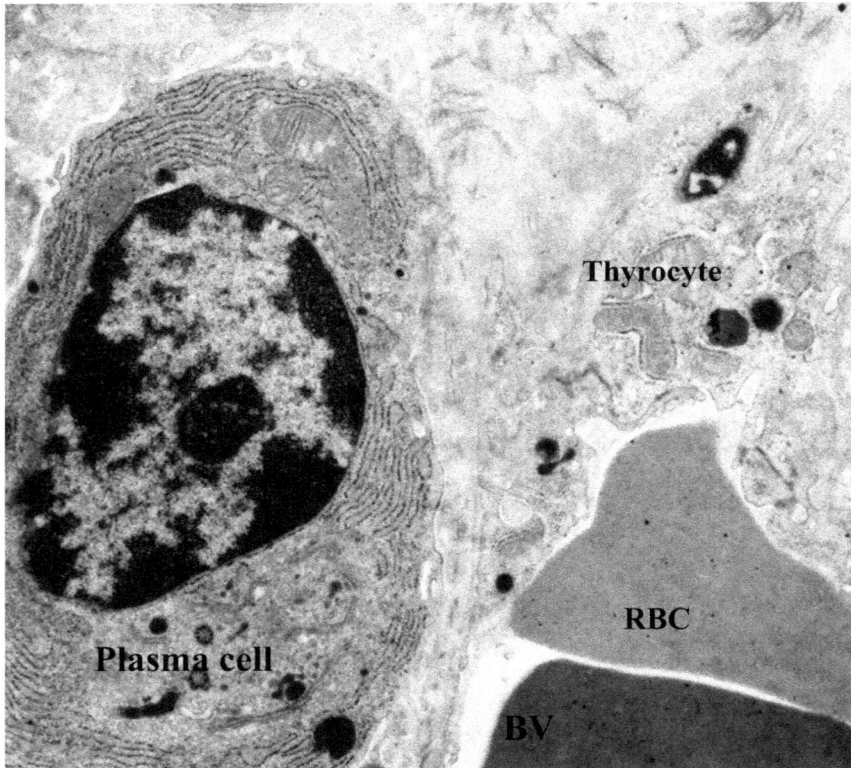

Fig. 5. The plasma cell producing antibodies in contact with thyrocytes. RBC-red blood cell, BV- Blood vessel. Transmission Electron Microscopy Magn. 15.00x

produced. The number of plasma cells in the thyroid was inversely proportional to time of treatment, which proved the immunomodulant activity of thyrostatic drugs [Ben-Skowronek et al., 2009].

In Graves' disease, the immunological deposits observed in the basal membrane of the thyroid follicles lead to thickening of this membrane and probably to changes in polarization of cell membranes. The thyrocytes in this region are columnar, with signs of increased activity (big nuclei; active, enlarged mitochondria; a big number of granules in the apical pole; long microvilli). [Ben-Skowronek et al., 2008,2009]. The antibody deposits do not damage thyrocytes but enhance their activity and metabolism by activation of the THS receptors, and lead to hyperthyroidism.

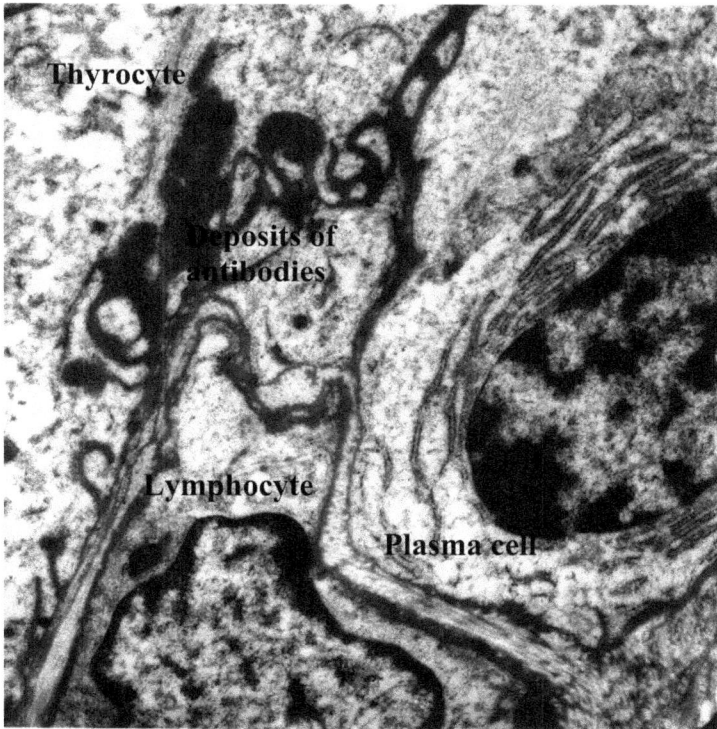

Fig. 6. The late phase of development of antibodies deposits in the basal membrane of the thyrocytes. Transmission Electron Microscopy Magn. 20 00x

Numerous reports have shown that Th-1 cell activating the antibody-dependent cellular cytotoxicity (ADCC) can be detected in Graves' disease, although the response is usually weak and not present in many patients [Guo et al., 1997, Metcalfe et al., 1997]. ADCC of thyroid cells is induced by anti TPO antibody positive sera, but other unknown antibody-antigen systems and methimazole therapy also contribute. Large granular lymphocytes – phenotypic NK cells - are rarely present in the lumen of the thyroid follicle. Here, degenerative changes in the thyrocytes were observed by electron microscopy [Ben-Skowronek et al., 2009].

Antibodies may be produced against the TSH receptor (TSH receptor stimulating antibodies – TS Ab, TSH binding inhibiton immunoglobulins – TBII, TSH stimulation blocking antibodies – TSBAb), against thyroperoxidase (TPO Ab), against thyroglobulin (TG Ab), against megalin [Marino et al., 1999], against the iodine symporter, against thyroid's DNA, against components of external eye muscles and fibroblasts, against parietal cells and against platelets [Weetmann, 2004].

The stimulating antibodies (TSAb) react with the TSH receptor and initiate activity of adenyl cyclase and phospholipase A2of the receptor, thus stimulating production of thyroid hormones and growth and division of thyrocytes [Orgiazzi et al.,1976, DiCerbo et al., 1999, Ewans et al.,1999, Morshed et al., 2009]. The blocking antibodies act like weak agonists of the TSH receptor [Lenzner et al., 2003, Schwarz-Lauer et al., 2002].

4. References

Arao T, Morimoto I, Kukinuma A, Ishida O, Zeki K, Tanaka Y, Ishikawa N, Ito K, Ito K, Eto S. (2000) Thyrocytes proliferation by cellular adhesion to infiltrating lymphocytes through the intercellular adhesion molekule-1/lymphocyte function-associated antygen-1 pathway in Graves'disease. J Clin Endocrinol Metab, 85,1: 382-389

Baecher-Allan C, Brown JA, Freeman GJ, Hafler DA. (2001) CD4+CD25 high regulatory cells in human peripheral blood. J Immunol., 167:1245–53.

Baecher-Allan C, Wolf E, Hafler DA. (2005) Functional analysis of highly defined, FACS-isolated populations of human regulatory CD4 + CD25 + T cells. Clin Immunol 115:10-18

Bagdi E, Krenacs l, Miller K, Isaacson PG. (2001) Follicular dendritic cells in reactive and neoplastic lymphoid tissues: a reevaluation of staining patterns of CD21, CD23, and CD35 antibodies in paraffin sections after wet heat-induced epitope retrieval. Appl Immunohistochem Mol Morphol 9:117-124.

Bagnasco M, Caretto A, Olive D, Pedini B, Canonica GW, and Betterle C. (1991) Expression of intercellular adhesion molecule-1 (ICAM-1) on thyroid epithelial cell in Hashimoto's thyroiditis but not in Graves' disease or papillary thyroid cancer. Clin Exp Immunol. 83:309–313.

Ben-Skowronek I, Szewczyk L., Sierocinska-Sawa J, Korobowicz E. (2007) The subsets of lymphocytes in autoimmunological and non-autoimmunological thyroid diseases in children. Endokrynol Ped 6 nr 3, s. 9-20.

Ben-Skowronek I, Sierocinska-Sawa J, Korobowicz E, Szewczyk L. (2008) Lymphocytes in peripheral blood and thyroid tissue in children with Graves' disease. World Journal of Pediatrics 4:274-282.

Ben-Skowronek I, Sierocinska-Sawa J, Korobowicz E, Szewczyk L. (2009), Interaction of Lymphocytes and Thyrocytes in Graves' Disease and Nonautoimmune Thyroid Diseases in Immunohistochemical and Ultrastructural Investigations. Horm Res 71,6 : 350-358

Bommireddy R, Babcock G, Singh RR, Doetschman T. (2008) TGFβ1 deficiency does not affect the generation and maintenance of CD4+CD25+FOXP3+ putative Treg cells, but causes the numerical inadequacy and loss of regulatory function. Clin Immunol, 127(2):206-213

Brigl M, Brenner MB. (2004). CD1: antigen presentation and T cell function. Annu. Rev. Immunol. 22 (1): 817–90.]

Bossowski A, Moniuszko M, Mrugasz M, Sawicka B, Dąbrowska M, Bodzenta-Łukaszczyk A. (2010). The assessment o CD4+CD25high, CD4+CD25+CD127low and CD4+FoxP3+ T cell n th peripheral blood of children with autoimmune thyroid diseases. Horm Res 73 (sppl 3): 47

Bossowski A, Stasiak –Barmuta A, Urban M. (2005). Relationship between CTLA-4 and CD28 Molecule expression on T Lymphocytes and Stimulating and Blocking Autoantibodies to the TSH-Receptor in children with Graves'disease. Horm.Res. 64,4: 189-197

Bossowski A, Urban M, Stasiak-Barmuta A. (2003). Analysis of changes in the percentage of B (CD19) and T (CD3) lymphocytes, subsets CD4, CD8 and their memory (CD45RO), and naive (CD45RA) T cells in children with immune and non-immune thyroid diseases. J Pediatr Endocrinol Metab, 16(1):63-70.

Bottazzo GF, Pujol-Borrell R, Hanafusa T, and Feldmann M. (1983). Role of aberrant HLA-DR expression and antigen presentation in induction of endocrine autoimmunity. Lancet 2: 1115–1119.

Cao D, Malmstrom V, Baecher-Allan C, Hafler D, Klareskog L, Trollmo C. (2003). Isolation and functional characterization of regulatory CD25brightCD4+ Tcells from target organ of patients with rheumatoid arthritis. Eur J Immunol , 33:215-223.

Catalfamo M, Seradell L, Roura – Mir C, Kolkowi E, Sospedra M, Vives-Pi M, Vargas-Nieto F, Pujol-Borrel R, Jaraquemada D. (1999). HLA-DM and invariant chain are expressed by thyroid folliocular cells, enabling the expression of compact DR molecules. Int Immunol, 11,2: 269-277.

Dedecjus M, Stasiołek M, Brzeziński J Selmaj K, Lewiński A (2010). Hormones Influence Human Dendritic Cells'Phenotype, Function, and Subsets Distribution. Thyroid 2010 Dec. 29[Epub ahead of print]

Deshun P, Shin YH, Gopalakrishnan G, Hennessey J, De Groot L. (2009). Regulatory T-cells in Graves-Disease. Clin Enocrinol, 71 (4) 587-593.

DiCerbo A, Di Paola R, Menzaghi C, Fillips VD, Tahara K, Corda D, et al. (1999). Graves'immunoglobulins activate phospholipase A by recognizing specific epitopes on thyrotropin receptor. J Clin Endocrinol Metab;84:3283-3292

Dustin ML, Rothlein R, Bhan AK, Dinarello CA, Springer TA. (1986). Induction of IL-1 and interferon, tissue distribution, biochemistry, and function of a natural adherence molecule (ICAM-1). J Immunol. 137:245–254.

Estienne V. Bisbarre N, Blanchin S, Durand-Gorde JM, Carayon P, Ruf J. (2004). An In vitro model based on cell monolayers grown on the underside of large-pore filters In bicameral chambers for studying thyrocyte-lymphocyte interactions. Am J Physiol Cell Physiol 287: C1763-C1768.

Estienne V, Duthoit C, Blanchin S , Montserret R, Durand-Gorde J-M, Chartier M, Baty D, Carayon P, and Ruf J. (2002) Analysis of a conformational B cell epitope of human thyroid peroxidase: identification of a tyrosine residue at a strategic location for immunodominance. Int. Immunol., 14(4): 359 - 366.

Estienne V, Duthoit C, Reichert M, Praetor A, Carayon P, Hunziker W, and Ruf J. (2002). Androgen-dependent expression of Fc RIIB2 by thyrocytes from patients with autoimmune Graves' disease: a possible molecular clue for sex dependence of autoimmune disease. FASEB J 16: 1087–1092.

Ewans C, Morgenthaler NG, Lee S, Llewellyn DH, Clinton-Bligh R, John R, Lazarus JH, Chatterjee VKK, Ludgate M. (1999). Development of a luminescent bioassay for thyroid stimulating antibodies. J Clin Endocrinol Metab; 84: 374

Guo J, Jaume JC, Rapoport B, Mc Lachlan SM. (1997). Recombinant thyroid peroxidase-specific Fab converted to immunoglobulin G (IgG) molecules: evidence for thyroid cell damage by IgG1, but not IgG4, autoantibodies. J Clin Endocrinol Metab 82:925-931

Janeway C.A, Jr Travers P, Walport M, and Shlomchik M.J. (2001). The Immune System in Health and Disease in: Immunobiology, 5th edition, New York: Garland Science.

Janeway CA, Medzhitov R. (2002) Innate immune recognition. Annu Re Immunol , 20:197

Kimura, H., M. Kimura, S. C. Tzou, Y. C. Chen, K. Suzuki, N. R. Rose, P. Caturegli. (2004). Expression of class II MHC molecules on thyrocytes does not cause spontaneous thyroiditis, but mildly increases its severity after immunization. Endocrinology 146: 1154-1162.

Kuby J., Kindt TJ.,Goldsby RA., Osborne BA. (2007). Kuby Immunology. New York: W.H. Freeman. , Janeway, Charles (2005). Immunobiology: the immune system in health and disease. New York: Garland Science. ISBN 0-8153-4101-6.

Lenzner C, Morgenthaler NG (2003) The effect of thyrotropin-receptor blocking antibodies on stimulating autoantibodies from patients with Graves' disease. Thyroid 13:1153–1161

Marelli-Berg FM, Weetman A, Frasca L, Deacock SJ, Imami N, Lombardi G, and Lechler RI. (1997) Antigen presentation by epithelial cells induces anergic immunoregulatory CD45RO+ T cells and deletion of CD45RA+ T cells. J Immunol 159: 5853–5861.

Marino M, Chiovato L, Friedlander JA, Latrofa F, Pinchera A and McCluskey RT. (1999). Serum antibodies against megalin (GP330) in patients with autoimmune thyroiditis. J Clin Endocrinol Metab. Jul;84(7):2468-74.

Martin A, Huber GK, and Davies TF. (1990). Induction of human thyroid cell ICAM-1 (CD54) antigen expression and ICAM-1-mediated lymphocyte binding. Endocrinology. 127:651–657.

Metcalfe RA, Oh YS, Stround C, Arnold K, Weetman AP. (1997). Analysis of antibody – dependent cell mediated cytotoxicuty in autoimmune thyroid disease. Autoimmunity 25:65-72

Morshed S.A, Latif R, Davies TF. (2009). Characterization of thyrotropin Receptor Antibody-Induced nSignaling Cascades. Endocrinol, 150(1):519-529

Nagayama Y, Horie I, Saitoh O, Nakahara M, Abiru N. (2007). CD4+CD25+ naturally occurring regulatory T cells and not lymphopenia play a role in the pathogenesis of iodide-induced autoimmune thyroiditis in NOD-H2h4 mice. J Autoimmun.29(2-3):195-202. Epub 2007 Sep 10.

Nakano A, Watanabe M, Iida T, Kuoda S, Matsuzuka F, Miyauschi A, Witani Y, (2007). Apoptosis induced decrease of intrathyroidal CD4+CD25+ regulatory T cells in autoimmune thyroid diseases.Thyroid ,17(1):25-31

Negrini, S., Fenoglio, D., Balestra, P., Fravega, M., Filaci, G. and Indiveri, F. (2006) Endocrine Regulation of Suppressor Lymphocytes. Ann Ny Acad Sci 1069: 377-385.

Orgiazzi J, Williams DE, Chora IJ, Solomon DH. (1976) Human thyroid adenyl cyclase stimulating activity in immunoglobulin G of patients with Graves'disease. J. Clin Endocrinol Metab 42:341

Piccirillo CA, Letterio JJ, Thornton AM, et al. (2002). CD4(+)CD25(+) regulatory T cells can mediate suppressor function in the absence of transforming growth factor beta1 production and responsiveness. J Exp Med. 196:237–246.

Piccirillo CA., Shevach E. (2003). CD4+CD25+Treg cells: naturally occurring but adaptable. Nature Revievs Immunology 3,3 online only (access 20.04.2011)

Piccirillo CA, Shevach EM. (2004). Naturalny occurring CD4+CD25+ immunoregulatory cells: central players In the arena of peripheral tolerance. Seminars in Immunoloy , 16:81-88.

Piccirillo CA, Thornton AM. (2004). Cornerstone of periferal tolerance naturally occurring CD4+CD25+ Tregulatory cells. Trends Immunol 25: 374-380.

Quadbeck B, Eckstein AK , Tews S, Walz M, Hoermann R,. Mann K, Gieseler M .(2002). Maturation of Thyroidal Dendritic Cells in Graves' Disease .Scand.J Immunol 55(6)612-620.

Rifa'i M, Kawamoto Y, Nakashima I, Suzuki H. (2004). Essential roles of CD8+CD122+ regulatory T cells in the maintenance of T cell homeostasis. J Exp Med; 200:1123-34.

Schwarz-Lauer L, Chazenbalk GD, McLachlan SM, Ochi Y, Nagayama Y, Rapoport B. (2002). Evidence for a simplified view of autoantibody interactions with the thyrotropin receptor. Thyroid 12:115-120

Shewach EM. (2006). From vanilla to 28 flavors: multiple varietes of T regulatory cells. Immunity 25: 195-201.

Springer TA. (1990). Adhesion receptors of the immune system. Nature. 346:425–434

Todd I, Pujol-Borrell R, Hammond LJ, McNally JM, Feldmann M, and Bottazzo GF. (1987). Enhancement of thyrocyte HLA class II expression by thyroid stimulating hormone. Clin Exp Immunol 69: 524–531.

Weetman AP. (2004). Autoimmune thyroid disease. Autoimmunity 37: 337-340

Weetman AP. (2010). Diseases associated with thyroid autoimmunity: explanations for the expanding spectrum. Clin Endocrinol (Oxf). [Epub ahead of print]

Wieczorek G., Asemissen A, Model F, Turbachova I, Floess S, Liebenberg V, Baron U, Stauch D. (2009). Quantitative DNA methylation analysis of FOXP3 as a new method for counting regulatory T cells in peripheral blood and solid tissue. Cancer Res 69 (2): 599–608.

Wu Z, Biro PA, Mirakian R, Hammond L, Curcio F, Ambesi-Impiobato FS, and Bottazzo GF. (1999). HLA-DMB expression by thyrocytes: indication of the antigen-processing and possible presenting capability of thyroid cells. Clin Exp Immunol 116: 62–69.

Zantut-Wittmann DE, Tambascia MA, da Silva Trevisan MA, Pinto GA, Vassallo J. (2001). Antithyroid drugs inhibit in vivo HLA-DR expression in thyroid follicular cells in Graves' disease. Thyroid 11:575-580

14

Hashimoto's Thyroiditis – Interactions of Lymphocytes, Thyroid Cells and Fibroblasts

Ben-Skowronek Iwona
Medical University Lublin
Poland

1. Introduction

Autoimmune Hashimoto's thyroiditis involves painless enlargement of the thyroid, which, in histopathological analysis, is characterised by diffuse lymphocytic infiltrations, fibrosis, and atrophic changes. It is a diffuse process, a combination of epithelial cell destruction, lymphocyte infiltrations, and fibrosis. The incidence of Hashimoto's thyroiditis ranges between 0,3 and 1,5 per 1000 persons. It is diagnosed 15-20 times more frequently in females than in males. The forms of Hashimoto's thyroiditis include: euthyroid goitre, and goitre in subclinical or clinical hypothyroidism, hypothyroidism without goitre, silent thyroiditis, postpartum thyroiditis, alternating hyperthyroidism and hypothyroidism [Weetman &McGregor 1994].

Hashimoto's thyroiditis is often associated with type I diabetes, coeliac disease and other autoimmune diseases. It is one of the components of the autoimmune polyglandular syndrome.

In histopathological investigations of Hashimoto's thyroiditis, the follicular epithelial cells in the thyroid are large and often eosinophilic; they are the so-called Hurthle or Askenazy cells packed with mitochondria. Lymphocyte clusters present between the follicles form typical lymphoid follicles in some sites. Infiltrations contain numerous plasma cells. In Hashimoto's thyroiditis, the immunological attack appears to be destructive, rather than stimulating, as in Graves' disease. Two variants of Hashimoto's thyroiditis have been reported so far: atrophic – related to gene HLA-DR3 inheritance, and hypertrophic – involving goitre enlargement associated with HLA-DR5 [Weetman, 2004]. A study of autoimmune thyroiditis in monozygotic twins demonstrated environmental factors inducing development of the disease [Brix et al., 2000]: high iodine intake, selenium deficiency, smoking, infectious diseases, e.g. hepatitis C, and some drugs [Duntas, 2008]. Prolonged exposure to iodine leads to enhanced iodination of thyroglobulin, which increases its antigenicity and initiates autoimmune processes in genetically predisposed individuals. Selenium deficiency causes a decrease in the activity of selenoproteins, including glutathione peroxidise, which leads to an increase in the concentration of hydrogen peroxide and development of inflammatory processes.

Classical histopathological descriptions of the thyroid in Hashimoto's thyroiditis emphasise the fact that the changes include destruction of thyrocytes, lymphocytic infiltration, and fibrosis.

2. The course of the immune response in Hashimoto's thyroiditis

2.1 Antigen presentation

Stimulation of the immune system depends on maturity of dendritic cells. Immature dendritic cells are characterized by expression of small numbers of co-stimulatory molecules and proinflammatory cytokines; they may also cause anergy. Maturing dendritic cells display significantly higher expression of MHC class II and co-stimulatory molecules, but low levels of proinflammatory cytokines. Only mature dendritic cells can induce regulatory T cells [Jonuleit et al., 2001; Menges et al., 2002; Gad et al., 2003; Wakkach et al., 2005]. Antigen presenting cells are more frequently found in Hashimoto's thyroiditis than in healthy thyroid glands or individuals with non-autoimmune thyroid diseases (simple goitre, non-toxic nodular goitre) [Ben-Skowronek et al., 2008, 2011]. No mature dendritic cells presenting MHC class II antigens have been found in thyroid preparations. The investigations conducted by Kimura et al. have indicated that MHC class II antigens may be expressed on thyrocytes in the autoimmune thyroid inflammation. Our own research has shown a positive reaction with the monoclonal antibody CD1a specific for dendritic cells in some thyrocytes. This is not sufficient to initiate the autoimmune response, but sufficient to sustain it [Kimura et al., 2004].

2.2 Development of immunological reaction in the thyroid gland

Lymphatic follicles appear inside the thyroid gland in the course of Hashimoto's thyroiditis. The study of Armengol et al. has demonstrated higher levels of lymphokines and their ligands responsible for lymphocyte migration, settlement, and formation of lymphoid follicles (lymphotoxin α, lymphotoxin β, CC chemokine ligand (CCL)), and CXC (CXCL 12, CXCL13) chemokine ligands). Moreover, in response to inflammatory cytokines, thyrocytes can produce CXCL12. Tissue stress caused by viral or bacterial inflammation is likely to lead to formation of lymphoid follicles in the thyroid [Armengol, et al., 2003]. Production of cytokine ligands for CXCL21, CXCL 22, and CXCL 13 by thyrocytes is correlated with the level of anti-thyroid antibodies, and thus, directly with the inflammatory response in the thyroid [Armengol et al., 2003].

From the physiological point of view, lymphoid follicles are small structures in which processes of somatic hypermutation, maturation of immune affinity receptors, switching of antibody isotypes (e.g. from IgM to IgG), and receptor control take place. Autoreactive T cells arise de novo in the germinal centres; here operates the mechanism sustaining tolerance - apoptosis of autoreactive lymphocytes [Pulendrav et al., 1997, Janevay et al., 2002]. In autoimmune diseases of the thyroid, muscles, and joints as well as in Sjögren's syndrome and autoimmune alveolitis, the ectopic lymphoid tissue is arranged in lymphoid follicles in non-lymphatic organs, which do not contain physiological, growing lymphoid tissue [Crawford et al.1983, Schroeder et al., 1996, Wallace et al.1996, Shione et al 1997, Stott et al 1998, Itoh et. al 2000, Sims et al,. 2001]. The function of this lymphoid tissue, sometimes defined as tertiary lymphoid tissue (primary tissues - thymus and bone marrow, secondary - lymphatic glands and organs), is unclear [Weetman et al. 1994, Ruddle et al. 1999, Armengol et al , 2001]. The structure of the ectopic lymphoid follicles in the thyroid is similar to that of typical lymphoid follicles in lymphoid organs: they consist of a germinal centre and a peripheral zone (mantle zone) containing lymphocytes B and T, and dendritic cells. An analysis of immunoglobulin gene rearrangement (RAG1 and RAG2) has confirmed the possibility of formation of high endothelial venules in lymphoid follicles and production of cytokines responsible for lymphocyte migration and settlement, which would trigger an autoimmune reaction [Armengol et al., 2001]. TG Ab, TPO Ab and TRAK anti-thyroid antibodies are produced in B cells in the lymphoid follicles [Armengol et al., 2001]. High levels of antibodies against thyroglobulin (TG Ab) and thyroperoxidase (TPO Ab) are detected in the serum of patients with Hashimoto's thyroiditis. These antibodies are regarded to have cytotoxic activity. However, investigations of thyroids of foetuses from mothers with Hashimoto's thyroiditis did not show the expected damage. Hypothyroidism was observed only in some children.

T cells originating from mice immunized with TPO strongly react with sequence 540-559; immunisation of mice with this peptide results in development of hypothyroidism and thyroiditis. Peptide 540-559 is probably a key factor in the immune response against TPO [Kawakami et al. 1992]. Natural *HLA-DR-associated peptides* have also been identified; they are present in the colloid, and some of them derive from thyroglobulin [Ng et al., 2006]. A larger proportion of lymphocytes binding to thyroglobulin are present in the thyroid than in peripheral blood [Heuer et al., 1996]. Being the major stimulatory antigen, thyroglobulin is indispensable for T cell response [Sugihara et al., 1993]. The severity of autoimmune reactions following immunization with thyroglobulin has been observed in transgenic mice producing IL-12 [Kimura et al.,2005].

Immune reactions involving T cells are controlled by certain T lymphocyte subpopulations: CD4 + Treg and natural killer lymphocytes are employed in the control of the magnitude and class of the immune response, while lymphocytes CD8 + are responsible for recognition for self- and non-self- antigens [Jang et al., 2006].

A slightly larger number of CD4 + cells have been observed in Hashimoto's thyroiditis than in non-autoimmune thyroid diseases; however, the number was statistically significantly lower than in Graves' disease [Ben-Skowronek et al., 2007,2008]. The studies of McLachlan suggest that the reduction in the number of Treg cells (particularly CD25) induces lymphocyte infiltration in the thyroid accompanied by transient or permanent hypothyroidism [Mc Lachlan et al., 2007].

Animal studies have shown that depletion of CD4 + CD25 + Treg in mice increases susceptibility to thyroiditis by enhancement of the immune reaction against thyroglobulin and exacerbates the existing thyroiditis, whereas an increase in the number of CD4 + CD25 + T cells restores resistance to thyroiditis [Morris et al., 2006,2007, Nagayama ey al. 2007]. It appears that an insufficient percentage of CD4 + T cells in Hashimoto's disease is the cause of the destructive autoimmune reaction in the thyroid.

Suppressor/cytotoxic lymphocytes CD8 + have been found among thyrocytes in thyroid follicles, in lymphatic infiltrations and in the lymphoid follicles of the mantle zone. Glycoprotein CD8 present on the surface of cytotoxic lymphocytes may bind to the class I MHC molecule, which leads to activation of T cells CD8+. This activation is also dependent on co-stimulatory proteins binding to antigen CD28 (the so-called two-signal model). Once activated, cytotoxic lymphocytes may secrete cytotoxins, and granzymes and granulysins. They perforate the cell membrane and form pores, which induces apoptosis of the target cell. Another pathway leading to apoptosis is activation of the Fas ligand [Iannacone et al., 2005,2006, Subramanian et. al., 2005]. Hypothyroidism in patients with autoimmune thyroiditis is associated with apoptosis of alveolar epithelial cells induced by cytokines. Expression of Fas ligand on thyrocytes of patients with Hashimoto thyroiditis and a weak reaction for Bcl-2 have been detected, which suggests cytokine-induced apoptosis [Kawakami et al., 1996, Mitsiiades et al.,1998, Stassi et al., 2002]. TPO-specific T cells cause destruction through cytotoxic mechanisms involving CD4+ and CD8 + cells or programmed Fas- TNF-alpha-induced apoptosis [Stassi et al., 2002]. In Hashimoto's disease, damaged thyrocytes in contact with CD8 + T lymphocytes may be observed in the light microscope. The electron microscopy has shown contact sites of lymphocytes with thyrocytes located in the thyroid follicular epithelium. Polarization of endolysosomes near the site of contact has been detected in the lymphocytes which displayed the T-cell phenotype of and CD8 + location. Similar observations of cultured CD8 + and dendritic cells in experimental conditions were conducted by Gardella et al. [Gardella et al., 2001]. The studies of Negrini et al. [Negrini et al.,2006] have indicated possible presence of the GITR (Glucocorticoid-Induced TNF-Like Receptor) antigen on the surface of CD8 + T cells, which would render them as regulatory Treg cells. Therefore, it is believed that cytotoxic T cells, K (killer) lymphocytes, NK (natural killer) cells, and regulatory (Treg) or suppressor T cells may play an important role in autoimmune thyroid damage. Some studies indicate the ability of T cells to transfer thyroid autoimmune processes, both in animals with experimental autoimmune thyroiditis and patients who have undergone bone marrow transplantation [Kawakami et al.,, 1992, Ng et al., 2006, Drabko et. al., 2006].

Active lymphocytes B CD79alfa+ and antibody-producing plasma cells were found in a small percentage of thyroids from healthy children (4,11%), in the colloid goitre (1,83%) and the nodular goitre (5,22%). The largest number of CD79 alpha+ lymphocytes was observed in thyroid specimens from patients with Hashimoto's thyroiditis (average 31,65%) In lymphatic infiltrates, plasma cells constituted almost half of the cells (46,67%), and amounted to 17,23% in the thyroid parenchyma. Foci of damaged thyroid follicles and numerous fibroblasts and collagen bands have been observed at the plasma cell accumulation sites. The thyroid glands in children with Hashimoto's thyroiditis displayed characteristics of lymphocyte activation, the so-called blastic transformation, consisting in an increase in the volume of the cell and, particularly, of the nucleus, appearance of nucleoli and an increase in the cytoplasm volume through enlargement of the rough endoplasmic reticulum, in which antibody production takes place [Ben-Skowronek et al., 2007].

Thyrocytes in Hashimoto's thyroiditis are cuboidal or flat. The thyroid cells exhibit damage. Cell nuclei are often folded; secretory vesicles are sporadically present in the apical pole (sometimes there are no vesicles); and swollen mitochondria are present in the basal pole. The swollen part of thyrocytes without microvilli or with single microvilli projects into the lumen of the follicle. The basal membrane is thickened. Plasma cells, lymphocytes and fibroblasts are visible among the thyroid follicles. At the lymphoid infiltration sites, the lymphoid cells separate the thyroid epithelium from the basal membrane of the capillary blood vessels. Lymphocytes are often in direct contact with plasma cells. Plasma cells filled with concentrically arranged layers of the rough endoplasmic reticulum adhere to the basal membrane of the thyroid follicle and the surrounding thyrocytes. The thick, electron dense basal membrane contains numerous collagen fibres. The adjacent cytoplasmic membrane does not exhibit characteristic folds. The fibrous basal membrane hinders blood flow in the capillary blood vessels and deformed erythrocytes can be seen in their lumen. The exchange of nutrients and oxygen between thyrocytes, the interstitium, and blood vessels is impeded [Fig. 1].

3. Apoptosis in autoimmune thyroid diseases

Apoptosis is a physiological form of cell death resulting from the need of multicellular organisms to maintain balance between dividing and dying cells. Typical morphological

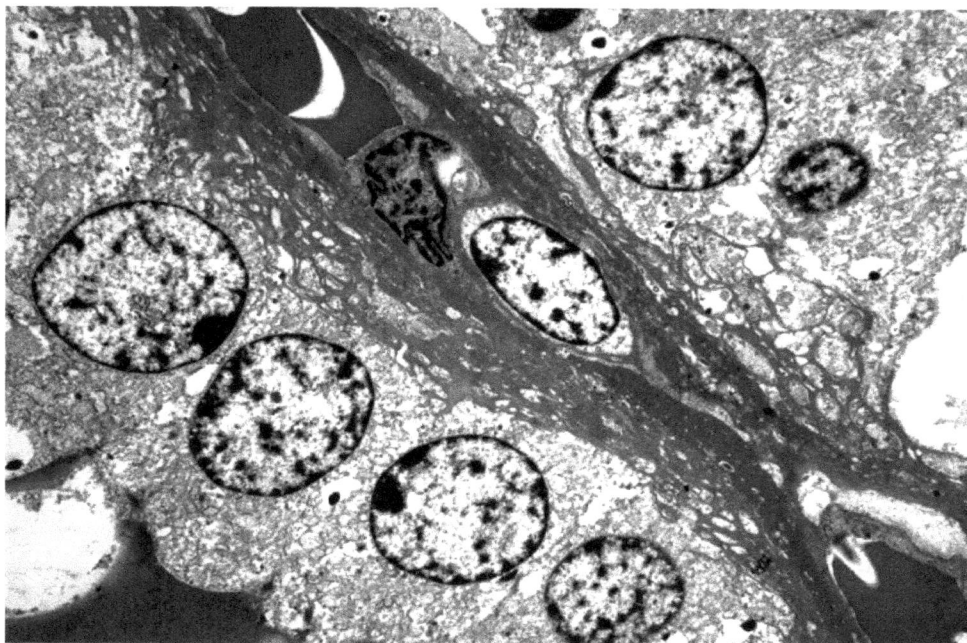

Fig. 1. A markedly thickened basal membrane of the thyroid follicle containing collagen fibres impedes thyrocyte contact with the capillary vessel lumen. In the basal membrane is present lymphocyte (phenotype lymphocyte T). The thyrocytes exhibit signs of damage of thyroid follicular cells– swollen mitochondria, dilated cisterns of the rough endoplasmic reticulum, absence of secretory granules, and atrophy of microvilli. Transmission Electron Microscope Magn. 10 000x.

changes in cells that received the signal to begin the apoptotic process include folding of the cell membrane, condensation of cytoplasm and cellular organelles, disappearance of the mitochondrial membrane, shrinkage of the nucleus, and condensation of chromatin [Yamazaki et al., 2000, Lorenz et al., 2005].
Apoptosis can be initiated by T cells through two pathways:

* by perforins secreted by lymphocytes into the junctions between lymphocytes and target cells; they perforate the cell membrane and form pores thus inducing osmotic lysis of the cell; simultaneously, granzymes B activate the caspase cascade, which leads to cell apoptosis;

* the Fas ligand and TNF-related apotosis induced ligand (TRAIL) secreted by lymphocytes stimulate the so-called death receptors on the cell surface causing activation of caspase cascade through caspase 8 and 10.

Lymphocytic infiltration and antibodies secreted by plasma cells lead to destruction of thyrocytes, but actively stimulate the production of collagen by fibroblasts. As a result, large amounts of collagen accumulate in the follicular and vascular basal membranes. In the final stage of the process, thyrocytes are destroyed via apoptosis. Typical signs of cell apoptosis are visible: chromatin condensation in the nuclei of thyroid epithelial cells, condensation of the cytosol and swelling of the mitochondria [Fig.2].

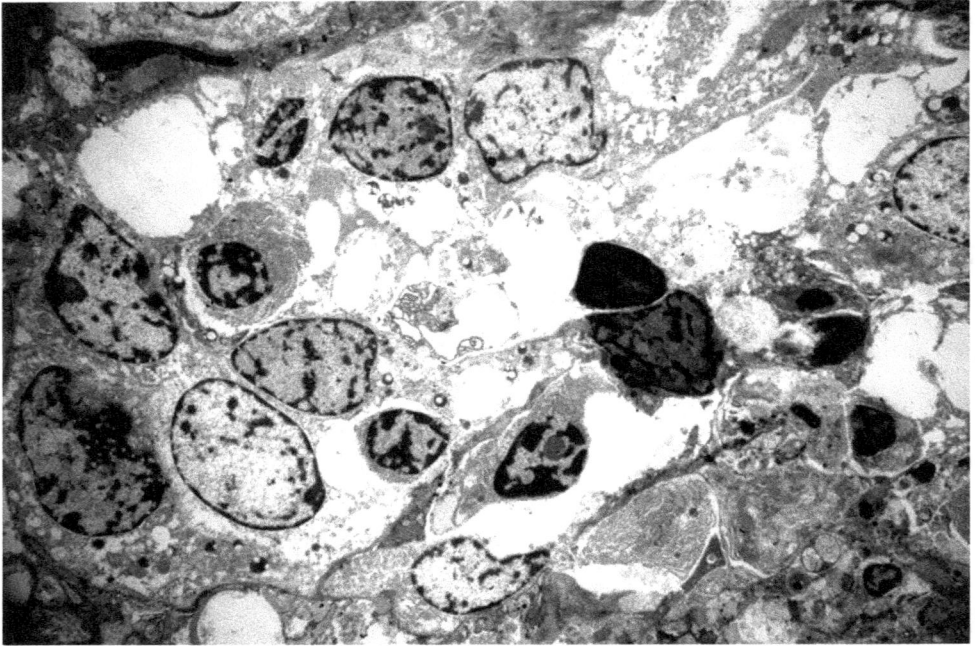

Fig. 2. The last phase of destruction of the thyroid in Hashimoto's thyroiditis. The thyrocytes are damaged due to apoptotic processes. Plasma cells and lymphocytes predominate in the interstitium. The fibroblast migrates to this place and produces collagen fibres. Transmission Electron Microscope. magn. 5000x.

Various phases of thyrocyte death were visible at the lymphocyte infiltration sites; apoptosis was caused by active plasma cells and lymphocytes of the large granular lymphocyte phenotype (LGL) [Fig.2] Ultrastructural investigations have revealed that the reaction between lymphocytes and plasma cells producing antibody results in thyrocyte damage, which, in turn, changes the permeability of cell membranes and intracellular membranes and leads to accumulation of water in the endoplasmic reticulum cisterns in the mitochondria and cytoplasm. Consequently, the cell is enlarged, microvilli disappear, and swollen mitochondria occupy the basal pole of thyroid cells causing cell staining with acidic dyes. At the same time, electron-dense substances (probably antibodies) are deposited in the follicular basal membrane. In response, large amounts of collagen are secreted around the damaged follicles. Communication between the lumen of capillary vessels and thyrocytes is impeded; hence, the transport of oxygen, nutrients, and substrates for production of thyroid hormones is inhibited. The thyrocyte metabolism is decelerated, and production of hormone and protein colloid is disrupted. Thyrocytes gradually die and exfoliate into the follicle lumen. Lymphocytes migrate to replace them and form lymphoid follicles. Fibroblast bands producing collagen fibres penetrate the site as well.

The contact between lymphocytes and thyrocytes in Hashimoto's thyroiditis forms an immunological synapse, which has been described as a specialized intercellular connection between T cells and antigen presenting cells [Paul et al., 1994, Dustin et al., 1999, Grakoui et al., 1999].

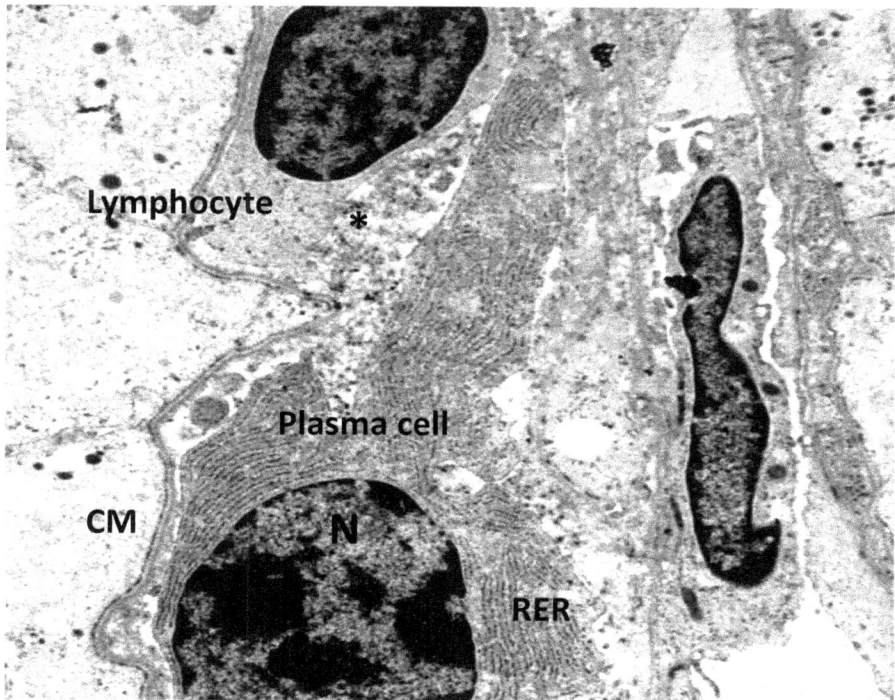

Fig. 3. Junction between the lymphocyte and plasma cell in Hashimoto's thyroiditis. Electron-dense (probably protein) substance is visible in the intercellular space. N – cell nucleus, RER - rough endoplasmic reticulum, L – lysosome, CM – cell membrane. Transmission Electron Microscope magnification 25 000x

The immunological synapse consists of a central zone containing antigen receptors and a surrounding ring of adhesion molecules [Dustin, 2002]. Lymphocytes form projections – lamellipodia – and form junctions with the cell membrane of thyrocytes. Presumably, it is at these sites that antigen presentation by thyrocytes occurs [Bromley et al., 2001]. Recent studies demonstrate different types of immunological synapses: cytotoxic [Dustin et al., 2010] and transitory (the so-called kinapses) [Dustin et al. 2007, 2010]. Observations of the interaction between lymphocytes and other thyroid cells in the course of AITD indicate possible formation of analogous junctions between thyrocytes and lymphocytes, i.e. cytotoxic synapses in Hashimoto's thyroiditis. This implies that lymphocytes secrete granzymes and other cytotoxic substances leading to cell damage.

The junctions of plasma cells with thyrocytes are large adhesion zones with thyrocyte apoptosis visible nearby [Fig.3]. The junctions between plasma cells and fibroblasts, however, are associated with production of collagen fibres. In Hashimoto's thyroiditis, numerous junctions between lymphocytes and plasma cells in the form of adhesion zones and spaces have been detected, into which medium electron-density substances (probably proteins) were secreted [Fig.3]; there are also synapses between young and mature lymphocytes T and B in the lymphoid follicles.

Such cell junctions occur mainly in the lymphoid nodes. Very tight junctions are visible between lymphoblasts and B cells, which are phenotypically similar to plasma cells. Immunological synapses have been found also between lymphocytes [Ben-Skowronek in press]

In Hashimoto's disease, activation of apoptotic processes is also associated with activation of Th1 cells, which enhance the activity of caspase and apoptosis through production of IFN-γ. While reduction in the number of CD4 + cell subsets in the thyroid parenchyma has been reported both in our own study and in animal models of the disease [Sugihara et al., 1993], an increase in the number of active CD4 + IL-4 + was observed in the peripheral blood [Maziotti et al., 2003]. However, no correlation has been found between the number of CD4 + T cells in the thyroid and the antiperoxidase antibody levels in serum [Watanabe et al., 2002, Pandit et al., 2003].

Antibody-dependent cell-mediated cytotoxicity (ADCC) plays an important role in development of Hashimoto's thyroiditis, whereas complement-dependent cytotoxicity (CDC) exerts a lesser effect. The thyroid peroxidase antigen evokes the reaction [Czarnocka et al., 1985, Estienne et al., 2002, Guo et al., 2005 Rebuffat et al., 2006, Ng et al., 2004, 2006]. TPO Ab has been detected in 90% of Hashimoto's thyroiditis patients [Rappaport et al., 2001]. Anti-TPO antibodies are various isotypes of the IgG antibodies. Anti-peroxidase antibodies TPOAb can damage thyrocytes through the ADCC and CDC mechanisms. The cytotoxic ADCC mechanism depends on the interaction between the target cell, antibody and effector cell. Monocytes, which due to FcγRI receptors are effector cells activated by TPOAb, can affect T cells and lead to destruction of thyrocytes [Rebuffat et al.,2008]. FcγRIII are present on Natural Killer cells and FcγRII on monocytes and neutrophils. All FcγR fragments are involved in the ADCC reaction [Rebuffat et al., 2008]. The investigations of Giancotti and Williams et al. suggest that integrins β2 may participate in cytotoxic reactions involving FcγR [Giancotti et al., 1999, Williams et al., 1999]. The study of Rebufatt et al. [Rebuffat et al., 2008], however, indicates involvement of two monocytic cell lines in this process.

It has not been sufficiently documented yet whether specific IgG antibody subclasses take part in thyrocyte damage [Metcalfe 1997, Guo 1997]. Xie L-D et al. investigated the occurrence of anti-TPO IgG subclasses and found that IgG1 was present in 70.2%, IgG2 in 35.1%, IgG3 in 19.6%, and IgG4 in 66.1% of patients; increased proportion of IgG2 predisposes to thyroid damage and hypothyroidism [Xie et al., 2008].

Metcalfe et al. found no correlation between the IgG subclasses and thyrocyte damage in vitro [Metcalfe et al., 1997], whereas Guo et al. demonstrated that thyrocyte damage is associated with subclass IgG1 [Guo et al., 1997]. Recent studies conducted by Rebuffat et al. [Rebuffat et al., 2010, Pappenwali et al., 2010] indicate that anti-TPO antibodies exhibit moderate activity in the ADCC process and can be used in the new methods of treatment of papillary thyroid cancer, the cells of which show expression of TPO.

Thyrocyte damage continues and is potentialized by the CDC reaction [Rebuffat et al., 2008]. Complement component C4, hyperexpressed on the surface of thyrocytes in Hashimoto's thyroiditis, participates in this reaction [Blanchin et al., 2003]. The key antigen here is thyroid peroxidase. The TPO ectodomain consists of a long module similar to myeloperoxidase, followed by a module similar to the complement control protein (CCP) and a module similar to the epidermal growth factor (EGF). The CCP contains a fragment that activates the complement. Therefore, TPO can activate the complement cascade without the help of immunoglobulins. Tg Ab antibodies do not fix the complement [Weetmann et al.,

2004] and probably are not directly involved in the CDC reaction, which is related to the fact that thyroglobulin is not expressed on the surface of thyrocytes.

Reduction or loss of intercellular communication in the final phase of Hashimoto's thyroiditis may lead to destruction of thyrocytes and hypothyroidism [Greek et al., 1996, Green et al., 1997, DiMatola et al., 2000]

• Fibrocytes and fibroblasts in autoimmune thyroid diseases

Fibrocytes and fibroblasts are frequently disregarded in analyses of autoimmune reactions in the thyroid. Ultrastructural studies have revealed significant participation of fibroblasts in the pathogenetic processes in Hashimoto's disease. They enter the space between the basal membrane and thyrocytes and produce substantial amounts of collagen, thus leading to thickening of the basal membrane and impeded contact between the capillary vessel lumen and thyrocytes [Fig. 1,2].

Influx and proliferation of lymphocytes in the thyroid as well as production of collagen is a response to inflammation processes and a stimulus for further thyrocyte damage through isolation thereof from oxygen and nutrients in the blood vessels. Progressive damage of thyrocytes leads to release of large amounts of autoantigen and triggers the inflammatory response. Own observations indicate a possible direct impact of plasma cells, lymphocytes and fibroblasts, since thyroids of Hashimoto's thyroiditis patients exhibit close contact between the groups of lymphocytes, plasma cells and fibroblasts.

4. References

Armengol MP, Cardoso-Smith CB, Fernandez M, Ferrer X, Pujol-Borrel R, Manel J. 2003 Chemokines determine local lymphogenesis and a reduction circulating CXCR4+T andCCR7B an T lymphocytes in thyroid autoimmune Diseases. J Immunol, 170:6320-6328

Armengol MP; Juan M; Lucas-Martin A; Fernandez-Figueras MT; Jaraquemada D; Gallart T; Pujol-Borrell R. 2001 Thyroid autoimmune disease: demonstration of thyroid antigen-specific B cells and recombination-activating gene expression in chemokine-containing active intrathyroidal germinal centers. Am J Pathol , 159(3): 861-73

Armengol, M. P., M. Juan, A. Lucas-Martín, M. T. Fernández-Figueras, D. Jaraquemada, T. Gallart, R. Pujol-Borrell. 2001. Ectopic lymphoid follicles in thyroid autoimmune glands are sites of active B cell expansion and maturation: relevance to pathogenesis. Am. J. Pathol. 159:861.

Ben-Skowronek I, Szewczyk L., Sierocinska-Sawa J, Korobowicz E. 2007 The subsets of lymphocytes in autoimmune and non-autoimmune thyroid diseases in children. Endokrynol Ped 6 (3), 9-20.

Ben-Skowronek I, Sierocinska-Sawa J, Korobowicz E, Szewczyk L. 2008 Lymphocytes in peripheral blood and thyroid tissue in children with Graves' disease. World Journal of Pediatrics 4:274-282.

Ben-Skowronek I, Szewczyk L, Ciechanek R, Korobowicz E. The interactions of lymphocytes, thyrocytes and fibroblasts in Hashimoto's thyroiditis – immunohistochemical and ultrastructural study. In press

Brix TH, Kyvik KO, Hegedus L. 2000 A population-based study of chronic autoimmune hypothyroidism in Danish twins. J Clin Endocrinol Metab. 85, 2 536-539.

Bromley SK, Burack WR, Johnson KG, Somersalo K, Sims TN, Sumen C, Davis MM , Shaw AS, Allen PM, and Dustin ML. 2001 The immunological synapse. Annual Review of Immunology Vol. 19: 375.

Crawford, D. H., S. M. McLachlan. 1983. The relationship between the Epstein-Barr virus and rheumatoid arthritis. Br. J. Rheumatol. 22:129.

Czarnocka B, Ruf J, Fernand M, Carayon P, Lissitzky S.1985 Purification of the human thyroid peroxidase and its identification as the microsomal antigen involved in autoimmune thyroid disease. FEBS lett. , 190,147-152

DiMatolaT, Mueller F, Fenzi G, Rosi G, Bifulco , Marzano LA, Vitale M. 2000 Serum withdrawal-induced apoptosis in thyroid cells is caused by loss of fibronectin-integrin interaction. J Clin Endocrinol Metab 85: 1188-1193.

Drabko K, Winnicka D, Gaworczyk A, Ben-Skowronek I, Skomra D, Kowalczyk JR. 2006 Donor origin of Graves' disase i BMT recipient: evidence from FISH studies of thyroid tissue. Bone Marrow Transplantation 37, 789-91.

Duntas LH 2008. Environmental factors and autoimmune thyroiditis. Nat Clin Pract Endocrinol Metab. 4(8):454-60.

Dustin ML, 2007 Cell adhesion molecules and actin cytoskeleton at immune synapses and kinapses . Curr Opin Cell Biol. 19(5): 529–533.

Dustin ML, Long EO, 2010 Cytotoxic immunological synapses .Immunological Reviews Special Issue: Cytotoxic CellsVolume 235, 1: 24–34. Dustin ML, Rothlein R, Bhan AK, Dinarello CA, Springer TA. 1986 Induction of IL-1 and interferon, tissue distribution, biochemistry, and function of a natural adherence molecule (ICAM-1). J Immunol. 137:245–254.

Dustin ML and Shaw AS. 1999 Perspectives Immunology. Costimulation: Building an Immunological Synapse Science . 283, 5402, 649 – 650.

Dustin ML, 2002 The immunological synapse . Arthritis Res Therapy 4 (Suppl3): 119-125.

Estienne V, Bisbarre N, Blanchin S, Durand-Gorde JM, Carayon P, Ruf J. 2004 An In vitro model based on cell monolayers grown on the underside of large-pore filters In bicameral chambers for studying thyrocyte-lymphocyte interactions. Am J Physiol Cell Physiol 287: C1763-C1768.

Estienne V, Duthoit C, BlanchinS , Montserret R, Durand-Gorde J-M, Chartier M, Baty D, Carayon P, and Ruf J. 2002 Analysis of a conformational B cell epitope of human thyroid peroxidase: identification of a tyrosine residue at a strategic location for immunodominance. Int. Immunol., 14(4): 359 - 366.

Gad, M., M. H. Claesson, A. E. Pedersen. 2003. Dendritic cells in peripheral tolerance and immunity. APMIS 111: 766-775.

Gardella S, Andrei C, Lotti L, Poggi A, Torrisi R, Zocchi R, Rubartelli A.2001 CD8+ T lymphocytes induct polarized exocytosis of secretory lysosomes by dendritic cells with release of interleukin 1β and cathepsin D. Blood, 90(7):2152-2159

Grakoui A, Bromley SK, Sumen C, Davis MM, Shaw AS, Allen PM, Dustin ML 1999 The immunological synapse: A molecular machine controlling T cell activation .Science 285:221-227.

Greek LM, LaBue M, Lazarus JP, Jennings JC. 1996 Reduced cell-cell communication in experimentally induced autoimmune thyroid disease. Endocrinol 137: 2823-2832.

Green LM, Lazarus JP, Song ,Stagg RB, LaBue M, Hilliker S. 1997 Elevation of protein kinase C in thyrocytes isolated from a Lews Rat model of autoimmune thyroiditis prevents assembly of immunodetecteable connexin 43 gap junction and reduces intercellular communication. Thyroid 7: 913-921.

Guo J, Jaume JC, Rapoport B, Mc Lachlan SM. 1997 Recombinant thyroid peroxidase-specific Fab converted to immunoglobulin G (IgG) molecules: evidence for thyroid cell damage by IgG1, but not IgG4, autoantibodies. J Clin Endocrinol Metab 82:925-931.

Guo J, McLachlan S. M., Pichurin P. N., Chen C.R., Pham N., Aliesky H. A., David C. S., and Rapoport B. 2005 Relationship between Thyroid Peroxidase T Cell Epitope Restriction and Antibody Recognition of the Autoantibody Immunodominant Region in Human Leukocyte Antigen DR3 Transgenic Mice. Endocrinology, 146(11): 4961 - 4967.

Heuer M, Aust G, Ode-Hakim S, Scherbaum WA. 1996 Different Cytokine mRNA Profiles in Graves' Disease, Hashimoto's Thyroiditis, and Nonautoimmune Thyroid Disorders Determined by Quantitative Reverse Transcriptase Polymerase Chain Reaction (RT-PCR) Thyroid., 6(2): 97-106.

Iannacone, M, Sitia, G,; Guidotti, L G. 2006 Pathogenetic and antiviral immune responses against hepatitis B virus. Future Virology 1: 189–96.

Iannacone, M, Sitia, G, Isogawa, M, Marchese, P, Castro, M G, Lowenstein, PR; Chisari, FV, Ruggeri V, Zaverio M et al. 2005 Platelets mediate cytotoxic T lymphocyte–induced liver damage. Nature Medicine 11 (11): 1167–9.

Itoh M, Takahashi T, Sakaguchi N, Kuniyasu Y, Shimizu J, Otsuka F, Sakaguchi S 1999 Thymus and Autoimmunity: Production of CD25+CD4+ naturally anergic and suppressive T Cells as a key function of the thymus in maintaining immunologic self-tolerance. J Immunol 162: 5317-5326.

Itoh, K., E. Meffre, E. Albesiano, A. Farber, D. Dines, P. Stein, S. E. Asnis, R. A. Furie, R. I. Jain, N. Chiorazzi. 2000. Immunoglobulin heavy chain variable region gene replacement as a mechanism for receptor revision in rheumatoid arthritis synovial tissue B lymphocytes. J. Exp. Med. 192:1151.

Janeway C.A, Jr Travers P, Walport M, and Shlomchik M.J. 2001 The Immune System in Health and Disease in: Immunobiology, 5th edition, New York: Garland Science.

Janeway CA, Medzhitov R. 2002 Innate immune recognition. Annu Re Immunol , 20:197

Jang H, Hess L. 2006 Regulation of immune response by T- cells . NEJM 354; 1166-1176.

Jonuleit, H., E. Schmitt, K. Steinbrink, A. H. Enk. 2001. Dendritic cells as a tool to induce anergic and regulatory T cells. Trends Immunol. 22: 394-400.

Karandikar NJ, Vanderlugt CL, Walunas TL, Miller SD, Bluestone JA. 1996 CTLA4: A negative regulator of autoimmune disease. J Exp Med 184:783-788.

Kawakami A, Eguchi K, Matsuoka N, Tsuboi M, Kawabe Y, Ishikawa N, Ito K, Nagataki S. 1996 Thyroid-stimulating hormone inhiibits Fas antigen-mediated apoptosis ofhuman thyrocytes in vitro. Endocrinology 137:316.

Kawakami Y, Fisfalen M-E, DeGroot LJ. 1992 Proliferative responses of peripheral blood mononuclear cells from patients with autoimmune thyroid diseases. J Immunol 148:2084–2089.

Kimura H., Tzou S.C, Rocci R, Kimura M, Suzuki K, Parlow A.F, Noel R. 2005 Interleukin12 driver primary hypothyroidism: the contrasting role sof two Th1 cytokines (IL-12 and IFN γ. Endocrinol 8; 3642-3651.

Kimura, H., M. Kimura, S. C. Tzou, Y. C. Chen, K. Suzuki, N. R. Rose, P. Caturegli. 2004. Expression of class II MHC molecules on thyrocytes does not cause spontaneous thyroiditis, but mildly increases its severity after immunization. Endocrinology 146: 1154-1162.

Lorenz M, Hermann M, Winkler T, Gaipl U, Kalden JR. 2000 Role of apoptosis in autoimmunity. Apoptosis 5:443-449.

Maziotti G., Sorvillo F., Naclerio C., Tarzati A., Cioffi M., Perna R., Valentini G., Farziati B., Amato G., Carella C. 2003 Type-1 response in peripheral CD4+ and CD8+ T-cells from patients with Hashimoto's thyroiditis; Eur. J. Endocrinol.:148(4), 383-388.

McLachlan SM, Nagayama Y, Pichurin PN, Mizutori Y, Chen CR, Misharin A, Aliesky Rapoport B. 2007 The link between Graves' disease and Hashimoto's thytroiditis: a role for regulatory T-cells. Endocrinology 148:5724-5733.

Menges, M., S. Rossner, C. Voigtlander, H. Schindler, N. A. Kukutsch, C. Bogdan, K. Erb, G. Schuler, M. B. Lutz. 2002. Repetitive injections of dendritic cells matured with tumor necrosis factor αinduce antigen-specific protection of mice from autoimmunity. J. Exp. Med. 195: 15-21.

Metcalfe RA, Oh YS, Stround C, Arnold K, Weetman AP.1997 Analysis of antibody – dependent cell mediated cytotoxicuty in autoimmune thyroid disease. Autoimmunity 25:65-72.

Mitsiiades N, Poulaki V, Kotoula V, Mastorakos G, Balafouta S, Koutras DA, Tsokos 1998 Fas/Fas ligand up-regulation and BCL-2 down-regulation may be significant in the pathogenesis of Hashimoto' thyroiditis. J Clin Endo Metab 83:2199

Morris GP, Chen L, Kong YC 2007 CD137 signaling function of CD4+CD25+ regulatory T-cells in induced tolerance to experimental immune thyroiditis. Cell Immunol 226:20-29.

Morris, G.P. and Kong, Y.M. 2006 Interference with CD4+CD25+ T cell-mediated tolerance to experimental autoimmune thyroiditis by glucocorticoid-induced tumor necrosis factor receptor monoclonal antibody. J. Autoimmunity, 26:24-31.

Nagayama Y, Horie I, Saitoh O, Nakahara M, Abiru N. 2007 CD4+CD25+ naturally occurring regulatory T cells and not lymphopenia play a role in the pathogenesis of iodide-induced autoimmune thyroiditis in NOD-H2h4 mice. J Autoimmun.29(2-3):195-202. Epub 2007 Sep 10.

Negrini S, Fenoglio D, Balestra P, Fravega M, Filaci G and Indiveri F. 2006 Endocrine Regulation of Suppressor Lymphocytes. Ann Ny Acad Sci 1069: 377-385.

Ng HP, Kung AWC 2006 Induction of Autoimmune Thyroiditis and Hypothyroidism by Immunization of Immunoactive T Cell Epitope of Thyroid Peroxidase Endocrinology, 147(6): 3085 - 3092.

Ng HP, BangaJP, and Kung AWC 2004 Development of a Murine Model of Autoimmune Thyroiditis Induced with Homologous Mouse Thyroid Peroxidase. Endocrinology, 145(2): 809 - 816.

Pandit AA, Vijay Warde M, Menon PS. 2003 Correlation of number of intrathyroid lymphocytes with antimicrosomal antibody titer in Hashimoto's thyroiditis. Diagn Cytopathol 28 (2):63-65.

Pappenwali C, Ehlers M, Schott M.2010 Advances in cellular therapy for the treatment of thyroid cancer. J Oncol ID 179491 in press

Paul WE, Seder RA 1994 Lymphocyte responses and cytokines. Cell 76:241-251.

Pulendrav B, van Driel R, Nossal GJ. 1997 Immunologicl toleranc in germinal centres. Immunol Today, 18:27.

Rapaport B, McLachlan SM 2001 Thyroid autoimmunity. Clin Invest 108:1253-1259.

Rebuffat SA, Bresson D, Nguyen B, and Peraldi-Roux S. 2006 The key residues in the immunodominant region 353-363 of human thyroid peroxidase were identified. Int. Immunol., 18(7): 1091 - 1099.

Rebuffat SA, Morin M, Nguyen B Castex F, Robert B, Peraldi-Roux S. 2010 Human recombinant anti-thyroperoxidase autoaibodies: in vitro cytotoxic activity on papillary thyroid cancer expressing TPO. Br J Cancer 102: 852-861.

Rebuffat SA, Nguyen B,Robert B, Castex F, Peraldi Roux S. 2008 Antiperoxidase Antibody-Dependent Cytotoxicity in Autoimmune Thyroid Disease. J Clin Endocrinol Metab, 93;3: 929-934

Ruddle, N. H.. 1999. Lymphoid neo-organogenesis: lymphotoxin's role in inflammation and development. Immunol. Res. 19:119.

Schroeder A, Greiner EA, Seyfert, A. Berek C. 1996. Differentiation of B cells in the nonlymphoid tissue of the synovial membrane of patients with rheumatoid arthritis. Proc. Natl. Acad. Sci. USA 93:221.

Shione H, Fujii Y, Okumura Y, Yakeuchi M, Inoue M, Matsuda H. 1997. Failure to down-regulate Bcl-2 protein in thymic germinal center B cells in myasthenia gravis. Eur. J. Immunol. 27:805.

Sims GP, Shiono H, Willcox N, Stott DI. 2001. Somatic hypermutation and selection of B cells in thymic germinal centers responding to acetylcholine receptor in myasthenia gravis. J. Immunol. 167:1935.

Stassi G, De Maria R 2002 Autoimmune thyroid disease: New model of cell health in autoimmunity. Nat Rev Immunol 2: 198-204

Stassi G, Di Liberto D, Todaro M, Zeuner A, Ricci-Vitiani L, Stoppacciaro A, Ruco L, Farina F, Zummo G and De Maria G. 2000 Control of target cell survival in thyroid autoimmunity by T helper cytokines via regulation of apoptotic proteins Nature Immunology 1, 483 – 488.

Stott D, Hiepe, M, Hummel, Steinhauser C. Berek. A. 1998. Antigen-driven clonal proliferation of B cell within the target tissue of an autoimmune disease. J. Clin. Invest. 102:938.

Subramanian S, Ramalingam K. 2005 Electron microscopic evidence on the participation Cytotoxic T Lymphocytes and Macrophages in Mtb adjuvant induced connective tissue inflammation and arthritogenesis in Rattus norvegicus. Asian Journal of Microbiology, Biotechnology and Environmental Sciences 7 (2): 227–233.

Sugihara S, Fuiwara H, Sherarer GM. 1993 Autoimmune thyroiditis In mice depleted of particular T cell subsets. Characterization of thyroiditis- inducing T cell lines and clones derived from thyroid lesions. J Immunol 150 (2),:683-694.

Wakkach, A., N. Fournier, V. Brun, J. P. Breittmayer, F. Cottrez, H. Groux. 2003. Characterization of dendritic cells that induce tolerance and T regulatory 1 cell differentiation in vivo. Immunity 18: 605-617.

Wallace, WEH, Howie SEM, Krajewaki AS. 1996. The immunological architecture of B-lymphocytes aggregates in cryptogenic fibrosing alveolitis. J. Pathol. 178:323.

Watanabe M, Yamamoto N, Maruoka H, Tamai H, Matsuzuka F, Miyauchi A, Iwatani Y. 2002 Independent involvement of CD8+CD25+ cells and thyroid autoantibodies in disease severity of Hashimoto's disease. Thyroid 12 (9):801-808

Weetman AP 2004 Autoimmune thyroid disease. Autoimmunity 37: 337-340

Weetman AP, McGregor AM. 1994. Autoimmune thyroid disease: further developments in our understanding. Endocr. Rev. 15:788.

Xie LD, Gao MR, Lu GZ,Guo XH.2008 Distribution of immunoglobulin G subclasses of anti-thyroid peroxidase antibody in sera from patients with Hashimoto's thyroiditis with different thyroid functional status. Clin Exp Immunol 154: 172-177.

Yamazaki H, Bretz J, Arscott PL, Baker JR. 2000 Apoptosis and the thyroid: the biology and potential implications for thyroid disease. Curr Opinion in Endocrinology and Diabetes;7(5):260-264.

Permissions

The contributors of this book come from diverse backgrounds, making this book a truly international effort. This book will bring forth new frontiers with its revolutionizing research information and detailed analysis of the nascent developments around the world.

We would like to thank Clio P. Mavragani, MD, for lending her expertise to make the book truly unique. She has played a crucial role in the development of this book. Without her invaluable contribution this book wouldn't have been possible. She has made vital efforts to compile up to date information on the varied aspects of this subject to make this book a valuable addition to the collection of many professionals and students.

This book was conceptualized with the vision of imparting up-to-date information and advanced data in this field. To ensure the same, a matchless editorial board was set up. Every individual on the board went through rigorous rounds of assessment to prove their worth. After which they invested a large part of their time researching and compiling the most relevant data for our readers. Conferences and sessions were held from time to time between the editorial board and the contributing authors to present the data in the most comprehensible form. The editorial team has worked tirelessly to provide valuable and valid information to help people across the globe.

Every chapter published in this book has been scrutinized by our experts. Their significance has been extensively debated. The topics covered herein carry significant findings which will fuel the growth of the discipline. They may even be implemented as practical applications or may be referred to as a beginning point for another development. Chapters in this book were first published by InTech; hereby published with permission under the Creative Commons Attribution License or equivalent.

The editorial board has been involved in producing this book since its inception. They have spent rigorous hours researching and exploring the diverse topics which have resulted in the successful publishing of this book. They have passed on their knowledge of decades through this book. To expedite this challenging task, the publisher supported the team at every step. A small team of assistant editors was also appointed to further simplify the editing procedure and attain best results for the readers.

Our editorial team has been hand-picked from every corner of the world. Their multi-ethnicity adds dynamic inputs to the discussions which result in innovative outcomes. These outcomes are then further discussed with the researchers and contributors who give their valuable feedback and opinion regarding the same. The feedback is then collaborated with the researches and they are edited in a comprehensive manner to aid the understanding of the subject.

Apart from the editorial board, the designing team has also invested a significant amount of their time in understanding the subject and creating the most relevant covers. They scrutinized every image to scout for the most suitable representation of the subject and create an appropriate cover for the book.

The publishing team has been involved in this book since its early stages. They were actively engaged in every process, be it collecting the data, connecting with the contributors or procuring relevant information. The team has been an ardent support to the editorial, designing and production team. Their endless efforts to recruit the best for this project, has resulted in the accomplishment of this book. They are a veteran in the field of academics and their pool of knowledge is as vast as their experience in printing. Their expertise and guidance has proved useful at every step. Their uncompromising quality standards have made this book an exceptional effort. Their encouragement from time to time has been an inspiration for everyone.

The publisher and the editorial board hope that this book will prove to be a valuable piece of knowledge for researchers, students, practitioners and scholars across the globe.

List of Contributors

Wellington K. Ayensu and Raphael D. Isokpehi
College of Science, Engineering & Technology, Jackson State University, Jackson, USA
Bioinformatics Section, Jackson State University, Jackson, USA

Ibrahim O. Farah
College of Science, Engineering & Technology, Jackson State University, Jackson, USA

Emmanuel O. Keku
Department of Public Health and Preventive Medicine, School of Medicine, St. George's University, St. George, Grenada, West Indies

Chris A. Arthur and Sophia S. Leggett
School of Health Sciences, College of Public Service, Jackson State University, Jackson, USA

Iñaki Álvarez
Immunology Unit, Department of Cell Biology, Physiology and Immunology, Institut de Biotecnologia i Biomedicina, Universitat Autònoma de Barcelona, Spain

Sujayita Roy and Paula M. Pitha
Krieger School of Arts & Sciences, Department of Biology, Johns Hopkins University, Department of Oncology, Johns Hopkins School of Medicine, United States of America

Bilyy Rostyslav and Yaroslav Tolstyak
Institute of Cell Biology, National Academy of Sciences of Ukraine, Lviv, Ukraine Danylo Halytsky Lviv National Medical University, Lviv, Ukraine

Havrylyuk Anna and Chopyak Valentina
Danylo Halytsky Lviv National Medical University, Lviv, Ukraine

Kit Yuriy, Stoika Rostyslav and Tomin Andriy
Institute of Cell Biology, National Academy of Sciences of Ukraine, Lviv, Ukraine

Fang-Ping Huang and Susanne Sattler
Division of Immunology and Inflammation, Department of Medicine, Imperial College London, Great Britain

Natalia Cherepahina, Murat Agirov, Jamilyia Tabaksoeva, Kusum Ahmedilova and Sergey
Suchkov First Moscow State Medical University, Russian State Medical University, Russia

Rizwan Ahmad
Department of Biochemistry, Oman Medical College, Sohar, Sultanate of Oman

Haseeb Ahsan
Department of Biochemistry, Faculty of Dentistry, Jamia Millia Islamia, New Delhi, India

Serena Schippa and Valerio Iebba
Public Health and Infectious Diseases dept., 'Sapienza' University of Rome, Italy

Naoko Kumagai, Megumi Maeda, Hidenori Matsuzaki, Suni Lee, Yasumitsu Nishimura and Takemi Otsuki
Department of Hygiene, Kawasaki Medical School, Kurashiki, Japan

Hiroaki Hayashi and Wataru Fujimoto
Department of Dermatology, Kawasaki Medical School, Kurashiki, Japan

Yoshie Miura
Division of Molecular and Clinical Genetics, Department of Molecular Genetics, Medical Institute of Bioregulation, Kyushu University, Higashi-ku, Fukuoka, Japan

Rajni Rani
National Institute of Immunology, New Delhi, India

Valentina Di Caro
Division of Immunogenetics, Department of Pediatrics, School of Medicine, University of Pittsburgh, USA Rimed Foundation, Italy

Nick Giannoukakis and Massimo Trucco
Division of Immunogenetics, Department of Pediatrics, School of Medicine, University of Pittsburgh, USA

E. Helen Kemp, Sherif Emhemad and Anthony P. Weetman
Department of Human Metabolism, The Medical School, University of Sheffield, Sheffield, United Kingdom

David J. Gawkrodger
Department of Dermatology, Royal Hallamshire Hospital, Sheffield, United Kingdom

Ben-Skowronek Iwona
Medical University in Lublin, Poland